Platelets
Cellular Response Mechanisms and their Biological Significance

Platelets

Cellular Response Mechanisms and their Biological Significance

Proceedings of an EMBO Workshop
held at The Weizmann Institute of Science,
Rehovot, Israel,
14 - 16 April, 1980

Edited by
A. Rotman, F.A. Meyer, C. Gitler, *and* **A. Silberberg,**
*The Weizmann Institute of Science,
Rehovot, Israel*

A Wiley-Interscience Publication

JOHN WILEY & SONS
Chichester · New York · Brisbane · Toronto

Copyright © 1980 by John Wiley & Sons Ltd.

All rights reserved.

No part of this book may be reproduced by any means, nor transmitted, nor translated into a machine language without the written permission of the publisher.

British Library Cataloguing in Publication Data:

EMBO Workshop on Platelets: Cellular Response Mechanisms and their Biological Significance, *Rehovot, 1980*
   Platelets
  1. Blood platelets—Congresses
  I. Rotman, A   II. European Molecular Biology Organisation
  612'.117   QP97   80–041257

ISBN 0 471 27896 3

Printed in Great Britain

Contributors

L.A. Amos, MRC Laboratory for Molecular Biology, Cambridge, England.

H.R. Baumgartner, Pharma Research Department, F. Hoffmann-La Roche & Co. Ltd., 4002 Basel, Switzerland.

M.C. Berndt, Department of Biochemistry, St. Jude Children's Research Hospital, Memphis, Tennessee 38101, USA.

G.V.R. Born, Department of Pharmacology, King's College, London WC2R 2LS.

D.J. Boullin, MRC Unit & University Department of Clinical Pharmacology, Radcliffe Infirmary, Oxford, and Nuffield Labs of Comparative Medicine, Institute of Zoology, Regents Park, London.

J.P. Caen, Unité 150 INSERM, Hôpital Lariboisière, Paris 10, France.

A.G. Castle, Department of Biochemistry, Royal College of Surgeons of England, London.

J.L. Costa, Clinical Neuropharmacology Branch, National Institute of Mental Health, Bethesda, Maryland 20205, USA.

N. Crawford, Department of Biochemistry, Royal College of Surgeons of England, London.

M.M.L. Davidson, Department of Pathology, McMaster University, Hamilton, Ontario, Canada L8N 3Z5.

T.C. Detwiler, Department of Biochemistry, S.U.N.Y. Downstate Medical Center, Brooklyn, New York 11203, USA.

D. Dupuis, Unité 150 INSERM, Hôpital Lariboisière, Paris 10, France.

A. Dvilansky, Department of Haematology, Soroka Medical Centre, Ben Gurion University of the Negev, Beer-Sheva, Israel.

H.H. Edwards, Department of Biochemistry, St. Jude Children's Research Hospital, Memphis, Tennessee 38101, USA.

G. Fleischer, Department of Haematology, Soroka Medical Centre, Ben Gurion University of the Negev, Beer-Sheva, Israel.

J.E.B. Fox, Department of Biochemistry, St. Jude Children's Research Hospital, Memphis, Tennesse 38101, USA and Department of Pathology, McMaster University, Hamilton, Ontario, Canada L8N 3Z5.

J.N. George, Division of Hematology, Department of Medicine, University of Texas Health Science Center at San Antonio, and the Veterans Administration Hospital, San Antonio, Texas 78284, USA.

J.M. Gerrard, University of Minnesota Health Sciences Center, Minneapolis, Minnesota, USA.

C. Gitler, Department of Membrane Research, The Weizmann Institute of Science, Rehovot, Israel.

R.J. Haslam, Department of Pathology, McMaster University, Hamilton, Ontario, Canada L8N 3Z5.

A. Hefez, Technion, Departments of Pharmacology and Psychiatry, Faculty of Medicine, Haifa, Israel.

H. Holmsen, Thrombosis Research Center, Temple University, Philadelphia, Pennsylvania, USA.

G.A. Jamieson, American Red Cross Blood Services, Bethesda, Maryland 20014, USA.

L.K. Jennings, Department of Biochemistry, St. Jude Children's Research Hospital, Memphis, Tennessee 38101, USA.

S.M. Jung, American Red Cross Blood Services, Bethesda, Maryland 20014, USA.

R. Käser-Glanzmann, Theodor Kocher Institute, University of Berne, Switzerland.

R. Kettler, F. Hoffmann-La Roche & Co. Ltd., Pharmaceutical Research Department, CH-4002 Basle, Switzerland.

T. Kunicki, Unité 150 INSERM, Hôpital Lariboisière, Paris 10, France.

F. Laub, Department of Membrane Research, The Weizmann Institute of Science, Rehovot, Israel.

A. Laubscher, Research Department of the University Clinics and Institutes, Cantonal Hospital Basel, Switzerland.

J.M. Launay, F. Hoffmann-La Roche & Co. Ltd., Pharmaceutical Research Department, CH-4002 Basle, Switzerland

Present address: Laboratoire de Biochimie, Hôpital St. Louis, Paris, France.

A. Livne, Department of Biology, Ben Gurion University of the Negev, Beer-Sheva, Israel.

E.F. Lüscher, Theodor Kocher Institute, University of Berne, Switzerland.

J.A. Lynham, Department of Pathology, McMaster University, Hamilton, Ontario, Canada L8N 3Z5.

R.M. Lyons, Division of Hematology, Department of Medicine, University of Texas Health Science Center at San Antonio, and the Veterans Administration Hospital, San Antonio, Texas 78284, USA.

J.M. Marcum, American Red Cross Blood Services, Bethesda, Maryland 20014, USA.

P. Massini, Theodor Kocher Institute, University of Berne, Switzerland.

F.A. Meyer, Polymer Department, Weizmann Institute of Science, Rehovot, Israel.

R.K. Morgan, Division of Hematology, Department of Medicine, University of Texas Health Science Center at San Antonio, and the Veterans Administration Hospital, San Antonio, Texas 78284, USA.

R. Muggli, Pharma Research Department, F. Hoffmann-La Roche & Co. Ltd., 4002 Basel, Switzerland.

D.L. Murphy, Clinical Neuropharmacology Branch, National Institute of Mental Health, Bethesda, Maryland 20205, USA.

I. Nathan, Department of Haematology, Soroka Medical Centre, Ben Gurion University of the Negav, Beer-Sheva, Israel.

A.T. Nurden, Unité 150 INSERM, Hôpital Lariboisière, Paris 10, France.

A. Ordinas, American Red Cross Blood Services, Bethesda, Maryland 20014, USA.

A.H. Parola, Department of Chemistry, Ben Gurion University of the Negev, Beer-Sheva, Israel.

E.I. Peerschke, Department of Pathology, New York University Medical Center, New York, USA.

D.R. Phillips, Department of Biochemistry, St. Jude Children's Research Hospital, Memphis, Tennessee 38101, USA.

G.B. Picotti, Institute of Pharmacology, School of Medicine, University of Milan, 20129 Milan, Italy.

D. Pidard, Unité 150 INSERM, Hôpital Lariboisière, Paris 10, France.

A. Pletscher, Research Department of the University Clinics and Institutes, Cantonal Hospital Basel, Switzerland.

M. Da Prada, F. Hoffmann-La Roche & Co. Ltd., Pharmaceutical Research Department, CH-4002 Basle, Switzerland.

H.R. Prasanna, Department of Biochemistry, St. Jude Children's Research Hospital, Memphis, Tennessee 38101, USA.

V. Pribluda, Department of Membrane Research, The Weizmann Institute of Science, Rehovot, Israel.

G.H.R. Rao, University of Minnesota Health Sciences Center, Minneapolis, Minnesota, USA.

A. Rotman, Department of Membrane Research, The Weizmann Institute of Science, Rehovot, Israel.

S.E. Salama, Department of Pathology, McMaster University, Hamilton, Ontario, Canada L8N 3Z5.

S.W. Tam, Department of Biochemistry, S.U.N.Y. Downstate Medical Center, Brooklyn, New York 11203, USA.

Th.B. Tschopp, Pharma Research Department, F. Hoffmann-La Roche & Co. Ltd., 4002 Basel, Switzerland.

J.G. White, University of Minnesota Health Sciences Center, Minneapolis, Minnesota, USA.

M.B.H. Youdim, Technion, Departments of Pharmacology and Psychiatry, Faculty of Medicine, Haifa, Israel.

M.B. Zucker, Department of Pathology, New York University Medical Center, New York, USA.

Contents

Contributors   v

Introduction   xi

PLATELET FUNCTION

Platelets in Haemostasis and Thrombosis   3
    G.V.R. Born

Interaction of Platelets with Subendothelium in Flowing Blood   17
    H.R. Baumgartner, R. Muggli, and Th.B. Tschopp

Drug Interactions with Platelets and Arteries : Their Role in Cerebrovascular Disorders and the Cerebral Vasospasm Syndrome   29
    D.J. Boullin

Determinants for Platelet Adhesion and Aggregation on Collagen   51
    F.A. Meyer

The Role of Calcium Ions in the Induction of Platelet Activities   67
    E.F. Lüscher, P. Massini, and R. Käser-Glanzmann

PLATELET MEMBRANE STRUCTURE AND RECEPTORS

Membrane Alterations Caused by Platelet Aggregation and Secretion   81
    J.N. George, R.M. Lyons, and R.K. Morgan

Lipid-Protein Interaction in Activated Platelet Membrane   95
    G. Fleischer, I. Nathan, A. Livne, A. Dvilansky, and A.H. Parola

Labelling and Separation of Platelet Membrane Proteins   107
    A. Rotman

Platelet Glycoproteins in Relation to Human Platelet Function   119
    A.T. Nurden, D. Dupuis, T. Kunicki, and J.P. Caen

Platelet Membrane Glycoproteins as Thrombin and Aggregation Receptors   131
    D.R. Phillips, L.K. Jennings, M.C. Berndt, H.R. Prasanna, J.E.B. Fox, and H.H. Edwards

The Platelet Thrombin Receptor   143
    T.C. Detwiler, and S.W. Tam

The Influence of Receptor Mobility and Association on High
    Affinity Binding of Thrombin to Platelets   151
    G.A. Jamieson, S.M. Jung, A. Ordinas, and J.M. Marcum

Specific Binding of Fibrinogen to Platelets : Relationship
    to Shape Change and Aggregation   157
    M.B. Zucker, and E.I. Peerschke

INTRACELLULAR PLATELET RESPONSE

Platelet Microtubule Subunit Proteins : Assembly and
    Disassembly Factors   171
    N. Crawford, L.A. Amos, and A.G. Castle

Platelet Activation and the Cytoskeleton Networks   189
    C. Gitler, V. Pribluda, F. Laub, and A. Rotman

Prostaglandins in Platelet Activation   201
    J.G. White, G.H.R. Rao, and J.M. Gerrard

Roles of Cyclic Nucleotides and of Protein Phosphorylation
    in the Regulation of Platelet Function   213
    *R.J. Haslam, S.E. Salama, J.E.B. Fox, J.A. Lynham,
    and M.M.L. Davidson*

Unique Specializations for the Subcellular Compartmentation
    of Amines in Pig and Human Platelets   233
    J.L. Costa, and D.L. Murphy

Mechanisms of Platelet Secretion   249
    H. Holmsen

PLATELET PHARMACOLOGY

Use and Limitation of Platelets as Models for Neurons :
    Amine Release and Shape Change Reaction   267
    A. Pletscher, and A. Laubscher

Serotonin, Histamine, Catecholamines, Norepinephrine, and
    Octopamine in Blood Platelets   277
    M. Da Prada, G.B. Picotti, R. Kettler, and J.M. Launay

Platelet Function and Monoamine Oxidase (MAO) Activity in
    Psychiatric Disorders   289
    M.B.H. Youdim, and A. Hefez

Discussion   307

Author index   311

Subject index   325

Introduction

This book contains 22 chapters, each written by one of the invited lecturers to an EMBO Workshop on: "Platelets - Cellular Response Mechanisms and Their Biological Significance" held at the Weizmann Institute of Science, April 14-16, 1980. The Workshop, organised by the Aharon Katzir-Katchalsky Center, covered various aspects of platelet physiology, biochemistry and pharmacology. These lectures were followed by extensive and informal discussions. The book is divided into 4 parts according to the following topics:

1. Platelet Function
2. Platelet Membrane Structure and Receptors
3. Intracellular Platelet Response
4. Platelet Pharmacology

The discussion pertaining to each part is summarized very briefly at the end of the book. Although this volume covers a wide range of topics, it is in a sense limited to the molecular and cellular events that take place during platelet activation. The main emphasis throughout was upon the interaction of platelets with stimulating agents such as ADP, collagen, and thrombin, the changes that take place in the cell membrane as a result of this interaction and the intracellular events that follow this activation. A relatively lower emphasis was placed on platelet pharmacology. Because of lack of time, many topics such as the role of platelets in inflammation and platelet immunology were not represented at all. With respect to the topics discussed, however, this book contains contributions written by the leading scientists in the field.

We would like to thank EMBO, the Katzir Center and the Weizmann Institute for their support. Our deep appreciation and thanks go to Mrs. R. Goldstein, the secretary of the Katzir Center and many other people at the Weizmann Institute for their help in organizing and running of the workshop.

Avner Rotman
Frank A. Meyer
Carlos Gitler
Alexander Silberberg

PLATELET FUNCTION

There are probably a variety of functions which the platelet is called upon to fulfil . Yet, the role of platelets in hemostasis, the arrest of blood flow as a result of injury, is probably the one function which, at present, is best known and accepted. This is indeed the function which is most thoroughly addressed here. This subject has, however, many aspects, since there are a variety of injuries to be considered in addition to responses to be expected from platelets in cases where the coagulation chain is induced by diseased vessel walls or prosthetic devices. In thrombus formation and embolism, on the other hand, it is desirable to interfere with the hemostatic process and bring it under medical control.

Treated are the general aspects of blood arrest, the interaction of platelets with subendothelium, the participation of platelets in thrombus formation, their interaction with collagen and the role of calcium in platelet activation. Basic issues, such as the dependence of platelet aggregation on the haemodynamic and biochemical environment of the cells or the mechanism of platelet aggregation through haemorrhage, are discussed. How does flow affect the interaction of platelets with the walls of the vessel and with red blood cells? What is the nature of the interaction between subendothelial structures and what, in particular, is the nature of the collagen-platelet interaction? What is the reactivity of damaged endothelial cells towards platelets? Is a "second messenger" involved in platelet activation? Are calcium ions this second messenger and, if not, what is the role of calcium ions in platelet activation?

Platelet Function

PLATELETS IN HAEMOSTASIS AND THROMBOSIS

G.V.R. Born

Department of Pharmacology, King's College,
London WC2R 2LS

When blood vessels are injured so that they bleed, circulating platelets adhere to the damaged vessel walls and aggregate together, whereby the haemorrhage is diminished or arrested. This interaction between platelets and vessel walls has, therefore, an easily demonstrable physiological function. There is much clinical and experimental evidence that deficiency or defects of circulating platelets is associated with "spontaneous" haemorrhages from small vessels. This suggests that platelets are somehow essential for the functional integrity of these vessels, but no mechanism has yet been established.

Claims are made that agents released from platelets are able to damage vessel walls, either acutely (Mustard, Packham & Kinlough-Rathbone, 1977   ) or by contributing to atherogenesis (Ross & Glomset, 1973). The evidence for these propositions is indirect and circumstantial and no such effects have been incontrovertibly established (see Walton, 1975). On the other hand, there is conclusive evidence that occlusive thrombi in arteries damaged by atherosclerosis contain platelets as a major if not the main component. The formation of platelet thrombi appears so similar to that of haemostatic plugs of platelets that analysis of the mechanism of the latter is likely to provide understanding of the former.

This contribution considers how the mechanism depends on the haemodynamic and biochemical environment in which platelets adhere to and aggregate on vessel walls.

DOES INTERACTION BETWEEN PLATELETS AND ARTERIAL WALLS CONTRIBUTE TO ATHEROGENESIS?

The old thrombogenic hypothesis of atherosclerosis (von Rokitansky, 1841; Duguid, 1948) has reappeared in modern costume as claims that <u>platelets</u> contribute to atherogenesis in three ways. First, through damaging arterial endothelial cells by releasing injurious agents, presumably where circulating platelets adhere (Mustard, et al., 1977). Secondly, through the release in such situations of a factor responsible for smooth muscle proliferation in the arterial wall (Ross & Glomset, 1973). Thirdly, through the formation of persistent mural thrombi which are organised into intimal thickenings (see, eg, Mustard & Packham, 1975).

Such evidence as there is for these propositions establishes none of them as relevant to atherosclerosis in animals or man (see Walton, 1975). Underlying all three claims is the assumption that a proportion of normal circulating platelets settle on arterial walls for long enough to release some of their contents. There is no observational basis for this assumption in normal arteries. Therefore it is assumed further that arterial endothelium is continuously subject to "damage" or "injury" of some kind as a precondition for the adherence of platelets. There is no convincing evidence for this generalisation, certainly not in man. The only experimental basis which could conceivably apply to human arteries is the higher replacement rate of endothelium around the openings of branches than elsewhere in guinea-pig aorta (Payling-Wright & Born, 1971). This is most simply explained by assuming a dependence of endothelial turnover on, *inter alia*, haemodynamic effects due to non-laminar blood-flow over such areas. But this should be thought of more correctly as a quasi-physiological effect and, even there, platelets are rarely if ever seen adhering to the walls. The turnover rate of endothelium is increased in experimental hypertension (Payling-Wright, 1972). This is compatible with hypertension as a "risk factor" for coronary heart disease. It seems more likely that this is because of an accelerating effect on plasma lipoprotein accumulation through inter-endothelial gaps (Stehbens, 1965; Caro, 1977) than due to an increase in the indiscriminate or even selective deposition of platelets on arterial walls. Indeed, there are other ways in which hypertension could accelerate atherosclerosis (see Caro, 1977).

INTERACTION BETWEEN PLATELETS AND VESSEL WALLS IN THROMBOGENESIS

Gross and histological appearances of arterial thrombi establish that the central mass consists mainly of aggregated platelets. What, therefore, is the mechanism responsible for rapid and extensive platelet aggregation in an atheromatous artery as an apparently random event in time (see Born, 1979)? Close serial sectioning of obstructed coronary arteries established some time ago that the platelet thrombus responsible is invariably associated with recent haemorrhage into an underlying atherosclerotic placque (Friedman & Byers, 1965; Constantinides, 1966). The haemorrhages occur through fissures or fractures in the placque; and it is a reasonable assumption that the sudden appearance of such a fissure or fracture is the random, individually unpredictable event affecting coronary arteries that has to be assumed to account for the clinical onset of acute coronary thrombosis (Born, 1979).

How does haemorrhage into a ruptured placque start off platelet thrombogenesis? This can be regarded as part of the general question of how platelets are caused to aggregate through haemorrhage, most effectively haemorrhage from arteries. Until recently this was commonly answered by assuming that the process depends on the adhesion of platelets to collagen which is exposed where damaged vessel walls are denuded of endothelium. Adhering platelets then release other agents including thromboxane A_2 and ADP which in turn are responsible for the adhesion of more platelets as growing aggregates. This explanation is unlikely to be correct, for the following reasons. First, haemostatic and thrombotic aggregates of platelets grow without delay and very rapidly, (Hugues, 1959). For example, when an arteriole 200 μm in diameter is cut into laterally, the rate of accession of platelets to the haemostatic plug is of the order of 10^4 per second (Born & Richardson, 1979). In contrast, although the adhesion of platelets to collagen itself is almost instantaneous the subsequent aggregation of platelets begins, even under optimal conditions for their reactivity, only after a delay or lag period of at least 15 to 30 sec (Wilner, Nossel & LeRoy, 1968). Secondly, platelets tend to aggregate as mural thrombi when anti-coagulated blood flows through the plastic vessels of artificial organs such as oxygenators or dialysers (Richardson, Galetti & Born, 1976) which contain no collagen nor anything else capable of activating platelets similarly. This implies that there are conditions under which platelets are activated in the blood by something other than collagen or other constituents of the walls of living vessels.

The placque on which a thrombus grows has usually narrowed the arterial lumen. At constant blood pressure the flow of blood is faster through the constriction than elsewhere in the artery. Therefore, high flow and wall shear rates are no hindrance to the aggregation of platelets as thrombi (Born, 1977). Indeed, the question arises whether the activation of platelets which precedes their aggregation depends in some way on such abnormal haemodynamic conditions.

Measurements of the haemodynamic forces required to activate platelets directly (Hellums & Brown, 1977) indicate that the blood flow over atherosclerotic lesions *in vivo* is unable to do so (Colantouni, Hellums, Moake & Alfrey, 1977). Therefore, the activation must be indirect. Now it has been known for many years that platelets can be activated by at least one agent, namely ADP, derived from the red cells which outnumber and surround the platelets in the blood. Indeed, the discovery of the activation of platelets by ADP which is highly specific among nucleotides and related substances began with the demonstration that the adhesion of platelets in columns of small glass beads depended on the presence of red cells and varied in proportion to their concentration (Hellem, 1960); the agent was identified as ADP (Gaarder et al., 1961)

This contribution is, therefore, mainly concerned with questions, most of them unanswered, about effects of the fluid dynamics in and around a vascular leak on the interactions of platelets with the walls of the vessel and with the red cells, and on the chemical agents responsible for making the platelet adhere and aggregate.

Most of what is known about these agents and their effects on platelets has come from *in vitro* experiments (for a recent review see Ciba Foundation, 1975) in which adhesion and aggregation can be correlated with biochemical changes by comparatively easy and highly reproducible methods (Born, 1962). The relevance of *in vitro* observations to platelet aggregation as seen *in vivo* during haemostasis is still uncertain. The main reason for this is probably that it is much more difficult to devise satisfactory quantative methods for investigating the process *in vivo* than *in vitro*; and the main cause of the difficulty is the astonishing rapidity with which platelets adhere and aggregate in a blood vessel after it has been injured, in spite of extremely rapid blood flow which would be expected to counteract these processes. The haemodynamic situation should be well imprinted on the mind, preferably by microcinematographic observation of the haemostatic process, when considering hypotheses to explain *in vivo* platelet aggregation in biochemical terms.

Haemodynamic conditions during arteriolar haemostasis

The effectiveness of platelet aggregation in plugging a leak is at least as effective in arterioles as in venules. As the haemodynamic situation should be more unfavourable to aggregate formation in arterioles than in venules, an explanation of arteriolar haemostasis is likely to account in principle also for that in venules. For that reason, the following considerations are limited to arterioles.

When an arteriole is cut, platelets are seen to adhere with great rapidity to the damaged vessel wall, while the red cells continue to rush by. The high flow velocity in relation to the small size of the vessels implies the presence in the fluid of strong mechanical forces acting normally and tangentially on and near the vessel walls. The cut causes a sudden diminution in the peripheral resistance to the flow; and if the inflow pressure remains constant the mean flow velocity increases. Thus the fluid-mechanical forces on platelets adhering and aggregating on the vessel wall become greater still. With increasing size the platelet aggregates tend to constrict the cut causing a further, although usually temporary, increase in flow velocity.

In spite of wall shear stresses of 10^4 to 10^5 dyn/cm^2, which are one or two orders of magnitude greater than anywhere in the normal circulation, platelets succeed in aggregating into haemostatically effective plugs. The blood-flow velocities that would be experinced by platelets closest to the vessel wall and therefore with the sites of damage can be calculated (Schmid-Schönbein, Rieger & Fischer, 1976). Human platelets have a major diameter of about 1,5 µm. In an arteriole of medium size the flow velocity of plasma and of any cells in it at a distance of 1 µm from the wall is of the order of 10-100 µm/ms. Therefore, a platelet flowing within a distance no greater than its own diameter would pass an injury site 100 µm long in at most 10 ms. In the absence of other influences, this would seem to be the time available for such a platelet to adhere to the damaged wall.

Activation time of platelets

The time just calculated as available to circulating platelets "at risk" for adhering to a wall lesion has to be compared with what is known about the time required for the activation of platelets into a condition in which it is highly probable that their collision with such a lesion would result in adhesion. That a process of activation is an essential prerequisite for adhesion and aggregation is inferred from the non-reactivity of normal circulating platelets.

As activation is indicated by adhesiveness, the change must involve one or more constituents of the platelets' outer surface. There is evidence that the essence is the exposure of surface receptors for fibrinogen, which has long been known to be an essential and specific plasma co-factor for platelet aggregation (Born & Cross, 1964; Cross, 1964). The activation time of platelets may then be defined as the interval between the encounter of platelets with an activating agent such as ADP and their ability to react with plasma fibrinogen.

Until recently, it seemed reasonable to suppose that the activation of platelets was accompanied by the gross morphological changes which are quantifiable morphometrically or photometrically *in vitro* (Born, 1970). A prominent component of this change is the extrusion of long thin spikes; and it seemed reasonable to assume that the ability of platelets, like that of other cells with fixed surface charges, to approach closely enough for adhesion is facilitated by the extrusion of pseudopodia. The first question is, therefore, whether anything approaching the gross morphological changes demonstrable *in vitro* invariable precedes adhesion and aggregation *in vivo*. However, recent electron microscopical observations indicate that platelets can adhere to vessel walls and to each other without any obvious deviations from their normal morphology (Born, 1977). Whether this is really so can be conclusively established only by quantitative statistical electron-microscopical methods of the kind that have established, for example, the reversibility of the shape-changing effects of ADP (Born, et al., 1978). If, therefore, activation is accompanied by changes in morphology they are apparently beyond the limits of resolution in time and emplitude of the *in vitro* photometric techniques so far employed. Minimal morphological changes should occur in very much less time than the time constant determined for the gross changes in shape.

At all events, activation as defined above is likely to precede the gross morphological changes which, at 37°, have a time constant of the order of 1 sec (Born, 1970). This is some two orders of magnitude greater than the time available for adhesion under conditions that are likely to obtain *in vivo*. The discrepancy is so great that the assumptions underlying the calculations have to be reconsidered on the basis of additional experimental evidence.

Platelet activation *in vivo*

That circulating platelets can be activated to adhere in much less time than that required by the gross shape changes is indicated by direct experimental observations. An arteriole can be irradiated by a laser in such a way that damage is limited to a few square micrometres of endothelium (Arfors, Cockburn & Gross, 1976). The site of damage is covered almost immediately with platelets that must have been activated in small fractions of a second.

Very similar events follow the application of the activating agent ADP by micro-ionophoresis to the outside of an arteriole or venule under conditions in which appropriate controls indicate complete absence of any evidence of damage to the endothelial layer (Begent & Born, 1970; Begent, Born & Sharp, 1972). Platelet aggregates grow in the vessel exactly opposite the tip of the micropipette, while the blood continues to flow rapidly and without noticeable disturbance over the site. This is explained most simply by assuming that sufficient ADP diffuses between the endothelial cells into the blood to reach platelets passing close to the wall and that this ADP activates them in a few milliseconds.

An extension of this technique has provided a basis for calculating an average activation time for circulating platelets. It was found that the size of platelet aggregates produced by the iontophoretic application of ADP increases exponentially. The rate constant of this increase depended on the mean blood flow velocity, determined in the same vessels at the same time, as shown in Fig. 1a (Begent & Born, 1970). The shape of the experimentally determined curve was simulated closely by the theoretical curve shown in Fig. 1b (Richardson, 1973) which was derived on the single assumption that platelets require an activation time of about 100 ms to 200 ms. This time is still one order of magnitude greater than that indicated by the earlier theoretical considerations, so that either this experimental derivation gives an over-estimate of the true activation time or the earlier considerations failed to take something into account that would allow flowing platelets more than a few milliseconds for activation. More time would, for example, be available if the blood flow near the vessel wall were non-laminar, so that platelets caught up in vortices, however small, might be exposed to localised activating conditions for longer than they would otherwise be. When branching vessels of the microcirculation are observed microscopically, platelets can often be seen trapped in vortices for variable times of up to several seconds. Such delays may occur in the immediate vicinity of major vessel wall lesions, whether caused by disease such as the sudden rupture of an atheromatous plaque (Constantinides, 1966; Friedman & Van den Bovenkamp, 1966) or by traumatic injury such as a puncture of transection. However, there is no evidence of even the smallest disturbances in the flow of blood in a normal vessel in which platelets are caused to adhere by ionophoretically applied ADP. Moreover, it seems most unlikely that any endothelial unevenness produced by laser injury would give rise to flow disturbances large enough to delay the passage of platelets.

Physical versus chemical activation of platelets

The major question is, therefore, the nature of the stimulus or stimuli which activate platelets so very rapidly under conditions in which they function haemostatically. One type of stimulus is primarily physical, ie, the effect of fluid-mechanical forces on the platelets. It has been established that platelets are activated by shear stresses greater than about 100 dyn/cm^2 and that the time required for activation varies inversely with applied shear stress (Colantouni, et al., 1977). However, even with shear stresses as great as those calculated for arteriolar lesions, only a very small proportion of platelets is activated in the time during which they are passing by.

Fluid-mechanical effects are, however, apparently able to activate platelets <u>indirectly</u> by acting on the red cells that surround and outnumber them in the blood. Clear evidence for this was provided by experiments in which blood was made to flow through branching channels in extracorporeal shunts (Rowntree & Shionoya, 1927; Mustard, Rowsell & Dounie, 1962). Chambers made of different plastic material were introduced into a shunt through which heparinised blood flowed from a carotid artery to a jugular vein of anaesthetised pigs. Deposits of platelets formed consistently on the shoulders of a bifurcation in the flow chamber but nowhere else in the channels. Clearly, therefore, this deposition did not depend on the properties of the materials from which the chambers were made. Furthermore, when the chambers were perfused not with blood but with platelet-rich plasma no deposit formed, showing that red cells were essential for the increased reactivity of the platelets that resulted in their mural deposition. The augmenting effect of red cells on the deposition of platelets can also be demonstrated with blood flowing through chambers of other geometrical conformations or other types of wall surface. For example, the endothelium can be removed by introducing a balloon catheter into rabbit aortas, exposing a subendothelial surface composed mainly of connective tissue; such a subendothelial surface can also be exposed to blood flowing in annular chambers of different diameters to provide a variety of shear rates at the blood-surface interface (Baumgartner & Haudenschild, 1972; Baumgartner, 1973; Turitto & Baumgartner, 1975). When blood was perfused over such a surface, platelets soon covered almost all of it and there were numerous platelet aggregates or thrombi on the adhering layer. When platelet-rich plasma was perfused instead of blood, very few platelets were deposited.

The increased deposition of platelets from flowing blood associated with the presence of the red cells could be caused by physical or chemical mechanisms or, of course, by both acting synergistically. A physical mechanism would depend essentially on an increase in the diffusivity of platelets caused by the flow behaviour of the erythrocytes. Indeed, the diffusivity of platelets in flowing blood has been estimated to be two orders of magnitude greater than that predicted for platelets diffusing in plasma (Turitto, Benis & Leonard, 1972; Turitto & Baumgartner, 1975). This is consistent with the enhanced radial fluctuations of erythrocytes and latex microspheres (2 μm in diameter) in flowing suspensions of red-cell ghosts (Goldsmith, 1972).

There is evidence also of a chemical mechanism for the increased adhesiveness of platelets in the presence of red cells, ie, through release of their ADP. The concentrations of ADP required are small (less than 10^{-6} M Milton, et al., 1979) so that its direct demonstration in plasma involved two important considerations : first, red cells are such a large reservoir of ATP and ADP that the slightest damage to them swamps the plasma with ADP; and, secondly, because the outer surfaces of the cells as well as the plasma contain enzymes that catalyse the rapid breakdown of ADP (Bolton & Emmons, 1967; Haslam & Mills, 1967 Parker, 1970). Therefore, the release of ADP into plasma has been inferred indirectly by demonstrating that the effect of red cells on platelets is prevented by the addition of enzyme systems capable of utilising ADP specifically. Thus, in the presence of the pyruvate kinase system, which removes ADP by enzymic phosphorylation to ATP, the difference in the adhesiveness to glass of platelets from whole blood or from platelet-rich plasma is abolished and so is the increase in platelet adhesiveness caused by adding red cells to platelet-rich plasma (Harrison & Mitchell, 1966). Similar results are obtained with added apyrase which catalyses the hydrolysis of ADP to AMP. Indirect evidence of this kind is analogous to the conclusion that abolition to atropine of, say, a secretion indicates that it is mediated physiologically by acetylcholine which, unless its destruction is prevented by an anticholinesterase, is too rapidly destroyed to be demonstrated directly.

It has recently become possible to demonstrate the appearance of free ADP in blood directly in concentration sufficiently high to activate platelets (Schmid-Schönbein, et al., 1979). In specially designed apparatus whole blood or resuspended cells are exposed to controlled, different shear stresses for known time periods. The apparatus is designed to cover the range of these variables presumed to be relevant to the *in vivo* situations. The experiments show that ADP appears in the plasma in concentrations above those required for platelet activation (0.1 to 1.0 μM) but in direct proportion to free haemoglobin, indicating that platelet activation can result from small degrees of haemolysis due to haemodynamic stresses such as occur during haemorrhage, whether external or through a placque fissure. It seems, moreover, that the appearance of free ADP is rapdi enough to account for *in vivo* aggregation. This process is much faster than the release of ADP from the platelets themselves or of thromboxane A_2 produced by them which, in any case, induces aggregation via ADP (personal communications from B. Samuelsson and A. Marcus).

Other experiments (Born, Bergquist & Arfors, 1976) provide further evidence that the indirect activation of platelets via erythrocytes is mediated chemically rather than physically. When a polyethylene tube 200 μm internal diameter is perfused with heparinised blood at

37°C, a small puncture is sealed off within two minutes or so by a haemostatic plus of platelets, just as in a living blood vessel. This "bleeding time" is prolonged when the blood contains chloropromazine in low concentrations which have no effect on platelets but which increase the resistance of erythrocytes to hypotonic haemolysis (Seeman, 1972). Under these conditions, therefore, the activation of platelets is inhibited by a membrane-stabilising drug acting on the accompanying red cells by diminishing either their physical collision-mediated effect, which seems improbable, or their release of platelet-activating agent, presumably ADP.

Recent discoveries about prostaglandins and related substances suggest another way in which fluid-mechanical forces could initiate chemical changes resulting in the haemostatic aggregation of platelets. The first step in the formation of thromboxane A_2 by platelets which it causes to aggregate (Hamberg, Svensson & Samuelsson, 1975; Svensson, Hamberg & Samuelsson, 1976) is the release of arachidonic acid from phospholipids in the cell membrane. This release is catalysed by the enzyme phospholipase A_2, which is normally inactive in platelets. How the enzyme is activated physiologically is not known, but perhaps activation is initiated by small distortions of the outer membrane of platelets passing through a field of fluid-mechanical forces greater than those in the normal circulation, for example, during arteriolar haemorrhage. Such fluid-mechanical activation of platelets would not involve the red cells which apparently do not contain the thromboxane-forming system.

Significance of the haemostatic reactivity of platelets

Platelets can be activated by an extraordinary variety of naturally occurring agents, including ADP, collagen, thrombin, arachidonic acid, thromboxane A_2, some prostaglandins, and several neurotransmitters including, at least in the dog, even acetylcholine. Human platelets, those of other mammals and the functionally homologous thrombocytes of birds (Belamarich & Simoneit, 1973) are activated by 5-hydroxytryptamine (serotonin) which is also accumulated in the platelets by mechanisms similar to those in tryptaminergic neurones. Because of these similarities, platelets are used increasingly as accessible models for nerve cells, with promising results.

The question remains why such extraordinary pharmacological reactivity should be associated with this type of circulating cell, the only certain function of which is in haemostasis. Local haemostasis must now be one of the few of the homeostatic mechanisms of the organism, if not the only one, in which neither the central nervous system nor the endocrine system is directly involved. The ability of platelets to be activated by so many different agents may, therefore, be an evolutionary adaptation to the comparative isolation in which they carry out their literally vital function.

REFERENCES

Arfors, K.E., Cockburn, J.S., and Gross, J.F., 1976. Measurement of growth rate of laser-induced intravascular platelet aggregation and the influence of blood flow velocity. Microvasc.Res., 11, 79-82.

Baumgartner, H.R., and Haudenschild, C., 1972. Adhesion of platelets to subendothelium. Ann.N.Y.Acad.Sci., 201, 22-36.

Baumgartner, H.R., 1973. The role of blood flow in platelet adhesion, fibrin deposition and formation of mural thrombi. Microvasc.Res., 5, 167-179.

Begent, N.A., and Born, G.V.R., 1970. Growth rate in vivo of platelet thrombi produced by iontophoresis of ADP, as a function of mean blood flow velocity. Nature, 227, 926-930.

Begent, N.A., Born, G.V.R., and Sharp, D.E., 1972. The initiation of platelet thrombi in normal venules and its acceleration by histamine. J.Physiol. (London), 223, 229-242.

Belmarich, F.A., and Simoneit, L.W., 1973. Aggregation of duck thrombocytes by 5-hydroxytryptamine. Microvasc.Res., 6, 229-234.

Bolton, C.H., and Emmons, P.R., 1967. Adenosine diphosphate breakdown by the plasma of different species and by human whole blood and white cells. Thromb.Diath.Haemorrh., 18, 779-782.

Born, G.V.R., 1962. Aggregation of blood platelets by adenosine diphosphate and its reversal. Nature, 194, 927-929.

Born, G.V.R., and Gross, M.J., 1963. The aggregation of blood platelets. J.Physiol., 168, 178-195.

Born, G.V.R., 1970. Observation on the change in shape in blood platelets brought about by adenosine diphosphate. J.Physiol., (London), 209, 487-511.

Born, G.V.R., Bergquist, D., and Arfors, K.E., 1976. Evidence for inhibition of platelet activation in blood by a drug effect on erythrocytes. Nature, 259, 233.

Born, G.V.R., 1977. Fluid-mechanical and biochemical interaction in haemostasis. Br.Med.Bull., 33, 193-197.

Born, G.V.R., Dearnley, R., Foulks, J.G., and Sharp, D.E., 1978. Quantification of the morphological reaction of platelets to aggregation inhibitors. J.Physiol., 280, 193-212.

Born, G.V.R., Dearnley, R., Foulks, J.G., and Sharp, D.E., 1978. Quantification of the morphological reaction of platelets to aggregating agents and of its reversal by aggregation inhibitors. J.Physiol., 280, 193-212.

Born, G.V.R., 1979. Arterial thrombosis and its prevention. Excerpta Medica., (Amsterdam) (in press).

Caro, C.G., 1977. Mechanical factors in atherogenesis, in Cardiovascular Flow Dynamics and Measurements (Hwang and Normann, eds.) pp.473-487. Univ.Park Press Baltimore.

Ciba Foundation Symp.: Biochemistry and Pharmacology of Platelets, Elsevier, Excerpta Medica, North-Holland, 1975.

Colantuoni, G., Hellums, J.D., Moake, J.L., Alfrey, C.P., 1977. The response of human platelets to shear stress at short exposure times. Trans.Am.Soc.Artif.Internal Organs, 23, 626-630.

Constantinides, P., 1966. Plaque fissures in human coronary thrombosis. J.Ather.Res., 6, 1-17.

Cross, M.J., 1964. Effect of fibrinogen on the aggregation of platelets by adenosine diphosphate. Thromb.Diath.Haemorrh., 12, 524-527.

Duguid, J.B., 1948. Thrombosis as a factor in the pathogenesis of aortic atherosclerosis. J.Pathol.Bact., 60, 57-61.

Friedman, M., and Byers, S.O., 1965. Aortic atherosclerosis interaction in rabbits by prior endothelial denudation. Arch.Pathol. 79, 345-356.

Friedman, M., and Van den Bovenkamp, G.J., 1966. Pathogenesis of a coronary thrombosis. Am.J.Pathol., 48, 19-44.

Gaarder, A., Jonsen, J., Leland, S., Hellem, A., and Owren, P.A., 1961. Adenosine diphosphate in red cells as a factor in the adhesiveness of human blood platelets. Nature, 192, 531-532.

Goldsmith, H.L., 1972. The flow of model particles and blood cells and its relation to thrombogenesis, in Progress in Hemostasis and Thrombosis (Spaet, ed.) Vol. 1, pp.97-139. Grune and Stratton, New York.

Hamberg, M., Svensson, J., and Samuelsson, B., 1975. Thrombozanes: New group of biological active compounds derived from prostaglandin endoperoxidases. Proc.Natl.Acad.Sci.USA., 72, 2994-2998.

Harrison, M.J.G., and Mitchell, J.R.A., 1966. The influence of red blood cells on platelet adhesiveness. Lancet, 2, 1163-1164.

Haslem, R.J., and Mills, D.C.B., 1967. The adenylate kinase of human plasma, erythrocytes and platelets in relation to the degradation of adenosine diphosphate in plasma. Biochem.J. 103, 773-784.

Hellem, A.J., 1960. The adhesiveness of human blood platelets in vitro. Scand.J. of Clin. and Laboratory Invest., 12, suppl. 51.

Hellums, J.D., and Brown, C.H., 1977. Blood cells damage by mechanical forces. in Cardiovascular Flow Dynamics and Measurements. (Hwang and Normann, eds.) pp.799-823. Univ.Park Press Baltimore Md. USA.

Hugues, J., 1959. Metamorphose visqueuse des plaquettes ét formation du clou hemostatique. Thromb.Diath.Haemorrh., 3, 34.

Milton, J.G., Yung, W., Glushak, C., and Frojmovic, M.M., 1979. Kinetics of ADP-induced human platelet shape change: Apparent positive cooperativity. Thromb.Haem., 42, 465.(Abstract).

Mustard, J.F., Murphy, E.A., Rowsell, H.C., and Downie, H.G., 1962. Factors influencing thrombus formation in vivo. Am.J.Med., 33, 621-647.

Mustard, J.F., and Packham, M.A., 1975. The role of blood and platelets in atherosclerosis and the composition of atherosclerosis. Thromb.Diath.Haemorrh., 33, 444.

Mustard, J.F., Packham, M.A. and Kinlough-Rathbone, R.L., 1977. Platelets and thrombosis in the development of atherosclerosis and its complications. Adv.Exp.Med.Biol., 102, 7-30.

Mustard, J.F., Moore, S., Packham, M.A., and Kinlough-Rathbone, R.L., 1977. Platelets, thrombosis and atherosclerosis. in Proceedings of the First International Atherosclerosis Conference. Prog. Biochem.Pharmacol. Basel.

Parker, J.C., 1970. Metabolism of external adenine nucleotides by human red blood cells. Am.J.Physiol., 218, 1568-1574.

Payling-Wright, H., and Born, G.V.R., 1970. Reactions of blood platelets and endothelium relevant to thrombosis. in Platelets Vessel Wall - Fibrin Deposition, Symp., 1969. (Schettler, ed.) pp.96-97. George Thieme, Stuttgart

Richardson, P.D., 1973. Effect of blood flow velocity on growth rate of platelet thrombi. Nature, 245, 103-104.

Richardson, P.D., Galletti, P.M., and Born, G.V.R., 1976. Regional administration of drugs to control thrombosis in artificial organs. Trans.Am.Soc.Artif.Intern.Organs, 22, 22-29.

Ross, R., and Glomset, J., 1973. Atherosclerosis and the arterial smooth muscle cell. Proliferation of smooth muscle is a key event in the genesis of the lesions of atherosclerosis. Science, 180, 1207-1210.

Rowntree, L.G., and Shionoya, T., 1927. Studies in experimental extracorporeal thrombosis. I. A method for the direct observation of extracorporeal thrombus formation. J.Exp.Med., 46, 7-12.

Schmid-Schönbein, H., Rieger, H., Fischer, T., 1976. in Blood Vessels; Problems arising at the border of natural and artificial vessels. (Effert and Meyer-Erkelenz, eds.) pp.57-63. Springer, Berlin.

Schmid-Schönbein, H., Born, G.V.R., Richardson, P.D., Cusack, N.J., Rieger, H., Forst, R., Rohling-Winckle, I., Blasberg, P., and Wehmeier, A., 1979. Biorheology (in press).

Seeman, P., 1972, The membrane actions of anaesthetics and tranquilizers. Pharmacol.Rev., 24, 583-655.

Stehbens, W.E., 1965. Intimal proliferation and spontaneous lipid deposition in the cerebral arteries of sheeps and skeers. J.Ather.Res., 5, 556-568.

Svensson, J., Hamberg, M., and Samuelsson, B., 1975. Proc.Natl. Acad.Sci.USA., 72, 2994-2998.

Turitto, V.T., Benis, A.M., and Leonard, E.F., 1972. Platelet diffusion in flowing blood. Ind.Eng.Chem.Fund., 11, 216-223.

Turitto, V.T., and Baumgartner, H.R., 1975. Platelet interaction with subendothelium in a perfusion system: Physical role of red blood cells. <u>Microvascular Res</u>., 9, 335-344.

Von Rokitansky, C., 1842. <u>Handbuch der pathologicken anatomie</u>. Vol. 2 : 534. Braunmuller and Seidel. Vienna, Austria. (1852 trans. by G.E. Day : 261 Sydenham Society London, England).

INTERACTION OF PLATELETS WITH SUBENDOTHELIUM IN FLOWING BLOOD

H.R. Baumgartner, R. Muggli and Th.B. Tschopp

Pharma Research Department, F. Hoffmann-La Roche & Co. Ltd.
4002 Basel, Switzerland

INTRODUCTION

The interaction of platelets with subendothelial connective tissue is thought to play an important role in the pathogenesis of thrombosis and arteriosclerosis. Subendothelium exposed to flowing blood in vivo is rapidly covered with platelets which release some of their constituents. Some of the released substances may induce various biologically significant reactions including platelet aggregation, plasma coagulation, vasoconstriction and smooth muscle cell proliferation. In order to investigate more carefully the interaction of platelets with subendothelium in vitro we developed annular perfusion chambers. The chambers were initially designed to mimic in vitro the sequence of events observed in vivo (Baumgartner, 1973). In the meantime the use of this new experimental tool has led to studies far beyond the initial scope. It emerged that in addition to the reactivity of subendothelium and platelets a number of other variables are important for the interaction of platelets with subendothelium. These include rheologic parameters, red cell concentration, factor VIII/von Willebrand factor and activities generated and released by the vessel wall.

The early results obtained in experiments with annular perfusion chambers were reviewed by Baumgartner and Muggli (1976). Weiss et al.(1978b) have discussed the results obtained with blood of patients with defects of platelet function and Turitto et al. (1979) have analyzed the rheologic aspects. The present paper updates our methodological approach and summarizes our present knowledge on the platelet reactive component(s) of subendothelium, on platelet reactivity and on the importance of rheologic parameters and red cells. The main focus is on more recent observations regarding the effects of anticoagulation, factor VIII/von Willebrand factor and platelet inhibitory activity generated by the vessel wall.

MATERIALS AND METHODS

Preparation of subendothelium. For exposure of subendothelium in vivo the endothelial lining is removed by means of a balloon catheter (Baumgartner, 1973). For exposure of subendothelium in annular perfusion chambers we currently use 4 preparations of everted rabbit aortae: (1) aortic segments prepared as described by Baumgartner (1973) and stored in Tris buffer at 4°C for 1-3 weeks ["stored vessels"]; (2) aortic segments prepared as "stored vessels" but without ballooning and used as quickly as possible for perfusion experiments ["fresh vessels"]; (3) aortic segments prepared as "fresh vessels", immediately frozen in liquid nitrogen, stored at -70°C and used after thawing under standardized conditions ["-70°C vessels"] and (4) aortic segments prepared as "fresh vessels" and subsequently treated with 10^{-3}M $HgCl_2$ in isotonic saline in order to block enzymatic activities ["$HgCl_2$ vessels"].

Exposure of subendothelium to flowing blood. Anticoagulated blood is usually recirculated from a reservoir at 37°C by a roller pump (Baumgartner et al., 1980a); native blood is either drawn from a vessel through the chamber at the selected flow rate (Baumgartner, 1976) or recirculated by using the chamber as extracorporeal shunt (Baumgartner, 1979). The wall shear rates obtained in annular flow chambers by perfusing blood at various flow rates were recently summarized (Turitto and Baumgartner, 1979).

Evaluation of platelet interaction with surfaces. Table 1 lists the parameters used to evaluate platelet-surface interactions after exposure to flowing blood in annular or flat chambers (Muggli et al., 1980).

TABLE 1. Quantitation of platelet interaction with surfaces.

Approach	Unit	Reference
Stereology on cross sections		
Contact platelets (C)	%*	(1)
Contact + spread platelets (C+S), adhesion	%*	(1)
Fibrin (F)	%*	(2)
Thrombi >5µm in height (T)	%*	(1)
Aggregation (100 T/S)	%**	(1)
Thrombus volume	$\mu m^3/\mu m^2$	(3)
Maximum thrombus height	µm	(3)
Microdensitometry "en face"		
Adhesion (D55)	%*	(4)
Thrombi (D33)	%*	(4)
Aggregation (100 D33/D55)	%**	(4)
Protein deposition	$\mu g/mm^2$	(4)
Deposition of [^{51}Cr]-platelets	cpm/mm^2	(5)

* percent of exposed surface covered with platelets or thrombi
** percent of spread platelets covered with thrombi

(1) Baumgartner und Muggli, 1976; (2) Baumgartner, 1976; (3) Baumgartner et al., 1980b; (4) Muggli et al., 1980, (5) Tschopp, 1977.

The correlation between corresponding values, such as thrombus volume and deposition of [^{51}Cr]-platelets (Tschopp, 1977) or protein- and [^{51}Cr]-platelet deposition (Muggli et al., 1980), was shown to be excellent. Analysis of sections by stereological techniques yields the most detailed and precise information, is - however - also most fastidious.

RESULTS AND DISCUSSION

Components of subendothelium. The subendothelium of aortae consists of a reticular network of collagen fibrils resting on the elastic lamina and embedded in amorphous basement membrane-like material. In addition, elastic microfibrils can be identified (Stemerman et al., 1971). The collagen fibrils are mostly composed of type III collagen molecules (Gay and Miller, 1978).

Amorphous basement membranes contain at least one collagenous protein and one or more noncollagenous glycoproteins. However, there is no general consensus with respect to the nature and number of its components, which may differ depending on the tissue and the anatomic location. From studies carried out on lens capsules and glomerular basement membrane collagen (Kefalides, 1975) the term "tpye IV collagen" is often used as equivalent to "basement membrane collagen". Other studies suggest a rich variety of collagen molecules (Gay and Miller, 1978; Trelstad and Carvalho, 1979). Information concerning the molecular organization and deposition of collagen molecules within basement membranes in the subendothelial tissue of vessels is incomplete and must be inferred from results obtained in studies with other tissues.

Among the noncollagenous elements, fibronectin (Stenman and Vaheri, 1978) and the glycoprotein laminin (Timpl et al., 1979) have been positively identified in subendothelium of vessel walls.

Reactivity of subendothelium and its components. On the subendothelial surface of rabbit iliac arteries in vivo surface coverage with platelets increases asymptotically to complete surface coverage (Baumgartner, 1973). Up to 100% of the surface is already covered with platelets after 10 min. The appearance of thrombi is transient with a peak of about 20% surface coverage at 10 min. After longer exposure times surface coverage with platelet thrombi declined, leading ultimately to a non-thrombogenic monolayer of spread and degranulated platelets. This time-curve of adhesion and platelet thrombus formation can be reproduced in the annular chamber with subendothelium of rabbit aortae (Baumgartner, 1973).

Each morphologically identifiable component differs with respect to its reactivity towards platelets (Baumgartner, 1974). Selective enzymic studies showed that the few platelets which adhere to elastin and microfibrils do so by simple cellular contacts. On the other hand, collagen fibrils trigger the release reaction, rapid transition from contact to spread platelets and the formation of platelet thrombi.

The role of amorphous basement membrane-like material is more difficult to assess. Electron microscopic studies of platelet-subendothelium interaction suggest that the stimulus provided by amorphous basement membrane-like material is strong enough to induce the formation of mural thrombi. On the other hand, glomerular basal lamina preparations limited platelet activation to adhesion when tested in vitro (Huang et al., 1974). In any case, the similarity of the time-curves of platelet adhesion on subendothelium and on an artificial surface composed exclusively of a mixture of soluble and fibrillar collagen (Fig. 1) indicates that the reactivity of subendothelium with respect to platelets resides chiefly in its collagenous components.

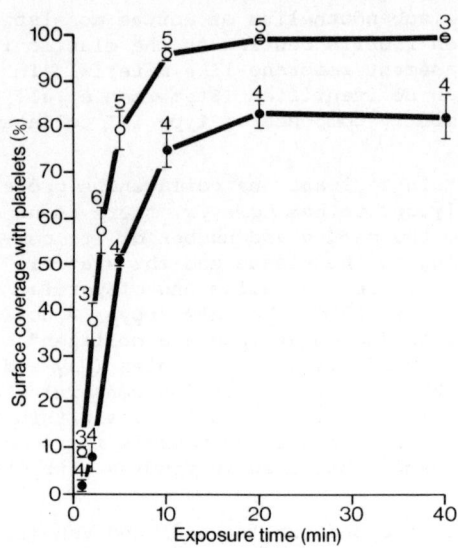

Fig. 1

Surface coverage with rabbit platelets as a function of the exposure time. Subendothelium exposed in the annular chamber at wall shear rates of 1,350 sec^{-1} (●, C+S). Artificial surface of a mixture of soluble and fibrillar collagen exposed in the flat flow chamber at wall shear rates of 1,000 sec^{-1} (○, D55).

Importance of platelet spreading for 100% surface coverage. Surfaces which do not trigger the spreading of platelets are saturated with platelets below 25% surface coverage (Leonard and Friedman, 1970; Baumgartner, 1974). The pattern of platelet deposition is non-random, in that around each platelet a distance of complete inhibition of adhesion is observed. The average minimum neighbour to neighbour distance is about 2.5 μm (Butruille, 1974) and can be ascribed to either electrostatic repulsion due to membrane surface charges or perturbation of local flow around previously adhered platelets.

Platelet reactivity. An important factor controlling the interaction of platelets with subendothelium is their reactivity. By studying patients with different platelet function disorders two main types of defective platelet-subendothelium interaction have emerged, i) defective platelet-surface interaction i.e. defective adhesion and/or ii) defective platelet-platelet interaction i.e. aggregation. The molecular abnormalities possibly responsible for some of these defects of platelet-subendothelium interaction have recently been identified and consist of abnormal glycoproteins of the platelet membrane.

Reduced platelet adhesion to subendothelium but normal adhesion-induced aggregation has been found in patients with von Willebrand disease (VWD) (see below) and in patients with the Bernard-Soulier syndrome (BSS) (Weiss et al., 1974). Platelets of both VWD and BSS do not aggregate in the presence of the antibiotic ristocetin (Howard and Firkin, 1971 ; Caen et al., 1973), which in VWD is due to the absence of factor VIII/VWF from plasma. Levels of factor VIII in plasma as well as in the platelet membrane of BSS are, however, normal (Caen et al., 1976). More recent studies found that the platelet membrane in BSS lacks glycocalicin and is deficient in glycoprotein I

(Nurden and Caen, 1978; Solum et al., 1977, Jamieson et al., 1979) indicating that both F VIII/VWF as well as glycocalicin are necessary for normal platelet adhesion to occur.

In vitro diagnostic criteria in patients with thrombasthenia include absent platelet aggregation, impaired clot retraction and decreased fibrinogen content of platelets (Weiss and Kochwa, 1968). Exposing subendothelium to flowing blood of two thrombasthenia patients at 800 sec^{-1} shear rate in the perfusion chamber showed normal platelet adhesion, but absent adhesion-induced platelet aggregation (Tschopp et al., 1975). Several workers found the platelets of these patients to contain decreased amounts of glycoprotein II and III (Nurden and Caen, 1978, Philips et al., 1975, Jamieson et al., 1979). In addition, an IgG antibody from the serum of a transfused thrombasthenia patient which was directed against a component of glycoprotein II (Levi-Toledano et al., 1978) induced upon perfusion a thrombasthenia-like aggregation defect when added to normal blood (Caen et al., 1977).

Adhesion-induced aggregation was also found to be deficient in patients with storage-pool disease (Weiss et al., 1975). The platelets of these patients have normal membrane glycoproteins (Jamieson et al., 1979) but contain and release decreased amounts of serotonin, ATP, ADP and Ca^{++} (Weiss, 1975) indicating that the membrane glycoproteins as well as the release reaction have to be normal for the sequence of platelet adhesion and aggregation to occur to the full extent.

<u>Shear rate dependence of platelet adhesion.</u> The wall shear rate is proportional to the ratio of blood flow velocity to vessel diameter. It is thus highest in arterioles or stenosed arteries and lowest in the large veins (Copley and King, 1976). Rheologic considerations indicate that the rate of platelet adhesion is predominantly transport controlled at shear rates up to 800 sec^{-1} (Turitto et al., 1979).

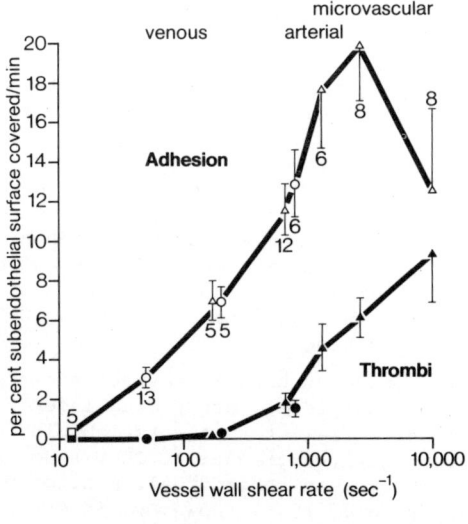

Fig. 2

Rates of coverage of subendothelium with platelets (adhesion), and with thrombi obtained at various wall shear rates in chambers of different annular diameters (d_e).

△ d_e = 0.7 ○ d_e = 2.4
□ d_e = 15.3 mm

(Data from Turitto and Baumgartner, 1979).

Thus, the frequency of platelet arrivals at the vessel wall determines the rate of adhesion at low shear. At higher shear rates platelet-surface reaction plays an increasing role for adhesion. Therefore platelet adhesion defects are more readily apparent at high than at low shear rates (Weiss et al., 1978b, Baumgartner et al., 1980a). The observation that the rates of adhesion were very similar at similar shear rates in chambers with different annular diameters despite markedly different blood flow rates is a strong argument in favour of a shear rate dependence of platelet adhesion. Thus at shear rates of 170 and 200 sec^{-1} adhesion was similar (Fig. 2) despite flow rates of 2.6 and 40 ml/min, respectively.

Thrombi do not form at very low shear rates. Their rate of formation increases sharply at approximately 650 sec^{-1} and continues to increase up to 10,000 sec^{-1} even though platelet adhesion is inhibited at the latter shear rate (Fig. 2). This decrease in adhesion is probably due to predominant consumption of platelets by the rapidly forming and growing thrombi. Thus comparatively few platelets reach the subendothelial surface at the highest shear rate.

Red blood cells markedly enhance platelet adhesion to subendothelium (Baumgartner et al., 1971). At a shear rate of 800 sec^{-1} the rate of platelet adhesion from whole blood was approximately 57 times that from platelet-rich plasma. Theoretical considerations indicate that this difference can be explained completely by the physical role of the red cells which enhance platelet transport towards the vessel wall (Turitto and Baumgartner, 1975). At much higher shear rates humoral factors possibly released by the red cells (Hellem, 1960) may also become important (Turitto and Weiss, 1980).

Effects of anticoagulation and drug-induced platelet inhibition. Our studies on the effects of anticoagulation are not yet completed. The results obtained in rabbits by using an annular chamber (d_e = 0.7 mm) as an extracorporeal shunt are summarized in Table 2. It appears that heparin (Liquemin ®) and the dicoumarol derivative, phenprocoumon (Marcoumar ®), have little, if any effect on platelet adhesion and thrombus formation on subendothelium; they prevent fibrin deposition. Thus platelets function normally at very low levels of the clotting factors II, VII, IX, X and in the presence of a strong thrombin and factor Xa antagonist. On the other hand thrombus volume and maximum thrombus height was reduced significantly in the presence of citrate, while adhesion was increased. These findings indicate that even low citrate concentrations inhibit thrombus growth, enhance thrombus breakdown and therefore, secondarily increase platelet adhesion (Baumgartner, 1979). Similar effects of citrate were observed with blood of human volunteers (Baumgartner et al., 1980b). Citrate at any concentration probably acts directly on platelets by chelating Ca^{2+} and thereby inhibiting platelet activation.

The effect of platelet inhibitory drugs is usually tested in citrated platelet-rich plasma obtained from individuals after drug ingestion. Aspirin and other non-steroidal antiinflammatory agents inhibit the platelet release reaction and subsequent aggregation. They also inhibit the formation of platelet thrombi on subendothelium after perfusion of citrated blood (Weiss et al., 1975). However, in the absence of citrate their inhibitory effect is much less pronounced or

Table 2. Effect of anticoagulation and vessel treatment on platelet adhesion and thrombus dimensions.

Anticoagulation	vessel-treatment	n	Adhesion C+S [%]	Thrombi T [%]	Thrombus volume [$\mu m^3/\mu m^2$]	Maximum thrombus height [μm]	Fibrin F [%]
none	stored[(1)]	29	38 (2)	14 (1)	10 (1)	86 (11)	43 (6)
none	$HgCl_2$	4	55 (5)	31 (5)	16 (5)	109 (15)	4 (3)
Phenprocoumon*	$HgCl_2$	4	63 (3)	31 (6)	15 (3)	111 (13)	0
Heparin (500U/kg)	stored[(2)]	15	53 (3)	19 (1)	7 (1)	86 (7)	0
Citrate (15mM)	stored[(3)]	34	66 (2)	13 (1)	2 (0.2)	23 (2)	0
Citrate (15mM)	$-70°C$	7	40 (4)	1 (1)	0.2 (0.1)	7 (2)	0
Citrate (15mM)	$HgCl_2$	12	65 (4)	10 (2)	2 (0.3)	22 (2)	0

Experimental conditions: Blood and vessel segments from rabbits, chamber with 0.7 mm annular diameter, flow rate 20 ml/min, shear rate 1300 sec^{-1}, exposure time 3 min. Values are means (SE).

*treatment for several days, Quick < 15%
Average time of storage in Tris at 4°C (1) 5.6 days
(2) 5.9 days
(3) 5.9 days

absent (Baumgartner, 1979). Citrate thus enhances the platelet inhibitory effect of these drugs. Whether this is an additive effect of two inhibitory actions remains to be demonstrated. Nevertheless, the effectiveness of compounds that inhibit platelet function is probably overestimated in the presence of citrate.

Factor VIII/von Willebrand Factor (F VIII/VWF) and platelet adhesion.
F VIII/VWF is synthesized by endothelial cells (Jaffe et al., 1974) and is part of the plasmatic factor VIII complex. Patients with von Willebrand disease (VWD) are deficient in plasmatic factor VIII and their blood vessel walls contain no factor VIII related antigen (F VIII R:AG) (Holmberg et al., 1974). A platelet function defect in VWD was postulated to explain the prolonged bleeding time, the decreased platelet retention in glass bead columns (Salzman, 1963) and the defective ristocetin-induced platelet aggregation (Howard and Firkin, 1971).

Borchgrevink reported in 1961 that platelet consumption was decreased in bleeding time incisions of VWD patients, but it was by use of the annular perfusion chamber that a defect of platelet adhesion to vascular subendothelium with blood of VWD patients was first demonstrated directly and quantitatively (Tschopp et al., 1974). The concept of factor VIII/VWF acting as cofactor for platelet adhesion was further supported by demonstrating that a F VIII/VWF - containing fraction from chromatographed cryoprecipitate corrected the adhesion defect in blood of patients with VWD (Weiss et al., 1978a). Furthermore, Sakariassen et al. (1979) exposed human artery segments to reconstituted blood containing F VIII/VWF and demonstrated a linear correlation between F VIII/VWF bound to the subendothelial surface and the extent of platelet adhesion in the system.

All experiments mentioned above were done at relatively low wall shear rates of 800 sec^{-1}. Under these conditions, platelet adhesion is mainly transport controlled, whereas at higher shear rates adhesion becomes increasingly dependent on platelet reactivity (Turitto and Baumgartner, 1979). Therefore, a greater adhesion defect was anticipated at high wall shear rates. Indeed, the adhesion defect found upon perfusion of citrated or native blood from VWD patients increased with increasing wall shear rates (Weiss et al., 1978b). A similar dependence of the magnitude of the adhesion defect on the shear rate was observed (Fig. 3) in perfused human or rabbit blood depleted of

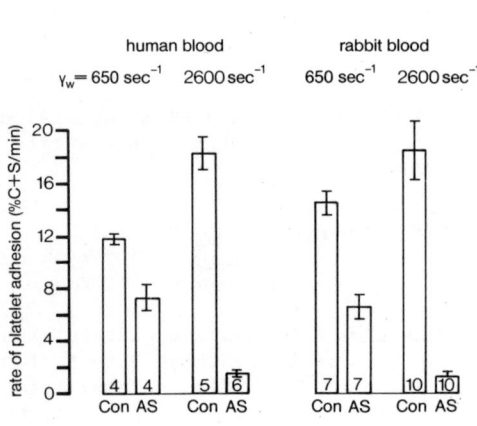

Fig. 3

Shear rate dependent inhibition of platelet adhesion by antisera to human F VIII/VWF or to rabbit F VIII complex. Citrated blood containing control- or antiserum (AS) was perfused over subendothelium at flow rates of 10 or 40 ml/min corresponding to the indicated wall shear rates (γ_w) for various times. The adhesion values obtained were normalized by exposure time in order to obtain the adhesion rate indicated.

F VIII/VWF by homologous or heterologous antisera to human F VIII/VWF or rabbit F VIII complex (Baumgartner et al., 1980a, Baumgartner and Tschopp, 1980).

These findings demonstrate that F VIII/VWF acts as a cofactor for platelet adhesion at high wall shear rates. Further studies, however, are needed to resolve the question whether F VIII/VWF in plasma, on the platelet membrane or in the vessel wall is responsible for the effect.

<u>Platelet inhbitory activity generated by the vessel wall</u>. Moncada et al. (1976, 1979) suggested that prostacyclin (PGI$_2$) which is generated by cells of the vessel wall has an important regulating function

in platelet vessel wall interaction. The question therefore arose whether the smooth muscle cells of vessel segments exposed in annular chambers generate sufficient amounts of prostacyclin to inhibit platelet-vessel wall interaction. Our studies related to this subject are still going on; at present they can be briefly summarized as follows. "Fresh vessels" and "-70°C vessels" do release sufficient amounts of platelet inhibitory activity to inhibit platelet adhesion and aggregation on the exposed subendothelial surface. Inhibition is more readily apparent at high wall shear rates (Baumgartner and Tschopp, 1979). Part of the released platelet-inhibitory activity can be neutralized by an antiserum against 5,6-Dihydroprostacyclin (kindly provided by Dr. Salvador Moncada). Hence at least part of the released platelet inhibitory activity is prostacyclin. On "fresh vessels" obtained from rabbits treated with Aspirin or on "fresh vessels" treated in vitro with unspecific enzyme inhibitors, such as mercurichloride, more platelets adhere and more thrombi form than on "fresh - or -70°C vessels". (Table 2). These observations indicate (1) that generation of inhibiting activity is inhibited by aspirin, thus lending further support to the prostacyclin hypothesis and (2) that generation requires enzyme activity which is destroyed by mercurichloride. On "-70°C vessels" of male rabbits less platelets adhere and less thrombi form than on those from female rabbits; a difference which is abolished by treatment of the vessels with mercurichloride in vitro. Thus vessels from males produce more inhibitory activity than vessels from females. During storage of vessel segments at 4°C their ability to generate and release platelet inhibitory activity diminishes progressively.

The vessel segments used in previous studies were usually stored in buffer at 4°C for several days up to 3 weeks. Based on our present knowledge it seems likely that these vessels produced variable but usually low amounts of platelet inhibitory activity. In future studies the vessel segments must be well characterized and standardized.

REFERENCES

Baumgartner, H.R., 1973. The role of blood flow in platelet adhesion, fibrin deposition and formation of mural thrombi. Microvascular Research, 5, 167-179.

Baumgartner, H.R., 1974. Morphometric quantitation of adherence of platelets to an artificial surface and components of connective tissue. Thrombosis et Diathesis Haemorrhagica, Supplementum, 60 39-49.

Baumgartner, H.R., 1976. Effects of anticoagulation on the interaction of human platelets with subendothelium in flowing blood. Schweizerische Medizinische Wochenschrift, 106, 1367-1368.

Baumgartner, H.R., 1979. Effects of acetylsalicylic acid, sulfinpyrazone and dipyridamole on platelet adhesion and aggregation in flowing native and anticoagulated blood. Haemostasis, 8, 340-352.

Baumgartner, H.R., and Muggli, R., 1976. Adhesion and aggregation: morphological demonstration and quantitation in vivo and in vitro in Platelets in Biology and Pathology (Ed. Gordon, J.L.) pp 23-60. Elsevier/North Holland, Amsterdam, New York, Oxford.

Baumgartner, H.R., Stemerman, M.B., and Spaet, T.H., 1971. Adhesion of blood platelets to subendothelial surface: distinct from adhesion to collagen. Experientia, 27, 283-285.

Baumgartner, H.R., and Tschopp, Th.B., 1979. Platelet interaction with aortic subendothelium in vitro: locally produced PG I_2 inhibits adhesion and formation of mural thrombi in flowing blood. Thrombosis and Haemostasis, 42, 6.

Baumgartner, H.R., and Tschopp, Th.B., 1980. Factor VIII/Willebrand factor and the interaction of blood platelets with subendothelium, in, Atherosclerosis V, Springer-Verlag, Berlin, Heidelberg (in press).

Baumgartner, H.R., Tschopp, Th.B., and Meyer, D., 1980a. Shear rate dependent inhibition of platelet adhesion and aggregation on collagenous surfaces by antibodies to human factor VIII/von Willebrand factor. British Journal of Haematology, 44, 127-139.

Baumgartner, H.R., Turitto, V.T., and Weiss, H.J., 1980b. Effect of shear rate on platelet interaction with subendothelium in citrated and native blood. II. Relationship among platelet adhesion, thrombus dimensions and fibrin formation. Journal of Laboratory and Clinical Medicine, 95, 208-221.

Borchgrevink, C.F., 1961. Platelet adhesion in vivo in patients with bleeding disorders. Acta Medica Scandinavica, 170, 231-243.

Butruille, Y., 1974. Stochastic interpretation of platelet adhesion on artificial surfaces. Thesis, Columbia University.

Caen, J.P., Michel, H., Bodevin, E., and Levy-Toledano, S., 1977. Adhesion and aggregation of human platelets to rabbit subendothelium. A new approach for investigation: specific antibodies. Experientia, 91-93.

Caen, J.P., Nurden, A.T., Jeanveau, C., Michel, H., Tobelem, G., Levi-Toledano, S., Sultan, Y., Valensi, T., and Bernard, J., 1976. Bernard-Soulier syndrome: a new platelet glycoprotein abnormality. Its relationship with platelet adhesion to subendothelium and with the Factor VIII von Willebrand protein. Journal of Laboratory and Clinical Medicine, 87, 586-596.

Caen, J., Levy-Toledano, V., and Sultan, Y., 1973. La dystrophie thrombocytaire hémorragipare (interaction des plaquettes et du facteur Willebrand). Nouvelle Revue Française d'Hématologie, 13, 595-602.

Copley, A.L., and King, R.G., 1976. Polymolecular layers of fibrinogen systems and the genesis of thrombosis. Thrombosis Research, Supplement II, 8, 393-408.

Gay, S. and Miller, E.J., 1978. Collagen in the physiology and pathology of connective tissue. Gustav Fischer Verlag, Stuttgart, New York.

Hellem, A.J., 1960. The adhesiveness of human blood platelets in vitro. Scandinavian Journal of Clinical and Laboratory Investigation, 12, Supplement 51.

Holmberg, L., Mannuci, P.M., Turesson, I., Ruggeri, S.M., and Nilsson, I.M., 1974. Factor VIII antigen in the vessel walls in von Willebrand's disease and hemophilia A. Scandinavian Journal of Hematology, 13, 33-38.

Howard, M., and Firkin, B.G., 1971. Ristocetin: A new tool in the investigation of platelet aggregation. Thrombosis et Diathesis Haemorrhagica, 26, 362-369.

Huang, T.W., Lagunoff, D., and Benditt, E.P., 1974. Nonaggregative adherence of platelets to basal lamina in vitro. Laboratory Investigation, 31, 156-160.

Jaffe, E.A., Hoyer, L.W., and Nachman, R.L., 1974. Synthesis of von

Willebrand factor by cultured human endothelial cells. Proceedings of the National Academy of Science of the United States of America, 71, 906-909.

Jamieson, G.A., Okumura, T., Fisback, B., Johnson, M.M., Egan, J.J., and Weiss, H.J., 1979. Platelet membrane glycoproteins in thrombasthenia, Bernard-Soulier syndrome, and storage pool disease. Journal of Laboratory and Clinical Medicine, 93, 652-660.

Kefalides, N.A., 1975. Basement membranes: structural and biosynthetic considerations. Journal of Investigative Dermatology, 65, 85-92.

Leonard, E.F., and Friedman, L.I., 1970. Thrombogenesis on artificial surfaces: a flow reactor problem. Chemical Engineering Progress, 66, 59-71.

Levy-Toledano, S., Tobelem, G., Legrand, Ch., Bredoux, R., Degas, L., Nurden, A., and Caen, J.P., 1978. Acquired IgG antibody occurring in a thrombasthenic patient: Its effect on human platelet function. Blood, 51, 1065-1071.

Moncada, S., Gryglewski, R., Bunting, S., and Vane, J.R., 1976. An enzyme isolated from arteries transforms prostaglandin endoperoxides to an unstable substance that inhibits platelet aggregation. Nature, 263, 663-665.

Moncada, S., and Vane, J.R., 1979. Arachidonic acid metabolites and the interactions between platelets and blood-vessel walls. New England Journal of Medicine, 300, 1142-1147.

Muggli, R., Baumgartner, H.R., Tschopp, Th.B., and Keller, H., 1980. Automated microdensitometry and protein assays as a measure for platelet adhesion and aggregation on collagen-coated slides under controlled flow conditions. Journal of Laboratory and Clinical Medicine, 95, 195-207.

Nurden, A.T., and Caen, J.P., 1978. Membrane glycoproteins and human platelet function. British Journal of Haematology, 28, 155-160.

Philips, D.R., Jenkins, C.S.P., Lüscher, E.F., and Larrieu, M.J., 1975. Molecular differences of exposed surface proteins on thrombasthenic platelet plasma membranes. Nature, 257, 599-560.

Sakariassen, K.S., Bolhuis, P.A., and Sixma, J.J., 1979. Human platelet adhesion to artery subendothelium is mediated by factor VIII-von Willebrand factor bound to the subendothelium. Nature, 279, 636-637.

Salzman, E.W., 1963. Measurement of platelet adhesiveness. A simple in vitro technique demonstrating an abnormality in von Willebrand's disease. Journal of Laboratory and Clinical Medicine, 62, 724-735.

Solum, N.O., Hagen, I., and Gjemdal, T., 1977. Platelet membrane glycoproteins and the interaction between bovine factor VIII related protein and human platelets. Thrombosis and Haemostasis, 38, 914-923.

Stemerman, M.B., Baumgartner, H.R., and Spaet, T.H., 1971. The subendothelial microfibril and platelet adhesion. Laboratory Investigation, 24, 179-186.

Stenman, S., and Vaheri, A., 1978. Distribution of a major connective tissue protein, fibronectin, in normal human tissues. Journal of Experimental Medicine, 147, 1054-1064.

Timpl, R., Rohde, H., Robey, P.G., Rennard, St.I., Foidart, J.M., and Martin, G.R., 1979. Laminin-a glycoprotein from basement membranes. Journal of Biological Chemistry, 254, 9933-9937.

Trelstad, R.L. and Carvalho, A.C.A., 1979. Type IV and type-A-B-collagens do no elicit platelet aggregation or the serotonin release reaction. Journal of Laboratory and Clinical Medicine, 93, 499-605.

Tschopp, Th.B., 1977. Aspirin inhibits platelet aggregation on, but not adhesion to collagen fibrils: an assessment of platelet adhesion and deposited platelet mass by morphometry and ^{51}Cr-labeling. Thrombosis Research, 11, 619-632.

Tschopp, Th.B., Weiss, H.J., and Baumgartner, H.R., 1974. Decreased adhesion of platelets to subendothelium in von Willebrand's disease. Journal of Laboratory and Clinical Medicine, 83, 296-300.

Tschopp, Th.B., Weiss, H.J., and Baumgartner, H.R., 1975. Interaction of thrombasthenic platelets with subendothelium: normal adhesion, absent aggregation. Experientia, 31, 113-116.

Turitto, V.T., and Baumgartner, H.R., 1975. Platelet interaction with subendothelium in a perfusion system: physical role of red blood cells. Microvascular Research, 9, 335-344.

Turitto, V.T., and Baumgartner, H.R., 1979. Platelet interaction with subendothelium in flowing rabbit blood: effect of blood shear rate. Microvascular Research, 17, 38-54.

Turitto, V.T., and Weiss, H.J., 1980. Red blood cells: their dual role in thrombus formation. Science, 207, 541-543.

Turitto, V.T., Weiss, H.J., and Baumgartner, H.R., 1979. Rheological factors influencing platelet interaction with vessel surfaces. Journal of Rheology, 23, 735-750.

Weiss, H.J., 1975. Platelet physiology and abnormalities of platelet function. New England Journal of Medicine, 293, 531-541 (part I), 580-588 (part II).

Weiss, H.J., Baumgartner, H.R., Tschopp, Th.B., and Cohen, D., 1978a. Correction by factor VIII of the impaired platelet adhesion to subendothelium in von Willebrand's disease. Blood, 51, 267-279.

Weiss, H.J., and Kochwa, S., 1968. Studies of platelet function and proteins in 3 patients with Glanzmann's thrombasthenia. Journal of Laboratory and Clinical Medicine, 71, 153-165.

Weiss, H.J., Tschopp, Th.B., and Baumgartner, H.R., 1975. Impaired interaction of platelets with subendothelium in bleeding disorders. New England Journal of Medicine, 293, 619-623.

Weiss, H.J., Tschopp, Th.B., Baumgartner, H.R., Sussman, I.I., Johnson, M.M., Egan, J.J., 1974. Decreased adhesion of giant (Bernard-Soulier) platelets to subendothelium. Further implications on the role of the von Willebrand factor in hemostasis. American Journal of Medicine, 57, 920-925

Weiss, H.J., Turitto, V.T., and Baumgartner, H.R., 1978b. Effect of shear rate on platelet interaction with subendothelium in citrated and native blood. I Shear rate-dependent decrease of adhesion in von Willebrand's disease and the Bernard-Soulier syndrome. Journal of Laboratory and Clinical Medicine, 92, 750-764.

DRUG INTERACTIONS ON PLATELETS AND ARTERIES: THEIR ROLE WITH CEREBROVASCULAR DISORDERS AND THE CEREBRAL VASOSPASM SYNDROME

D.J. Boullin

MRC Unit and University Dept of Clinical Pharmacology, Radcliffe Infirmary, Oxford, and Nuffield Labs of Comparative Medicine, Inst of Zoology, Regents Park, London.

INTRODUCTION

Blood platelets participate in 3 classes of physiological reaction: platelet aggregation, adhesion to endothelial surfaces and the platelet release reaction leading to blood clot formation.

The discovery of the anti-aggregatory and vasodilator prostaglandin prostacyclin (PGI_2) and its synthesis by arterial endothelium has highlighted the interactions between platelets and vessel walls. Most investigations of the physiology, pharmacology and pathology of platelets and arteries are made separately and in isolation.

In this chapter I want to draw attention to three aspects of platelet function which appear to play a role in cerebrovascular disorders. These are:

1. Platelet adhesion to vessel endothelium and subendothelial structures, platelet aggregation and participation in thrombus formation; also platelet shape change which may be a separate physiological phenomenon from platelet aggregation.

2. Production of vasoconstrictor substances by platelets.

3. Ability of platelets to produce substances causing tissue proliferation.

In addition I shall highlight the dual actions of some potent chemicals which act on platelets but also act on blood vessels. All my remarks will be made with cerebrovascular diseases in mind.

With regard to our own work which I shall outline in due course, we find that cerebrospinal fluid (CSF) collected from patients with a variety of cerebrovascular disorders not only has constrictor activity _in vivo_ and _in vitro_ in animal models which simulate certain aspects of cerebrovascular disorders, but also has effects on normal platelet physiology.

The importance of defects in platelet physiology in relation to cerebrovascular disorders is now becoming increasingly apparent. Substances released from platelets are involved in the pathogenesis of transient ischaemic attacks (Asano, Tamura, Mii and Sano, 1978) and there are increases in circulating platelet aggregates in various cerebrovascular disorders (Dougherty, Levy and Weksler, 1979). In the case of migraine, Hanington (1978) believes that disorders in platelet function play a major role.

Apart from changes in platelet aggregation and adhesion, it seems highly probable that the platelets are involved in some of the histopathological changes in arterial structure which occur in association with cerebrovascular disorders.

One of the salient features of cerebrovascular disease is reduced cerebral blood flow which is a result of pronounced and prolonged constriction of cerebral arteries. This phenomenon may be termed the cerebral vasospasm syndrome, and has been the subject of extensive study for some years (see Boullin, 1980).

The cerebral vasospasm syndrome is most well-known in association with subarachnoid haemorrhage due to spontaneous rupture of cerebral arterial aneurysms. The frequency of the association is due to the fact that patients with subarachnoid haemorrhage commonly undergo cerebral angiography to visualise the intra-cranial circulation so that the skull may be opened and the ruptured aneurysm clipped. Now, it has been known for some years that the cerebral vasospasm syndrome is not confined to subarachnoid haemorrhage, but also occurs after head injury and meningitis (see Hughes, 1980); certain extreme forms of migraine such as basilar artery migraine also seem to involve the syndrome in an attenuated form. The reason that the cerebral vasospasm syndrome is not normally seen in other cases than subarachnoid haemorrhage reflects the fact that it is not looked for; these cases seldom have carotid angiography.

Apart from prolonged arterial constriction, pathological abnormalities are a recently discovered feature of spastic arteries obtained from patients with the cerebral vasospasm syndrome. These changes involve large and small arteries shown by angiography to have been in spasm during life and include stripping and necrosis of the endothelial layer, with subsequent subendothelial thickening. The infiltration appears to involve blood cells although platelets are not specifically identified (see Hughes, 1980).

Because of the pronounced endothelial damage, I believe that the cerebral vasospasm syndrome may involve <u>prostacyclin deficiency</u> at the sites of arterial constriction. Although there is no direct evidence for this, prostacyclin synthetase is present in human cerebral arteries (Boullin, Bunting, Blaso, Hunt and Moncada, 1979; Jarman, Du Boulay, Kendall and Boullin, 1979).

The cause of the histopathological changes is not established but platelets may be the prime culprits.

It is well-known that platelets adhere to subendothelial tissues, most particularly collagen, and platelet deposits build up. Platelets can secrete an unidentified factor which stimulates the production of arterial smooth muscle cells (Ross, Glomset, Kariya and Harker, 1974). These factors do not promote growth of endothelial cells (Thorgeirsson and Robertson, 1978) but may be involved in formation of the atheromatous plaque. The release mechanism of this cell proliferative factor or a similar one occurs during the release reaction from α-granules, in parallel with the release of 5-HT, ADP and platelet factor IV (Witte, Kaplan, Nossel, Lages, Weiss and Goodman, 1978).

Two links now appear: First the link between platelets and the subendothelial changes that occur in association with the cerebral vasospasm syndrome; second, a link with prostacyclin. The question now arises as to whether prostacyclin may play any normal role in preventing the histopathological changes and smooth muscle cell proliferation in maintaining the integrity of the arterial endothelium (Cazenave, Dejana, Kinlough-Rathbone, Richardson, Packham and Mustard, 1979). It is possible that prostacyclin normally inhibits release of these factors, and release only occurs when there is endothelial damage.

ENDOTHELIUM, PROSTACYCLIN AND ANGIOTENSIN

Vascular endothelium is the site of synthesis of a variety of vasoactive substances. I wish to draw attention to two of these: prostacyclin and angiotensin. Prostacyclin is synthesised from arachidonic acid and endoperoxides in the vascular endothelium (Baenziger, Dillender and Majerus, 1977; Weksler, Marcus and Jaffe, 1977). Most importantly platelets do not provide endoperoxides to the vascular endothelium for prostacyclin synthesis (Hornstra, Haddeman and Don, 1979). Thus the fate of the endoperoxides in platelets and vessel walls is quite different; platelets synthesise vasoconstrictor and proaggregatory thromboxanes, only the endothelium synthesises the vasodilator and antiaggregatory prostaglandin prostacyclin.

Clearly, therefore, we may expect a physiological balance between vasodilator and vasoconstrictor prostaglandins generated by platelets and vessel walls. The physiological control of cerebral arterial calibre can be predicted to involve a balance between these opposing systems (see Boullin, 1980). Furthermore, defects in the endothelium wall favour the constrictor thromboxanes at the expense of prostacyclin. Thus the cerebral vasospasm syndrome which involves arterial constriction, endothelial damage and subendothelial thickening can be expected to lead to prostacyclin deficiency. However the situation is very complicated because the endothelium is not only the site of prostacyclin synthesis but also prostacyclin catabolism. The conventional view that prostacyclin is metabolised to 6-keto $PGF_{1\alpha}$ (Moncada and Vane, 1978) may be incorrect. Only a proportion may be metabolised by this route.

Recent work shows that PGI_2 is metabolised to 6:15 diketo $PGF_{1\alpha}$ by a 5-hydroxy-prostaglandin dehydrogenase present in vascular endothelium. Thus measurement of 6-keto $PGF_{1\alpha}$ may not give a true index of prostacyclin catabolism (Wong, Sun and McGiff, 1978). These observations must be pursued further before their significance can be determined, but obviously removal of the endothelial layer, as occurs in the course of prolonged arterial spasm, may be expected to dramatically reduce prostacyclin synthesis, swinging the balance in favour of constrictor prostaglandins and thromboxanes.

The extra-pulmonary vascular endothelium is also the site of synthesis of angiotensin II, at least in umbilical cord cell cultures (Hial, Gimbrone, Peyton, Wilcox and Pisano, 1979).

The role of angiotensins in the cerebral circulation is not properly understood, but I will refer to it again below in consideration of our own findings related to the aetiology of the cerebral vasospasm syndrome in cerebrovascular disorders. Angiotensin may also play a major role in the cerebral vasospasm syndrome.

ANIMAL MODELS FOR CEREBROVASCULAR DISORDERS

This is an extensive topic that cannot be covered here in depth as it has been discussed recently (Boullin, 1980). Most animal models developed for examination of the aetiology of the cerebral vasospasm syndrome are suitable for studying the effects of substances on arterial calibre without investigating platelet function.

However the obvious link between platelets and arteries brought about by the discovery of prostacyclin has led to the development of further models which may be useful for investigation of cerebral vasospasm. Rosenblum and El-Sabban (1978a) traumatized pial arteries and venules in mice by needle penetration and then studied platelet aggregation and arterial diameter simultaneously in untraumatized vessels a short distance away. They observed aggregation in venules but constriction in both arterioles and venules. As the effects were blocked by aspirin they considered prostaglandins were involved. This seems to be the case because Rosenblum and El-Sabban (1978b) showed that the prostacyclin synthetase inhibitor tranylcypromine enhanced aggregation as measured in the mouse experiments. Thus prostacyclin synthesis seems to play a direct antithrombotic role in the circulation. In their model involving ultra-violet light falling on sodium fluorescein treated microvessels Rosenblum and El-Sabban (1977) demonstrate the three facets of pathology associated with human cerebral vasospasm:

> Arterial constriction
> Endothelial damage
> Platelet aggregation

The mouse model involves blood loss from the damaged vessels adjacent to the vein under study and this blood could diffuse to the site of the undamaged vessels investigated. In any event platelet aggregation and vasoconstriction are shown to go hand-in-hand. The role of platelets in cerebral vasospasm is a vitally important problem that I shall refer to again.

To investigate the aetiology of cerebral vasospasm we required a larger model than a mouse. We prefer to use large primates because of their basic similarities in their cerebral circulation to man. But due to rarity and expense we have now used small rodents. These have the advantage that effects on platelets and cerebral arteries can be observed simultaneously in vivo. Our recent results, which are described below, definitely implicate both platelets and arterial walls in the aetiology of human cerebral arterial constriction.

THE RAT VASOSPASM/THROMBOSIS MODEL

It is rather surprising that the rat has not been used before as a model in studies of disorders of the cerebrovascular circulation. Previous work has been confined to microembolisation with arachidonic acid or ADP infusions (Furlow and Bass, 1976). We have found the rat to be a suitable model for investigation of both thromboembolic phenomena and also for changes in the calibre of the major cerebral arteries (Aitken, Boullin and Du Boulay, 1980). The procedure is outlined in Table 1. Thromboembolic phenomena are studied by observing arterial occlusion.

Effects on cerebral arterial calibre can be observed directly in animals pre-treated with prostacyclin, to eliminate formation of platelet emboli.

TABLE 1. Rat thromboembolism/vasospasm model

Procedure	Rat cerebral angiography
1. Anaesthesia	Arteries visualised on angiograms:
2. Carotid cannulation with prostacyclin	Stapedial (S)
3. Carotid angiography	Internal carotid (IC)
4. CSF or drug injection into carotid	Middle cerebral (M)
	Anterior cerebral (A)
5. Further angiography	
	Vertebro-basilar system (B)

Effects without Prostacyclin. In untreated animals occlusion of intracranial arteries occurs when rapidly aggregating human platelets in plasma are injected intra-arterially. There is complete blockage of some vessels so that they are no longer visible on subsequent angiograms and the blood is diverted along other arteries which are commonly dilated (Fig. 1).

In the internal carotid artery in Fig. 1 a filling defect can be observed in the lower portion of the vessel (at arrow); this is due to the formation of thrombii (see enlarged angiogram, Fig. 1).

Less dramatic events are observed with lower doses of ADP and aggregating platelets. Fig. 2 shows the effects when 2 nmols/ml ADP and rapidly aggregating platelets are injected; there is severe

Thromboembolism of rat cerebral arteries produced by ADP and rapidly aggregating platelets

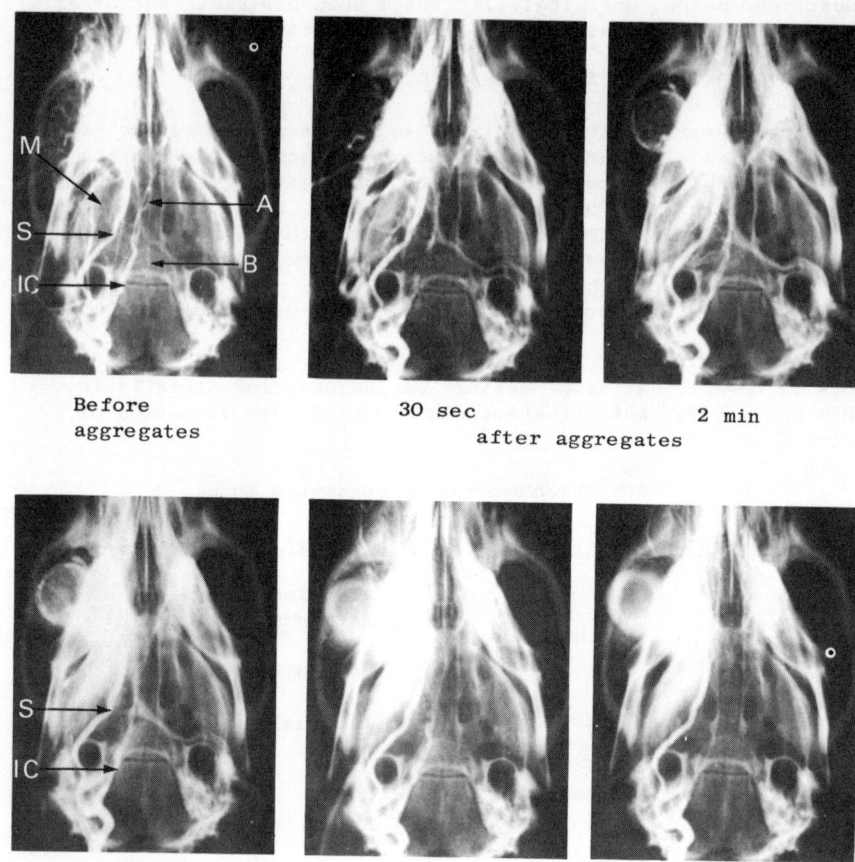

Before aggregates   30 sec   2 min
after aggregates

5 min   30 min   60 min
after aggregates

Fig. 1. 6 Serial angiograms before and up to 60 min after intracarotid injection of 20 nmols adenosine diphosphate (ADP) in 1 ml normal human platelet rich plasma. Arteries visualised are middle cerebral (M); stapedial (S); anterior cerebral (A); and basilar (B). Note prolonged occlusion of M, A, B and terminal portions of IC 30 sec to 60 min after injection. There is a large thrombus 30 min after aggregation (lower centre angiogram) which is shown enlarged below:

Enlarged view of lower centre angiogram of previous figure (30 min after platelet aggregation)

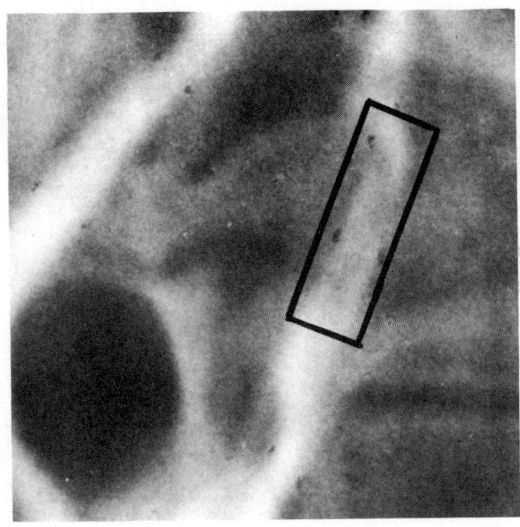

S is on the left and IC on the right. The boxed area indicates thrombii.

constriction of S and IC 10 min after injection, but the effect is largely gone after 20 min.

Angiographic Spasm Caused by Platelet Adhesion and Arterial Narrowing.
Generally following injection of either platelet aggregating agents or arterial vasoconstrictor drugs the number of arteries visualised on angiography was less. In particular, M, A and B were often invisible. Furthermore in the case of those arteries still visible the calibre was usually narrower. What appeared to be arterial narrowing was seen with both aggregating agents such as ADP alone (without the addition of human platelets) and vasoconstrictor drugs. Indeed the effects of aggregating agents and vasoconstrictor substances were indistinguishable.

For example, injection of either 5-HT or vasospastic CSF taken from patients with the cerebral vasospasm syndrome produced virtually identical arterial narrowing. These effects were superimposed on a pattern of spontaneous occlusion lasting up to 20 minutes, which occurred in the absence of pretreatment with prostacyclin.

Now the actual mechanism of human arterial narrowing in the cerebral vasospasm syndrome has been debated for many years. Is it due to

Transient thromboembolism of rat cerebral arteries produced by ADP and rapidly aggregating human platelets

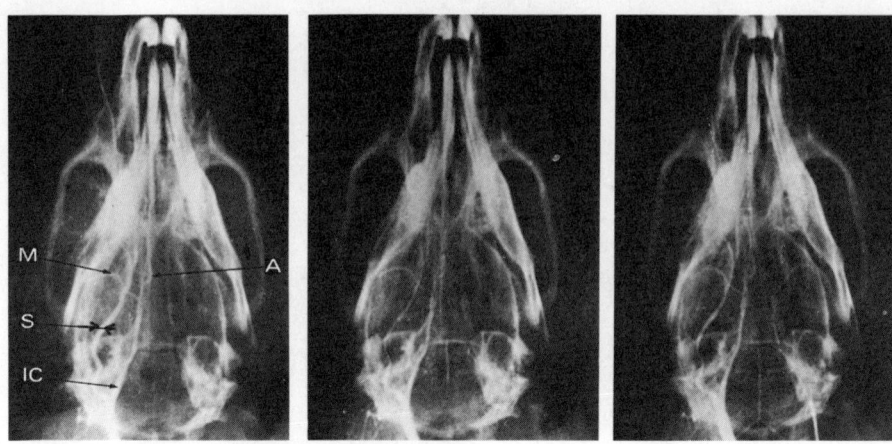

Before ADP   10 min   20 min
time after ADP and platelets

Fig. 2. 3 Angiograms showing changes in arterial calibre 10 and 20 min after intra-carotid injection of 2 nmols ADP in 1 ml rapidly aggregating normal human platelet rich plasma. Note the constriction of S and IC 10 min after injection (centre angiogram), with partial reversal of the spasm after 20 min (right angiogram). These effects should be compared with those of Fig. 5.

architectural narrowing of the vessel lumen resulting from histological changes in the structure of the arterial wall? Or is it due to vessel contraction brought about by vasoactive substances? The third possibility is adherence of platelets to the endothelial surface. This is, of course, heresy. But Gringrich and Hoak (1979) have observed platelets adhering to endothelium by the scanning elution microscope. Adhesion is also likely to occur to anoxic endothelium after some kind of head injury.

Consequently I believe that platelet adherence to the damaged vascular endothelium of cerebral arteries may be one of the factors responsible for the cerebral vasospasm syndrome in man. Luminal narrowing following platelet adhesion would, of course, result in lowered cerebral blood flow, and as we have shown in Fig. 2, changes in the calibre of rat cerebral arteries after injection of rapidly aggregating platelets and ADP produce angiographic spasm. Because of the irregular occlusion seen without administration of either aggregating or vasoconstrictor substances, we decided to carry out all further experiments in the presence of prostacyclin. Even so, it will become apparent that, even with prostacyclin, spasm produced by vasospastic substances including 5-HT and vasospastic CSF cannot be distinguished angiographically. These experiments are described below.

EFFECTS IN THE PRESENCE OF PROSTACYCLIN

Because of the spontaneous but transient occlusion of some arteries, we routinely administered prostacyclin (30-250 ng/kg) during common carotid artery catheterisation. This prevented thromboembolism for up to 3 hours. Platelets taken from rats given 30-250 ng/kg prostacyclin do not aggregate to ADP for up to 3 hours after prostacyclin injection - which thus exerts a heparin-like effect. Prostacyclin can substitute for heparin in extra-corporeal circulation techniques (Woods, Ash, Weston, Bunting, Moncada and Vane, 1978).

When 5-HT is injected in the absence of prostacyclin, both occlusion and vasoconstriction are observed. On the other hand, 5-HT injected after prostacyclin produces transient constriction of intracranial and extracranial arteries without any evidence of occlusion (Fig. 3).

Administration of prostacyclin prevents all but very gross thromboembolic phenomena so that effects upon arterial calibre can be studied in isolation. Fig. 4 shows the effects of a large dose of prostacyclin (3 µg/kg; 8 nmols/kg). The overall initial effect is constriction of cerebral vessels (M, A, IC and B) with dilatation of S but 30 and 60 min after injection all vessels are dilated, particularly S and IC. Lower doses, below 100 ng/kg, produce dilatation without prior constriction. Effects of CSF can be studied after prostacyclin-induced dilatation for up to 5 hours without occlusion of vessels.

Vasospastic CSF was collected from patients with subarachnoid haemorrhage and angiographic evidence of cerebral vasospasm, which we define as greater than 50% overall constriction of IC, M and A in man (see Boullin, 1980). 1 ml of this CSF after filtration was injected into experimental animals as described below. Further details of this characterisation of the CSF are given in earlier publications (for references see Boullin, 1980).

Vasospastic CSF produced rapidly developing spasm after injection of 1 ml into the carotid artery (Fig. 5). The diameters of S and IC were sufficient for quantitative data to be obtained (Fig. 6).

Interestingly, vasospastic CSF produced segmental spasm of S which compares with human segmental vasospasm (Fig. 7). We may speculate that there is some factor in vasospastic CSF that has preferential affinity for certain receptors in cerebral arteries in rats and in man after aneurysm rupture.

ANGIOTENSIN AND CEREBRAL VASOSPASM

Regarding the factors in CSF which produce vasospasm, we have recently isolated angiotensin I and angiotensin II from pooled

Transient constrictor effects of 5-HT on rat cerebral arteries

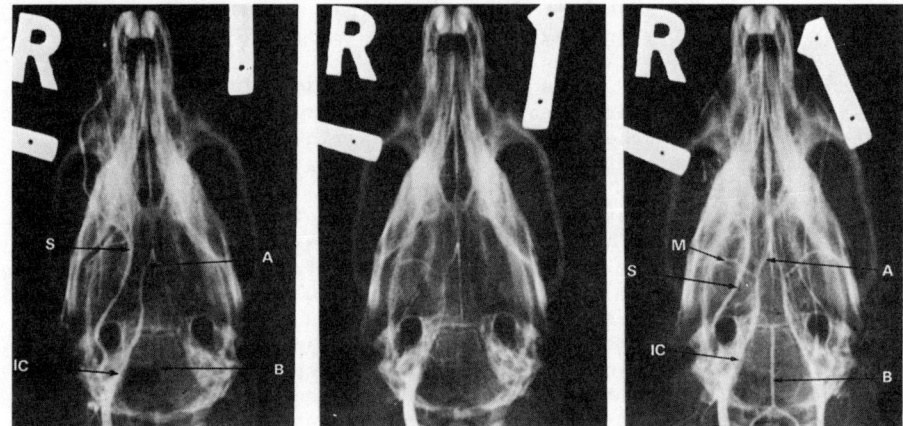

Before 5-HT   3 min   10 min
Time after 5-HT

Fig. 3. The series of 3 angiograms shows the transient constrictor effects of 5-HT in a rat not pretreated with prostacyclin. Prior to 5-HT (left angiogram) S, A and IC are clearly visible; M can just be visualised (see labelling of right angiogram). 3 Min after 30 nmols/kg 5-HT (centre angiogram), all vessels are constricted. 10 Min after 5-HT (right angiogram) the constrictor effects have largely disappeared. These effects should be compared with those produced by ADP and platelet aggregates shown in Fig. 2.

samples of vasospastic CSF obtained from 9 patients with angiographic evidence of vasospasm. The isolation procedures are given in Table 2.

We have not assayed normal CSF but Severs, Changaris, Kapsha, Neil, Petro, Reid and Sunny-Long (1977) report values which are one-fiftieth of ours. Reid and Moffatt (1978) find higher values in normal CSF of dogs, but again these are much lower than our values.

Vasoconstrictor effects of a high dose of prostacyclin

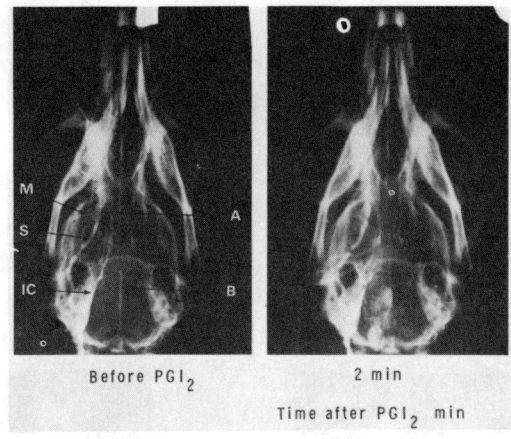

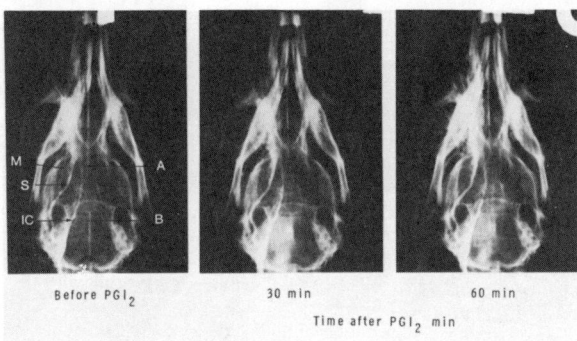

Fig. 4. Before prostacyclin injection all vessels normally seen on angiography were visible (left angiograms). 2 Min after injection of a high dose of prostacyclin 3 μg/kg (8 nmols/kg) M, A and B were not visible (upper right angiogram). S and IC showed severe segmental constriction in places. We draw the conclusion that this is constriction rather than embolic occlusion because of the potent antithrombotic effects of prostacyclin and the fact that the rat shown had previously received 210 ng/kg (600 pmols/kg) prostacyclin prior to administration of the dose illustrated here. Subsequent angiograms at 30 and 60 min (centre and lower left) both showed dilatation of S and IC.

Effect of vasospastic CSF on rat cerebral arteries

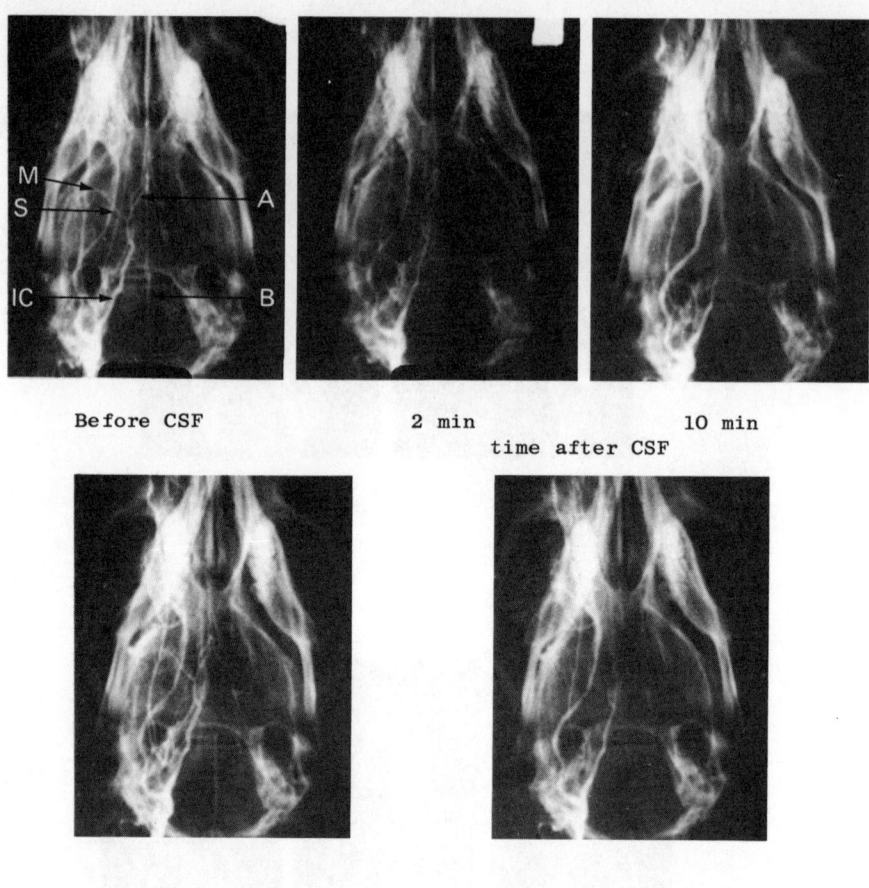

Fig. 5. Spasm of rat cerebral arteries following close intra-arterial injection of vasospastic CSF taken from a patient with subarachnoid haemorrhage and angiographic evidence of the cerebral vasospasm syndrome. The 5 angiograms show the effects of CSF 2-60 min after injection. 1 ml CSF was injected over a 2 min period into the common carotid artery. Prior to injection all vessels normally seen on angiography were visible (M, S, IC, A and B, upper left angiogram). 10 Min after injection, M, A and B were in severe spasm, as was the terminal portion of IC (upper right angiogram). These effects persisted for 30 min after injection, but after 60 min the spasm had largely disappeared, with the circulation and calibre of vessels comparable to that seen prior to CSF injection (lower angiograms).

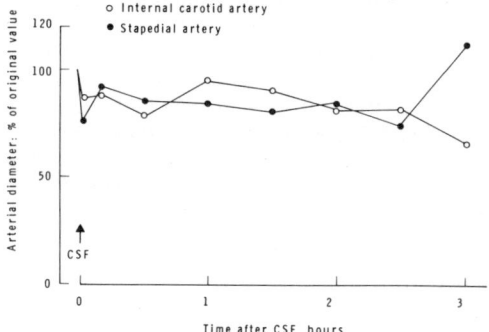

Fig. 6. Diameter of rat stapedial and internal carotid arteries following injection of vasospastic CSF at zero time (abscissa). Ordinate gives the % change in arterial calibre of S and IC in relation to the calibre of the vessels as measured on the initial pre-CSF angiogram by the method used with human angiograms (see Du Boulay, 1980). Values are the mean obtained in 3 experiments.

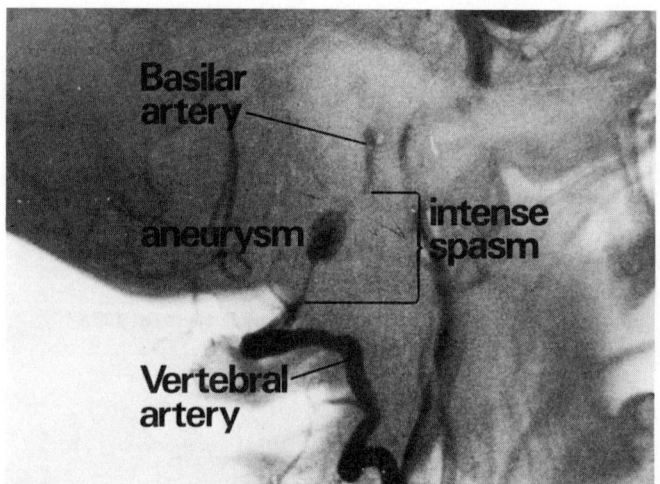

Fig. 7. Angiogram of 56-year-old female showing basilar aneurysm and region of segmental spasm (marked intense spasm).

TABLE 2. Identification of angiotensin in vasospastic CSF from patients with the cerebral vasospasm syndrome

120 ml Pooled vasospastic CSF ⟶ Bioassay
↓
Lyophilised concentrated 10:1 ⟶ Bioassay
↓
6 ml concentrated CSF
Cation exchange chromatography

(calibrated for mol wts 300-70,000)

elution with 0.5 mM phosphate buffer pH 7.6
↓
120 fractions collected
↓
Spectrophotometry 254 nm

Fractions 24 to 31 - Hb*
65 to 71 - Substance X ⟶ Bioassay
(approx mol wt = 1100)
↓
Fractions combined to number 60 ⟶ Bioassay
lyophilised
Fractions 33 to 35 - Substance X
↓
Fraction 34
↓
Preparative thin layer chromatography

(Silica Gel)
Acetic acid: water: 9:1
Rf 0.63 ⟶ Bioassay
↓
Radioimmunoassay for:

Angiotensin I   Angiotensin II

CSF concentrations   11.5 pmols/ml   306 fmols/ml

*Hb 1 haemoglobin

▲Fractions were bioassayed on human isolated basilar arteries and on the isolated rat stomach fundus preparation

Rat Cerebral Vasospasm Produced by Angiotensin I
(Labelling of arteries as described in the text)

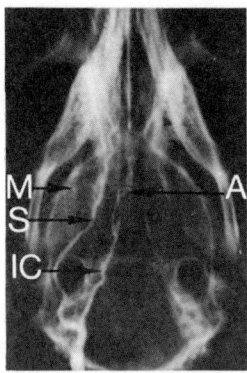 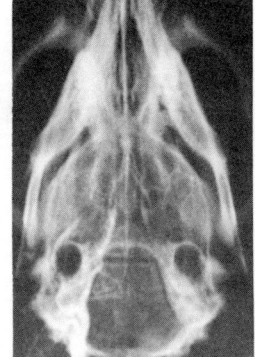 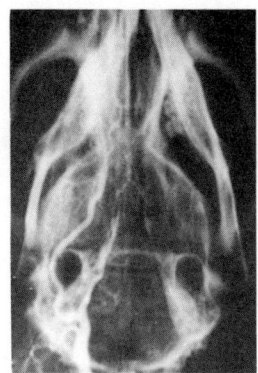

Before Angiotensin I   2 min   20 min
After Angiotensin I

Fig.8. 3 Angiograms show calibre of cerebral arteries before, 2 and 20 min after intra-carotid injection of 100 pmols/kg angiotensin I. Note severe segmental constriction of S in centre angiogram with dilatation 20 min after injection.

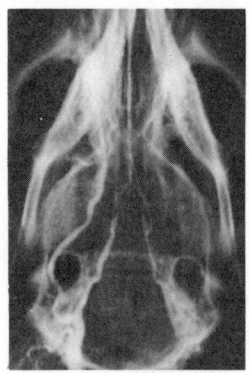 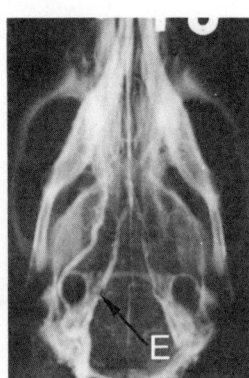 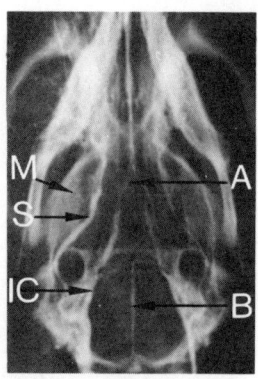

Before Angiotensin I   2 min   30 min
After Angiotensin I

3 Angiograms show effects before, 2 and 30 min after 200 pmols/kg angiotensin I given as above. Note segmental spasm of IC at point marked E in centre angiogram and prolongation of effects for 30 min (right angiogram). Results obtained in rats pretreated with 30 mg/kg prostacyclin as described in the text.

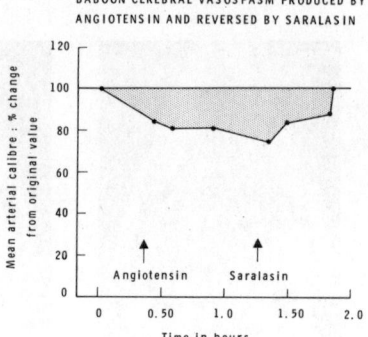

Fig. 9. Diameter of baboon arteries (M, IC and A) following intra-carotid injection of 0.75 nmols/kg angiotensin I. Ordinate gives the mean % change in diameter of above arteries (each increased at 4 different places) in relation to the original diameter of the vessels on the first angiogram (see Du Boulay, 1980).

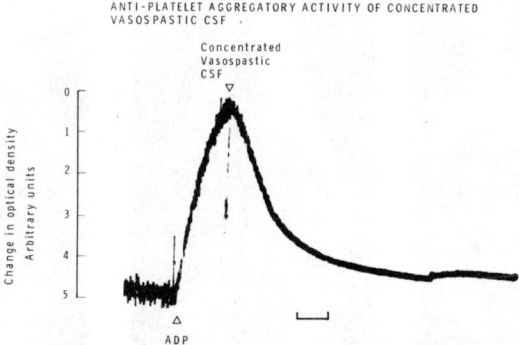

Fig. 10. Platelet aggregation measured at 37°C. Change in optical density of platelet rich plasma measured in arbitrary units of increasing density (ordinate) plotted against time (min scale indicated on abscissa). ADP 20 nmols/ml added as indicated at point when aggregation was approaching maximum. 20 µl 100:1 concentrated vasospastic CSF almost completely reversed ADP induced aggregation. 100:1 concentrated normal CSF did not have this effect (not shown).

Intra-carotid angiotensin I produces pronounced vasospasm including segmental spasm (Fig. 8). Similar effects are observed in baboons (Fig. 9) and this spasm is reversed by the angiotensin II antagonist saralasin (sarcosine 1-alanine-8-angiotensin II). Saralasin does not completely antagonise vasospastic CSF-induced vasospasm in these models, so that angiotensin does not account entirely for clinical vasospasm. Some other yet unidentified substances are involved.

ANTIAGGREGATORY SUBSTANCES IN CSF

Angiotensin I and angiotensin II do not have antiaggregatory properties, but we have found that vasospastic CSF concentration 100:1 has potent antiaggregatory properties - 5-50 µl of this concentrated material prevents or reverses ADP-induced aggregation of human platelets (Fig. 10). Accordingly it seems quite clear that CSF has actions on platelets as well as on cerebral vessels. I have already pointed out the essential similarity between angiographic effects produced by rapidly aggregating platelets (Fig. 2) and vasospastic CSF (Fig. 5). One cannot be sure that angiographic spasm, or reduced cerebral blood flow for that matter, is entirely due to arterial constriction and not due to architectural narrowing caused by platelet deposition or other thromboembolic factors. The importance of platelets in the development of cerebral vasospasm is further emphasised by the actions of catecholamines and 5-HT.

Catecholamines and 5-HT. Catecholamine and 5-HT concentrations are elevated in cerebrovascular disorders in CSF and in the general circulation (Benedict and Loach, 1978), in head trauma and subarachnoid haemorrhage.

Using platelet rich plasma obtained from normal subjects without evidence of cerebrovascular disorders, we find in vitro noradrenaline (NA) augments platelet shape change and platelet aggregation produced by 5-HT. Subthreshold doses of NA, too low to produce aggregation alone, greatly increase 5-HT-induced shape change and aggregation.

These interactions with NA involving platelet aggregation occur in the dose range 0.1 to 1.0 µmol/l, which is in the range found in patients with subarachnoid haemorrhage. Consequently localised platelet aggregation is likely to occur in those cerebrovascular disorders where plasma catecholamines are elevated and there is constriction of cerebral arteries. In disorders associated with the cerebral vasospasm syndrome, platelet deposition in regions of denuded or necrotic endothelium may be predicted to occur due to two causes: first, prostacyclin deficiency resulting from decreased synthesis or accelerated catabolism; second, exposure of collagen-containing subendothelial layers, as explained in the Introduction.

CONCLUSION

Blood platelet responses are likely to play a major role in the aetiology of cerebrovascular disorders so that it is unrealistic not to investigate changes in platelet function in disorders which are associated with decreased cerebral blood flow and angiographically-

TABLE 3. Various elements involved in the cerebral vasospasm syndrome

Vasoconstrictor properties	Proaggregatory properties	Antiaggregatory properties	Vasodilator properties
5-HT	5-HT	Prostacyclin	Prostacyclin
Catecholamines	Catecholamines	Unidentified CSF factors	Unidentified CSF factors
Prostaglandins generally and prostacyclin in high doses	Prostaglandins generally		
Prostaglandin endoperoxides thromboxanes arachidonic acid	Prostaglandin endoperoxides thromboxanes arachidonic acid		
Unidentified CSF factors			

determined arterial narrowing.

Table 3 indicates some of the elements involved in the generation and/or maintenance of the cerebral vasospasm syndrome. This simple scheme highlights the fact that few chemicals have a single action. Unidentified vasodilator factors have not been mentioned previously here (see Boullin, Du Boulay and Rogers, 1978; Boullin, 1980), but it is quite clear that numerous substances act both on platelets and arteries before and after metabolic transformation to other substances, which may in turn possess different, but still dual, actions.

Recent work indicates that the cerebral vasospasm syndrome occurs in a variety of cerebrovascular disorders and is not merely a feature of subarachnoid haemorrhage. Changes in platelet physiology have been more extensively investigated than changes in arterial calibre due to the invasive and hazardous nature of cerebral angiography but evanescent changes in platelet physiology occur in transient ischaemic attacks and in migraine where platelet function is more commonly investigated.

Much work on platelet function concentrates upon _in vitro_ aggregation phenomena. This is a _force majeure_ situation from the clinical viewpoint since sophisticated scanning electron microscope methodology for investigating platelet adhesion to endothelial and subendothelial surfaces (Cazenave, Blondowska, Richardson, Kinlough-Rathbone, Packham and Mustard, 1979) cannot be applied clinically.

However, studies on platelet shape change may show another aspect of platelet physiology because shape change is modulated by 5-HT and influenced by the catecholamines (Boullin, 1979), two classes of substances implicated in the aetiology of cerebrovascular disorders.

Our own work shows that angiotensin may play a role in cerebrovascular disease by acting as a vasospastic substance generated by vascular endothelium. Other substances still remain to be identified and these can cause inhibition of platelet aggregation and also cerebral arterial dilatation (Boullin, Du Boulay and Rogers, 1978).

REFERENCES

Aitken, V., Boullin, D.J. and Du Boulay, G.H., 1980. Actions of prostacyclin and cerebrospinal fluid on rat cerebral arteries in vivo. J. Physiol. (In press).

Asano, T., Tamura, A., Mii, K. and Sano, K., 1978. The role of humoral agents released by platelet aggregation in the pathogenesis of transient ischaemic attacks. Neurol. Med. Chir. (Tokyo), 18, 59-66.

Baenziger, N.L., Dillender, M.J. and Majerus, P.W., 1977. Cultured human skin fibroblasts and arterial cells produce a labile platelet inhibitory prostaglandin. Biochim. Biophys. Res. Comm., 78,

Benedict, C.R. and Loach, A.B., 1978. Clinical significance of plasma adrenaline and noradrenaline concentrations in patients with subarachnoid haemorrhage. J. Neurol. Neurosurg. Psychiat., 41, 113-117.

Boullin, D.J., Du Boulay, G.H. and Rogers, A.T., 1978. Aetiology of cerebral arterial spasm following subarachnoid haemorrhage: evidence against a major involvement of 5-hydroxytryptamine in the production of acute spasm. Br. J. Pharmacol., 6, 203-215.

Boullin, D.J., 1979. Blood platelets as a model for brain neurones: relevance to psychiatric disorders, in Neuro-psychopharmacology (Eds. Saletu et al), pp 283-302. Pergamon Press, Oxford.

Boullin, D.J., Bunting, S., Blaso, W.P., Hunt, T.M. and Moncada, S., 1979. Responses of human and baboon arteries to prostaglandin endoperoxides and biologically generated and synthetic prostacyclin: their relevance to cerebral arterial spasm in man. Brit. J. Clin. Pharmac., 7, 139-147.

Boullin, D.J., 1980. Cerebral Vasospasm. John Wiley, Chichester.

Cazenave, J.P., Blondowska, D., Richardson, M., Kinlough-Rathbone, R.L., Packham, M.A. and Mustard, J.F., 1979. Quantitative radioisotopic measurement and scanning electron microscopic study of platelet adherence to a collagen control surface and to subendothelium with a rotating probe device. J. Lab. Clin. Med., 93,

Cazenave, J.P., Dejana, E., Kinlough-Rathbone, R.L., Richardson, M., Packham, M.A. and Mustard, J.F., 1979. Prostaglandins I_2 and E_1 reduce rabbit and human platelet adherence without inhibitory serotonin release from adherent platelets. Thromb. Res., 15, 273-279.

Dougherty, J.H., Levy, D.E. and Weksler, B.B., 1979. Platelet activation in acute cerebral ischaemia. Serial measurements of platelet functions in cerebrovascular disease. Lancet, i, 821-824.

Du Boulay, G.H., 1980. Angiography - the radiologist's view, in Cerebral Vasospasm by D.J. Boullin, pp 47-79. Wiley, Chichester.

Furlow, T.W. and Bass, N.H., 1976. Arachidonate induced cerebrovascular occlusion in the rat: The role of platelets and aspirin in stroke. Neurology (Minneap.), 26, 297-304.

Gringrich, R.D. and Hoak, J.C., 1979. Platelet-endothelial cell interactions. Seminars in Hematology, 16, 208-220.

Hanington, E., 1978. Migraine: A blood disorder? Lancet, ii, 501-3.

Hial, V., Gimbrone, M.A., Peyton, J.P.Jr., Wilcox, G.M. and Pisano, J.J., 1979. Angiotensin metabolism by cultured human vascular endothelial and smooth muscle cells. Microvasc. Res., 17, 314-329.

Hornstra, G., Haddeman, E. and Don, J.A., 1979. Blood platelets do not provide endoperoxides for vascular prostacyclin production. Nature, 279, 66-68.

Hughes, J.T., 1980. Pathological changes associated with cerebral vasospasm, in Cerebral Vasospasm by D.J. Boullin, pp 171-206. John Wiley, Chichester.

Jarman, D.A., Du Boulay, G.H., Kendall, B. and Boullin, D.J., 1979. Responses of baboon cerebral and extracerebral arteries to prostacyclin and prostaglandin endoperoxide in vitro and in vivo. Journal of Neurology, Neurosurgery & Psychiatry, 42, 677-686.

Moncada, S. and Vane, J.R., 1978. Prostacyclin, platelet aggregation, and thrombosis, in Platelets: A Multidisciplinary Approach (Eds. de Gaetano and Garattini), pp 239-258. Raven Press, New York.

Reid, I.A. and Moffat, M., 1978. Angiotensin II concentration in cerebrospinal fluid after intraventricular injection of angiotensinogen or renin. Endocrinology, 103, 1494-1498.

Rosenblum, W.I. and El-Sabban, F., 1977. Platelet aggregation in the cerebral microcirculation. Effect of aspirin and other agents. Circ. Res., 40, 320-327.

Rosenblum, W.I. and El-Sabban, F., 1978a. Platelet aggregation and vasoconstriction in undamaged microvessels on cerebral surface adjacent to brain traumatized by a penetrating needle. Microvasc. Res., 15, 299-307.

Rosenblum, W.I. and El-Sabban, F., 1978b. Enhancement of platelet aggregation by tranylcypromine in mouse cerebral microvessels. Circ. Res., 43, 238-241.

Ross, R., Glomset, J., Kariya, B. and Harker, L., 1974. A platelet-dependent serum factor that stimulates the proliferation of arterial smooth muscle cells in vitro. Proc. Nat. Acad. Sci., 71, 1207-1210.

Severs, W.B., Changaris, D.G., Kapsha, J.M., Neil, L.C., Petro, D.J., Reid, I.A. and Sunny-Long, J.W., 1977. Presence and significance of angiotensin in cerebrospinal fluid, in Central Actions of Angiotensin and Related Hormones (Eds. Buckley and Ferrario), pp 225-245. Pergamon Press, Oxford.

Thorgeirsson, G. and Robertson, A.L., 1978. Platelet factors and the human vascular wall: variations in growth response between endothelial and smooth muscle cells. Atherosclerosis, 30, 67-78.

Weksler, B.B., Marcus, A.J. and Jaffe, E.A., 1977. Synthesis of prostaglandin I_2 (prostacyclin) by cultured human and bovine endothelial cells. Proc. Nat. Acad. Sci. (USA), 74, 3922-3926.

Witte, L.D., Kaplan, K.L., Nossel, H.L., Lages, B.A., Weiss, H.J. and Goodman, DeW.S., 1978. Studies on the release from human platelets of the growth factor for cultured human arterial smooth muscle cells. Circ. Res., 42, 402-409.

Wong, P.Y-K., Sun, F.F. and McGiff, J.C., 1978. Metabolism of prostacyclin in blood vessels. J. Biol. Chem., 253, 5555-5557.

Woods, H.F., Ash, G., Weston, M.J., Bunting, S., Moncada, S. and Vane, J.R., 1978. Prostacyclin can replace heparin in haemodialysis in dogs. Lancet, ii, 1075-1077.

DETERMINANTS FOR PLATELET ADHESION AND AGGREGATION
ON COLLAGEN

Frank A. Meyer

Polymer Department, Weizmann Institute of Science,
Rehovot, Israel

ABSTRACT

Both physical and chemical determinants are present on collagen fibers which together are responsible for platelet adhesion leading to platelet activation (aggregation/release). These determinants are the curvature of the fiber and certain aspects of the surface chemistry of collagen associated with the triple helix conformation. In cases where not all determinants are present, platelet adhesion may still occur but this does not then result in activation.

The role of shape has been investigated by adsorbing soluble triple helical collagen to glass fibers of graded curvature. To very thick fibers or to a flat surface (infinite curvature) platelets adhere but aggregation does not occur. Only when the fiber diameter becomes less than that of the platelet ($\sim 2\mu$) will adhesion-induced aggregation occur. A flat surface with adsorbed soluble collagen although possessing the same chemistry as the fine fibers with soluble collagen adsorbed to them does not induce platelet aggregation because the curvature is not high enough. The finding that soluble collagen adsorbed to fine fibers induces platelet aggregation shows that the long range order of the collagen molecules on the surface is not important. An increase in surface attractiveness with curvature is a general phenomenon and is also seen in cases where only adhesion occurs and which do not lead to aggregation presumably because the surface chemistry is not sufficiently attractive. This refers to non-collagen surfaces or to denatured collagen-covered surfaces.

The chemical determinants recognized by platelets on the triple helical surface involve some general features of collagen composition in particular the high proline/hydroxyproline content. Arginine is also recognized but possibly in a more selective context. It is not known whether other determinants, as well, are involved. However, the carbohydrates, telopeptides, amino, carboxyl and hydroxyl groups do not seem to have a role. The involvement of the imino acids, in particular, distinguishes platelet recognition of collagen chemistry from surfaces of other chemistries. The triple helical conformation may be required to provide a high concentration or particular spatial configuration of the chemical determinants on the surface.

The platelet membrane component(s) directly involved in mediating the interaction with collagen have yet to be identified.

Neither glucosyl transferase nor fibronectin seems to be involved. Studies with rabbit platelets indicate that glycoproteins I, II and III, also, are not involved. On the other hand, a platelet membrane protein strongly bound to collagen can be isolated from platelets adherent to collagen, but its involvement in the biologic interaction remains to be demonstrated.

INTRODUCTION

The physiological response of platelets to damaged vessel walls is largely attributed to exposed collagen fibers. The first observable event is the adhesion of platelets to collagen. As a consequence, adherent platelets become activated, i.e. undergo the release reaction and become sticky to circulating platelets. By a chain process, thought to be mediated through the release of ADP and prostaglandin derivatives (Mustard and Packham, 1977), aggregates build up on the surface.

Much can be learnt about the mechanism of the platelet/collagen interaction from *in vitro* studies. Events *in vitro* follow the same sequence (adhesion followed by activation) as in the physiological situation. This justifies the use of the *in vitro* systems. Even washed platelets in divalent ion-free suspensions will adhere to collagen fibers and release (Brass, Faile and Bensusan, 1976). It is thus presumed that the physiological interaction is likely to differ from that *in vitro* more with respect to quantitative aspects than with respect to the basic mechanisms involved. Such differences, nevertheless may be very significant. *In vivo*, factors such as flow conditions, the presence of plasma proteins, red cells and non-collagenous vessel wall constituents may modulate the intensity of the interaction.

The platelet/collagen interaction is specific in the sense that platelets rapidly adhere and activate on collagen. Other surfaces, in comparison, are of considerably lower affinity (Packham et al., 1969; Baumgartner and Muggli, 1976) and more often than not although some adhesion may occur, activation does not follow suit. The affinity for collagen is known to be a consequence both of physical structure and chemistry (Michaeli and Orloff, 1976; Beachey, Chiang and Kang, 1979; Gordon, 1979). In this presentation the factors involved in platelet adhesion and platelet activation induced by adhesion to collagen fibers will be discussed especially with reference to recent data obtained in our laboratory.

COLLAGEN: STRUCTURE AND CHEMISTRY

Collagen (Bornstein and Traub, 1979) in its native state is an assembly of three-stranded rod-shaped molecules (3000 Å x 15 Å) of 295,000 molecular weight. The molecules are packed longitudinally in head-to-tail fashion and laterally in a quarter-stagger arrangement, i.e. with parallel molecules regularly displaced by a quarter of their length with respect to their neighbors, to give a microfibril involving some four or five molecules packed around the microfibril axis. Microfibrils in turn are packed to build up macroscopic fibrils* whose diameter can range from about 50Å to several thousand Angstroms. Stability of the structure is due in part to the quarter-staggering which maximizes hydrophobic and charge interactions as well as by intra- and inter-molecular crosslinks that form with time.

Small amounts of soluble collagen representing monomers and low levels of crosslinked monomers which have not yet been crosslinked into the fibril can be extracted particularly from young tissues with neutral salt solutions or with acid. Such collagen solutions are stable, however, at physiological pH and ionic strength soluble collagen will self-assemble after a nucleation phase to reconstitute fibrils. The rate at which this occurs depends on concentration and temperature. Fibrils with different molecular packing arrangement can also be constituted under specific circumstances.

The collagen molecule involves three polypeptide chains (α-chains) of equal length with ends in register twisted together in a triple helix. Each collagen chain has glycine in every third position along its length, large quantities of proline and uniquely, hydroxyproline, are also present. These two features favor the triple helix conformation over others. In this conformation glycine is on the inside, the other amino acids are on the surface with their side chains pointed regularly to the outside. Small peptide regions of different composition (telopeptides) are present at both ends of the chain. These are not involved in the triple helix and are susceptible to proteolytic enzymes. Carbohydrate in small amounts, present as galactose or as a disaccharide of glucose and galactose, covalently linked to hydroxylysine is also found. The triple helix of the collagen molecule is normally quite stable but slightly elevated temperatures ($\sim$45°) cause chain separation and a helix to coil transition which can be reversed upon cooling. Modification of the collagen molecule, e.g. the charge groups, can lead to lower melting temperatures. Collagen chains can be cleaved at methionyl residues with cyanogen bromide to give a limited number of peptides. At low temperatures these, too, can form triple helices.

Recent chemical studies of collagens derived from various tissues have shown at least five genetically distinct types of molecule based on differences in amino acid composition and sequence and in carbohydrate content. Of these, types I, II and III are the most abundant. Types IV and V are found in basement membranes and fetal tissues respectively. Collagen in vessel walls is restricted to types I, III and IV. Triple helical collagen sequences also exist in other proteins, e.g. the Cl_q component of complement.

PHYSICAL DETERMINANTS ON COLLAGEN

It is a well-established fact that the physical state of collagen is important for platelet activation to occur. The collagen fibril will induce platelet activation but soluble collagen will not

---

* In the collagen literature these are termed "fibrils" whereas "fibers" refer to an organization of fibrils such as occurs in tissue.

do so unless it has polymerized (Muggli and Baumgartner, 1973; Jaffe and Deykin, 1974; Brass and Bensusan, 1974). The extent of the interaction of platelets with soluble collagen seems to be limited to binding. This is demonstrated by a reduced interaction with collagen fibers in the presence of soluble collagen in the platelet suspension (Gordon and Simons, 1977; Meyer and Weisman, 1978; Chesney et al., 1979) and by direct binding studies(Kay et al., 1977). In other studies (Gordon and Dingle, 1974), direct binding could not be demonstrated but these are open to the criticism that weak interactions may not have survived the separation procedures employed.

The physical features of the native collagen fiber that cause platelets to adhere and activate have been probed using a variety of particulates formed from soluble collagen (Balleisen, Marx and Kuhn, 1976; Muggli, 1978; Wang et al., 1978b; Barnes and MacIntyre, 1979).

In our studies we have used glass surfaces to which soluble collagen has been physically adsorbed from solution to give a monomolecular adsorbed layer (Meyer and Weisman, 1978; Meyer and Frojmovic, 1979; Bettelheim and Priel, 1979). This approach is based on a general property of macromolecules. Most macromolecules adsorb "irreversibly" from solution to most surfaces and form a dense monolayer about one macromolecular diameter thick. In our studies, adsorption was performed by introducing clean glass surfaces into stable solutions of soluble collagen that had been centrifuged before use. The surfaces were then rinsed several times with the solvent used to make up the collagen solution and used immediately without drying. The amount of collagen adsorbed is some 1 to 2 mg/m^2 (Bettelheim and Priel, 1979; A. Silberberg, priv.comm.). 1 mg/m^2 corresponds to the amount expected for a single layer of molecules lying flat on the surface and entirely covering it. There are indications, however, that this is not the structure of collagen on the surface, rather a good part of the molecule extends into the solution giving a diffuse layer containing solvent (Bettelheim and Priel, 1979). The molecules are irreversibly adsorbed to the surface, i.e. do not desorb when placed in physiologic ionic media. However, in the presence of plasma, replacement by plasma proteins occurs. Platelet interaction with such surfaces, therefore, was studied using washed platelets (rabbit) suspended in Tyrode's solution. Surfaces were introduced into the stirred platelet suspension, removed, and the interaction with the surface assessed directly by visualization in the light microscope.

We (Meyer and Weisman, 1978) have shown that platelets will adhere rapidly to a plane glass surface with adsorbed soluble collagen, but that adhesion does not lead to the formation of platelet aggregates even after a very long exposure to the platelet suspension. In comparison if native collagen fibers is the surface instead of individually adsorbed soluble collagen, platelets adhere much more rapidly and after two minutes platelet aggregates form on the fiber surface. Since chemically and structurally at the molecular level the two surfaces are very similar, this suggests that a mechanogeometrical factor may be involved. To test this the interaction of platelets with fine glass fibers (0.5 to 2.0µ diam.) to which soluble collagen has been adsorbed was studied (Meyer and Weisman, 1979;1980). Fig.1a and 1b show that there is indeed a marked difference in the interaction when platelets adhere respectively to a plane

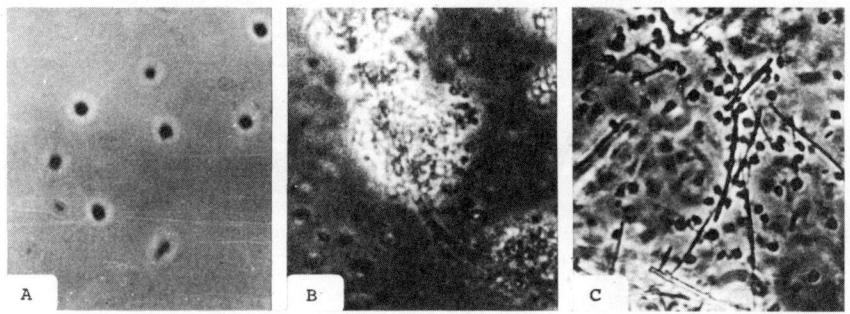

Fig. 1. Interaction of washed rabbit platelets in Tyrode's solution with surfaces. A. Soluble collagen adsorbed to a plane glass surface, x 1080. B. Soluble collagen adsorbed to glass fibers, x 660. C. Bare glass fibers, x 660. Glass fibers (borosilicate) ranging from 0.5 to 2.0μ in diameter were obtained by sonicating glass microfiber filters (Grade GF/F, Whatman, Inc., Kent, England). Adsorption was performed with neutral salt soluble collagen prepared from tendons of lathyritic chicks (Meyer and Weisman, 1978). Interaction in 0.3 ml of platelet suspension (Meyer and Weisman, 1978) was performed for four minutes at room temperature in the cuvette of a Payton aggregometer using a stir speed of 600 r.p.m. Fibers (80 μg) were added in suspension in one-tenth volume and the plane surface was immersed while held by forceps. Interaction was assessed directly by phase contrast microscopy of the plane surface or on a drop withdrawn from the platelet suspension with fibers. A control plane surface with deposited native collagen fibers, instead of adsorbed soluble collagen, induced platelet aggregation.

and to a fiber glass surface with adsorbed soluble collagen. It may be seen that on the latter surface platelet adhesion leads to platelet aggregation. Further observations indicated that the critical fiber diameter where adhesion goes over to activation is probably less than the diameter of the platelet since on 2μ fibers only adherent platelets were seen. For smaller-sized fibers, the size of the platelet aggregate seemed to increase as fiber diameter decreases. Quantitation of this effect was made difficult by the tendency of fibers with aggregates on them to clump. To a control preparation of bare glass fibers without adsorbed soluble collagen, platelets adhere but adhesion does not result in platelet aggregation (Fig.1c). This also occurs on glass fibers to which denatured soluble collagen or albumin has been adsorbed.

These results show that adhesion to a macroscopic surface of triple helical collagen does not normally lead to activation. For activation to be induced on this surface it must, besides being based on triple helical collagen, be of a sufficiently high curvature. This is provided for in collagen fibers in their native state. Activation, moreover, is not dependent on the organization of the collagen molecules on the surface (it being very different on

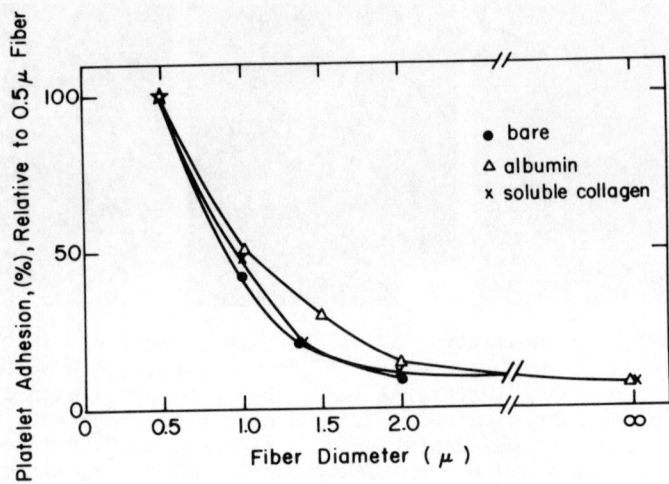

Fig. 2. Rate of adhesion of platelets as a function of fiber diameter on bare glass, and on albumin and soluble collagen adsorbed to glass. The ordinate is the number of platelets (per unit surface area) adhering to a surface after 4 min. relative to that found on a 0.5µ diameter fiber of the same surface chemistry and is expressed as a percentage. The experiment was performed as described for Fig.1 except that platelets were suspended in Tyrode's solution without the divalent cations (Meyer and Frojmovic, 1979). Fibers (greater than 100µ in length) were sized in the microscope according to diameter and the number of platelets adhering to ten fibers of the same diameter counted and averaged. On plane surfaces (infinite diameter) adhesion was quantitated by averaging the platelet counts on five separate areas selected from the middle of the surface (Meyer and Weisman, 1978).

the glass surfaces we have used and in the native fibers). This conclusion is in accord with other findings using collagen fibrils assembled in solution from soluble collagen under conditions which alter the molecular packing arrangement in the fiber (Balleisen, Marx and Kuhn, 1976; Muggli, 1978; Wang et al., 1978b; Barnes and MacIntyre, 1979). Wang et al. (1978b) have shown that the minimum fiber length required to induce activation is some 9000Å. The minimum fiber diameter is not known but fibrils in the range of 45 to 90Å are active (Brooks and Simons, 1978).

Using the surfaces in our study above, it could be demonstrated that the attractiveness of a surface for platelets increased with curvature to the same relative extent on all the surfaces (Meyer and Weisman, 1979, 1980). Only on a triple helical collagen surface, however, did adhesion go over to activation. This was demonstrated in an experiment where the number (after 4 mins.) of platelets adhering to a surface of given chemistry was determined as a function of fiber diameter. The experiment was performed with washed platelets suspended in Tyrode's solution without divalent cations so that adhesion could be quantitated also on otherwise activating collagen surfaces. The results are shown in Fig.2. The rate of adhesion on all surfaces increases markedly as the diameter of the fiber becomes less than 2µ but the relative changes are the same.

Differences in the interaction of platelets with these surfaces as a function of fiber diameter was also in evidence when the morphology of the adherent platelet was investigated (Meyer and Weisman, 1979, 1980). It was found that platelets adherent to plane surfaces flatten and spread themselves out with time whereas platelets adherent to single fine fibers tend to stand off the surface and do not collapse onto it. This was the case whether the surface was of glass, or of albumin or soluble collagen adsorbed onto glass.

It would appear that platelet interaction with a surface is increased as surface curvature increases such that if the chemistry of the surface is sufficiently attractive adhering platelets will activate. Such a combination of favorable morphology and surface chemistry exists on the collagen fiber. On a surface where only one of these is present, platelets may still adhere (though less effectively) but adhesion does not lead to activation. This is seen on a surface where the chemistry is favorable but the geometric form is not, e.g. on soluble collagen adsorbed to a plane surface, or where the geometric form is favorable but chemistry is not, e.g. on bare glass fibers or on albumin or denatured soluble collagen adsorbed to glass fibers. Other fibers in the last category may include elastin and microfibrillar glycoprotein (Ordinas et al., 1975; Barnes and MacIntyre, 1979) and collagen fibers whose surface chemistry has been made less attractive by denaturation or by other modifications. Whether the combination of an unfavorable surface chemistry on extremely fine fibers would induce platelet activation remains an open question.

The chemical determinants responsible for collagen being attractive must be related to the chemistry of the surface of the triple helix since denatured collagen does not support platelet activation. Moreover, they must be rather specific to triple helical collagen since the non-collagenous protein surfaces even as fibers do not induce activation. On the other hand, types I, II, III, IV and V soluble collagen and Cl_q all induce platelet activation when multimerized (Balleisen et al., 1975; Barnes, Gordon and MacIntyre, 1976; Cazenave et al., 1976; Santoro and Cunningham, 1977; Barnes and MacIntyre, 1979), suggesting that the essential chemical determinants are present in each of these cases despite the considerable variations in carbohydrate content, amino acid composition and sequence of the individual triple helices.

CHEMICAL DETERMINANTS ON COLLAGEN

Our studies (Meyer and Weisman, 1978; Meyer and Frojmovic, 1979) indicate that the high proline and hydroxyproline content of collagen is recognized by platelets. This was demonstrated when the ability of various polypeptides to compete with collagen for binding sites on the platelet membrane was tested. It was found that pre-incubation of platelet suspensions with soluble materials containing high contents of proline and/or hydroxyproline caused a reduction in the rate of platelet adhesion to surfaces based on triple helical collagen.

The soluble materials tested were used at a concentration of 100 µg/ml. At this concentration soluble collagen in the platelet suspension produced a marked inhibition in the rate of adhesion. Inhibitory activity was still evident when soluble collagen was used which had been treated with periodate or pepsin to remove the carbohydrates and the telopeptides respectively. Denatured soluble collagen, peptides from collagen obtained with cyanogen bromide, synthetic polypeptides $(Gly-Pro-Ala-Gly-Pro-Pro)_n$, $(Gly-Pro-Pro)_n$, $(Pro_2Gly)_2$ and the homopolypeptides, polyproline and polyhydroxyproline (but not proline or hydroxyproline), all gave effects similar to those of intact soluble collagen.

Platelets thus recognize a high proline and hydroxyproline content in a polypeptide independently of the amino acid sequence and the molecular conformation. An aspect of platelet adhesion to collagen as distinguished from adhesion to other surfaces is thus the involvement of proline and hydroxyproline whose presence in appreciable amounts is unique to collagen. A specific membrane site is involved since polyhydroxyproline did not influence the rate of platelet adhesion to a surface on which albumin or globulin had been adsorbed.

Low concentrations of ADP in platelet suspensions under conditions where aggregation is not induced also cause a reduction in the rate of platelet adhesion to collagen (Meyer and Frojmovic, 1979). The possibility that ADP is released by the proline/hydroxyproline-containing test materials and the decreased adhesion seen with these is due to an ADP dependent binding site could be ruled out. However, it turns out that ADP has an indirect effect on the proline/hydroxyproline binding site of the platelet. Upon attaching to its receptor on the platelet membrane, ADP induces a time-dependent temporary blockage of the proline/hydroxyproline site. This is a local effect and does not involve the disc-to-sphere shape change that is induced by ADP (Meyer, Weisman and Frojmovic, 1979, 1980).

The rate of adhesion to collagen is maximally inhibited by polyhydroxyproline to an extent of some 60% (Meyer and Frojmovic, 1979) and is not further reduced by addition of polyproline (personal observation). Hence, still other chemical determinants are likely to be present on collagen. It is unlikely that glycine is involved since this amino acid is in the interior of the collagen triple helix. Competitive inhibition studies (Meyer and Weisman, 1978; Meyer and Frojmovic, 1979) with homopolypeptides based on other amino acids present on the triple helical surface, e.g. alanine, glutamic acid, aspartic acid, lysine and arginine suggest that these amino acids, too, are not involved. Clearly, however, higher concentrations of homopolypeptides in the platelet suspension may show some involvement of these amino acids. Polylysine and polyarginine, in particular, which by themselves cause platelet aggregation at 100 µg/ml could only be tested at much lower concentrations.

The chemical determinants on collagen mediating interaction with platelets have also been investigated by others. The approach that has been used involves testing the ability of collagen, after specific enzymic or chemical modification, to induce aggregation and/ or release in platelet suspensions. Where no effect of modification is seen, it is probably safe to conclude that the particular chemical feature being tested for is not involved in interaction with platelets. Where an effect is seen, the possibility that this is because of reasons other than that due to the specific chemical modification needs to be taken into consideration. It is now recognized that modification may influence the reactivity of collagen by affecting its physical state and that this may mask the effect of the specific chemical alteration. For example, modification may affect the triple helix conformation or may influence fiber formation, dimensions and molecular packing arrangements particularly where soluble collagen has been used. In addition, where bulky blocking groups have been introduced sites other than those being modified may become masked through steric effects. It is also possible that modification may affect the state of dispersion of collagen fibers in the platelet suspension which also can influence the extent of the platelet response (Muggli and Baumgartner, 1973; Brooks and Simons, 1978; Kronick and Jimenez,1980).

Recent studies have been designed to minimize the above effects which often were responsible for the results obtained in early modification studies. Thus it is now generally accepted that collagen carbohydrates (Santoro and Cunningham, 1977; Gordon and Simons, 1977) and telopeptides (Wojtecka-Lukasik et al., 1967; Santoro and Cunningham, 1977; Chesney et al., 1979) are not involved in the platelet/ collagen interaction. In these studies soluble collagen, after treatment with periodate or with pepsin, was allowed to polymerize to form fibers prior to testing with platelets. Other studies implicating collagen carbohydrates in the interaction probably are the result of an effect on fiber formation and/or on the stability of the helix.

Recently, Wang et al. (1978a) have tested the effect of other collagen modifications using a reconstituted fiber preparation that had been crosslinked to prevent possible denaturation or molecular rearrangements during the modification procedures. It was shown that crosslinking did not interfere with the activity of collagen and that manipulation of amino, carboxyl and hydroxyl groups on collagen did not influence platelet response. On the other hand, arginine could be shown to be involved. Modification of arginine led to a collagen preparation with a decreased ability to induce aggregation and release. The extent of the effect was dependent on how much arginine had been modified and for the maximal treatment used, no aggregation or release occurred. This effect does not seem to be due to the introduction of a bulky blocking group since deguanidation also was effective. The state of dispersion of the fibers after arginine modification was not checked. However, it is unlikely that this was

a factor since other collagen preparations where charge also was
affected, e.g. by modification of amino or carboxyl groups, gave a
normal platelet response. Wang et al. (1978) propose that those arginine residues in position Y of the tripeptide unit Gly-X-Y of collagen, in particular, may be specifically involved.

It is likely, therefore, that these arginine residues contribute to the overall chemical attractiveness of the collagen triple
helical surface. Presumably their modification lowers the attractiveness of the surface to such an extent that activation is no longer induced. The interaction of such fibers with platelets may be similar
to that seen in our study for the fibers of unfavorable surface chemistries, i.e. some adhesion may still occur, in this case involving
proline/hydroxyproline, but this does not lead to activation.

The role of specific collagen sequences have also been investigated by testing the ability of cyanogen bromide peptides and
subfragments to induce aggregation and/or release (Katzman, Kang and
Beachey, 1973; Puett et al., 1973; Balleisen, Marx and Kuhn,1976;
Michaeli and Orloff, 1976; Fauvel, Legrand and Caen, 1978; Fauvel et
al., 1979; Beachey, Chiang and Kang, 1979). Since these materials
are neither in triple helix form nor organized into a fiber, their
relationship to the collagen/platelet interaction remains to be demonstrated. Moreover, there is controversy over whether they possess
activity and, where activity is claimed, over which particular peptide. Further studies using individual peptides that have been re-
natured and organized into a fiber may help elucidate to what extent
specific sequences are involved in the platelet/collagen interaction.

In summary, the chemical features of the triple helical collagen surface that seem to be recognized by platelets and have so far
been identified involve the proline/hydroxyproline and arginine residues. Other aspects of chemistry may yet be involved but these do not
seem to be the carbohydrates, the telopeptides or the amino, carboxyl
and hydroxyl groups (including the hydroxyl of hydroxyproline).
Platelets in recognizing the imino acids probably recognize a prominent general feature on the collagen surface. Recognition of arginine,
however, is likely to be more specific in the sense that arginine is
a relatively minor amino acid in the surface composition and only
certain arginines may be involved.

The involvement of the imino acids in the platelet/collagen
interaction confers a degree of specificity to this interaction and
sets it aside from platelet interactions with other surfaces. Recognition of the imino acids, in particular, may provide the collagen
surface with the additional measure of attractiveness that causes
adherent platelets to activate.

It is not known whether it is simply the extent to which the
collagen surface is occupied by proline/hydroxyproline and arginine
residues or whether it is their spatial organization on the surface
which is determining. Available evidence does not exclude the possibility that a more specific type of recognition is involved where these
amino acids form part of a particular sequence(s) which is recognized
when in the triple helical conformation. All three cases are influence
by denaturation and could explain the difference in platelet reactivity of collagen in the two conformational states. Denaturation
involves an unfolding of the helix such that glycine comes out from

the interior of the molecule. The concentration of amino acids formerly on the surface is thereby diluted and their organization is perturbed.

MEMBRANE COMPONENTS MEDIATING INTERACTION WITH COLLAGEN

The components and features of the platelet surface responsible for mediating the interaction with collagen have yet to be identified. It had been proposed that glucosyl transferase on the platelet surface mediates adhesion by forming an enzyme-substrate complex with incomplete disaccharide groups on collagen (Jamieson, Urban and Barber, 1971). This suggestion has since become untenable because collagen carbohydrates are not involved in the platelet/collagen interaction (Gordon and Simons, 1977; Santoro and Cunningham, 1977). Moreover, the preferred substrate for the enzyme is denatured rather than native collagen (Menashi, Harwood and Grant, 1976). Bensusan et al. (1978) have proposed that fibronectin may be the collagen receptor on platelets. However, fibronectin does not appear to be present on the platelet surface (Hynes et al., 1978) and an intracellular localization for it has been indicated (Zucker et al., 1979). Moreover, the affinity of fibronectin is for denatured collagen rather than for native collagen (Rouslahti and Engvall, 1978). Recently, it has been shown that fibronectin at best has only a limited role in the platelet/collagen interaction (Santoro and Cunningham, 1979).

In our studies (Lahav and Meyer, 1980), changes were effected in the components on the rabbit platelet membrane using proteolytic enzymes. The ability of such modified platelets to adhere to collagen was then tested. Fig.3 shows the effect of the enzyme treatments on the platelet membrane components as monitored by gel electrophoresis after labeling by the lactoperoxidase-iodination technique (Phillips, 1972). Most of the label in the intact platelet is taken up by three components which are the three major membrane glycoproteins of the rabbit platelet, i.e. GPI, GPII and GPIII (Nurden, Butcher and Hawkey, 1977; Greenberg et al., 1979a,b). It is seen that thrombin has no effect on these components. However, trypsin causes the removal of GPI and GPII, while chymotrypsin removes not only GPI and GPII, but GPIII as well. The labeling of other platelet membrane components was not high enough for the effect of proteases on these to be established.

The adhesion to collagen of platelets after enzyme modification is shown in Table 1. In order to eliminate possible effects on adhesion arising from ADP (Meyer and Frojmovic, 1979) released during the thrombin and trypsin treatments (Greenberg et al., 1979b), experiments were also performed in the presence of 1 mM AMP. In the presence of AMP adhesion in all cases is seen to be similar to that of control indicating that the three major membrane glycoproteins do not play a role in platelet adhesion to collagen. Our results also support the view that fibronectin is not involved. In other cell systems, trypsin treatment readily leads to the loss of surface fibronectin (Yamada, Yamada and Pastan, 1977), however, this treatment when applied to platelets did not affect adhesion in the absence of effects of released ADP.

An attempt to isolate platelet membrane components mediating platelet binding to collagen has been made (J. Lahav, personal comm.) using a collagen fiber affinity column (Lahav, 1979). Platelets,

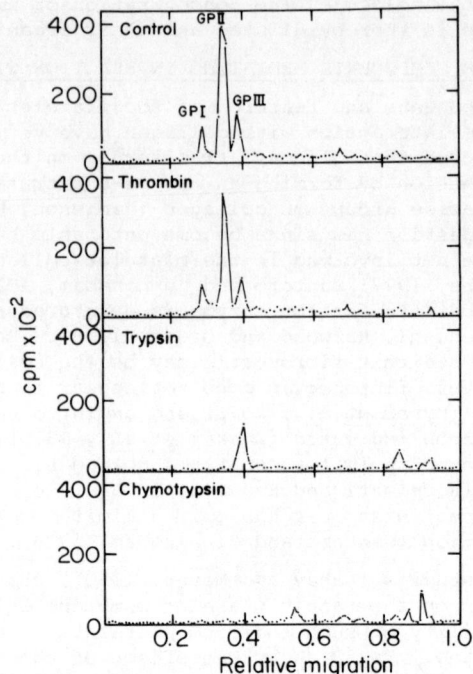

Fig.3. SDS-PAGE electrophoresis of platelet membrane components radiolabeled by the lactoperoxidase-iodination technique (Phillips, 1972) after treatment of intact rabbit platelets with enzymes. Washed platelets (500,000/µl) in divalent cation-free Tyrode's solution (Meyer and Frojmovic, 1979) containing 0.038% EGTA were treated at 37° with thrombin (0.06 U/ml) for 10 min, with trypsin (12.5 U/ml) for 30 min, or with chymotrypsin (98 U/ml) for 10 min. Electrophoresis was performed on linear gradient gels (5 to 20% acrylamide) using 5×10^7 platelets that had been solubilized in a 1% SDS solution containing 10% mercaptoethanol. Gels stained with the periodic acid-Schiff reagent indicated that the major iodinated components were the membrane glycoproteins, GPI, GPII and GPIII, of the untreated rabbit platelet (Control).

labeled by the lactoperoxidase-iodination technique, were introduced onto the column. Non-adherent platelets were eluted and the adherent platelets lysed with 0.5% Triton X-100, followed by 0.3% SDS. Electrophoresis of the eluates indicated that the Triton lysate mostly contains the major glycoproteins and, the SDS eluate, the membrane proteins. Subsequent elution with 8 M NaCl did not release further material. However, digestion of the collagen in the column with purified collagenase resulted in the elution of a single labeled membrane component. This protein has a molecular weight of some 80,000 Daltons and is not one of the major membrane glycoproteins.

TABLE 1. Adhesion of enzyme-treated rabbit platelets to collagen fibers. Enzyme treatments were performed as in Fig.3, in the presence and absence of 1 mM AMP. Adhesion was performed as previously described (Meyer and Frojmovic, 1979) and is expressed as the rate of adhesion relative to that of a control as a percentage.

Enzyme treatment	Adhesion (%)*	
	[AMP] = 0	[AMP] = 1 mM
Control (no enzyme)	100	109±11
Thrombin	116±9	102±11
Chymotrypsin	100±9	99± 5
Trypsin	47±8	102± 7

*Mean ±SEM of five experiments

Its marked affinity for collagen suggests that it may be an important surface component mediating platelet interaction with collagen. Presumably this membrane protein was not degraded when platelets were treated with the proteases used in the previous study since such modified platelets were fully capable of adhering to collagen. This is not unreasonable in view of the relative resistance to proteolysis of membrane proteins on the platelet (Phillips, 1972; Nachman and Ferris, 1972; Nurden and Caen, 1975). Further studies, however, are required to demonstrate the involvement of this isolated membrane protein in the biologic adhesion of platelets to collagen.

ACKNOWLEDGEMENTS

The author wishes to thank Prof. A. Silberberg for helpful discussions and comments. This work was performed in part under contract NO1-HV-5-2907 from the Devices and Technology Branch, Division of Heart and Vascular Diseases, National Heart and Lung Institute.

REFERENCES

Balleisen, L., Gay, S., Marx, R., and Kuhn, K., 1975. Comparative investigation of the influence of human and bovine collagen types I, II and III on the aggregation of human platelets. Klin. Wschr., 53, 903-905.

Balleisen, L., Marx, R., and Kuhn, K., 1976. Platelet-collagen interaction. The influence of native and modified collagen (Type I) on the aggregation of human platelets. Haemostasis, 5, 155-164.

Barnes, M.J., Gordon, J.L., and MacIntyre, D.E., 1976. Platelet aggregating activity of type I and type III collagens from human aorta and chicken skin. Biochem.J., 160, 647-651

Barnes, M.J., and MacIntyre, D.E., 1979. Platelet-reactivity of isolated constituents of the blood vessel wall. Haemostasis, 8, 158-170.

Baumgartner, H.R., and Muggli, R., 1976. Adhesion and aggregation: morphological demonstration and quantitation in vivo and in vitro, in Platelet in Biology and Pathology (Ed. Gordon), pp.23-60, North-Holland, Amsterdam.

Beachey, E.H., Chiang, T.M., and Kang, A.H., 1979. Collagen-platelet interaction. Int.Rev.Conn.Tiss.Res., 8, 1-21.

Bensusan, H.B., Koh, T.L., Henry, K.G., Murray, B.A. and Culp, L.A., 1978. Evidence that fibronectin is the collagen receptor on platelet membranes. Proc.Natl.Acad.Sci.U.S.A., 75, 5864-5869.

Bettelheim, F.A., and Priel, Z., 1979. Adsorption of biopolymers on solid surfaces. J.Coll.Interf.Sci., 70, 395-398.

Bornstein, P., and Traub, W., 1979. The chemistry and biology of collagen, in The Proteins (Eds. Neurath and Hill), Third edition, vol. IV, pp. 411-632, Academic Press, New York.

Brass, L.F. and Bensusan, H.B., 1974. The role of collagen quaternary structure in the platelet: collagen interaction. J.Clin.Invest., 54, 1480-1487.

Brass, L.F., Faile, D., and Bensusan, H.R., 1976. Direct measurement of the platelet:collagen interaction by affinity chromatography on collagen/Sepharose. J.Lab.Clin.Med., 87, 525-534.

Brooks, C., and Simons, E.R., 1978. Collagen age and platelet aggregation. Gerontology, 24, 169-178.

Cazenave, J.P., Assimeh, S.N., Painter, R.H., Packham, M.A., and Mustard, J.F., 1976. Cl_q inhibition of the interaction of collagen with human platelets. J.Immunol., 116, 162-163.

Chesney, C. Mcl., Pifer, D., Dabbous, M.K., and Brinkley, B., 1979. The role of the telopeptide region of collagen in the platelet-collagen interaction. Thrombos.Res., 14, 445-461.

Fauvel, F., Legrand, Y.J., and Caen, J.P., 1978. Platelet adhesion to type I collagen and alpha $I(I)_3$ trimers:involvement of the C-terminal alpha I(I)CB6A peptide. Thrombos.Res., 12, 273-285.

Fauvel, F., Legrand, Y.J., Kuhn, K., Bentz, H., Fietzek, P.P., and Caen, J.P., 1979. Platelet adhesion to type III collagen: involvement of a sequence of nine amino acids from α_1(III)CB4 peptide. Thrombos.Res., 16, 269-273.

Gordon, J.L., 1979. Mechanism of platelet-collagen interaction. Nature, 278, 13-14.

Gordon, J.L., and Dingle, J.T., 1974. Binding of radiolabelled collagen to blood platelets. J.Cell Sci., 16, 157-166.

Gordon, R.K., and Simons, E.R., 1977. The function of collagen carbohydrates in initiation of platelet aggregation. Thrombos Res., 11, 155-161.

Greenberg, J.P., Packham, M.A., Guccione, M.A., Harfenist, F.J., Orr, J.L., Kinlough-Rathbone, R.L., Perry, D.W., and Mustard, J.F., 1979a. The effect of pretreatment of human or rabbit platelets with chymotrypsin on their responses to human fibrinogen and aggregating agents. Blood, 54, 753-765.

Greenberg, J.P., Packham, M.A., Guccione, M.A., Rand, M.L., Reimers, H.J., and Mustard, J.F., 1979b. Survival of rabbit platelets treated in vitro with chymotrypsin, plasmin, trypsin, or neuraminidase. Blood, 53, 916-927.

Hynes, R.O., Ali, I.U., Destree, A.T., Mautner, V., Perkins, M.E., Senger, D.R., Wagner, D.D., and Smith, K.K., 1978. A large glycoprotein lost from the surfaces of transformed cells. Ann.N.Y.Acad.Sci., 312, 317-342.

Jaffe, R., and Deykin, D., 1974. Evidence for a structural requirement for the aggregation of platelets by collagen. J.Clin.Invest., 53, 875-883.

Jamieson, G.A., Urban, C.L. and Barber, A.J., 1971. Enzymatic basis for platelet collagen adhesion as the primary step in haemostasis. Nature, 234, 5-7.

Katzman, R.L., Kang, A.H., and Beachey, E.H., 1973. Collagen-induced platelet aggregation; involvement of an active glycopeptide fragment (α1-CB5). Science, (Wash.D.C.), 181, 670-672.

Kay, W.W., Swanson, R., Chong, G., Kurylo, E., and Bharadwaj, B.B., 1977. Binding of collagen by canine blood platelets. Thrombos. Haemostas., 37, 309-320.

Kronick, P. and Jimenez, S.A., 1980. The size of collagen fibrils that stimulate platelet aggregation in human plasma. Biochem.J., 186, 5-12.

Lahav, J. 1979. A column for isolation of platelet membrane components involved in collagen recognition, in Molecular Mechanisms of Biological Recognition (Ed. Balaban), pp.119-129. Elsevier/ North-Holland, Amsterdam.

Lahav, J., and Meyer, F.A., 1980. On the role of the major membrane glycoproteins in platelet adhesion to collagen. Submitted for publication.

Menashi, S., Harwood, R., and Grant, M.E., 1976. Native collagen is not a substrate for the collagen glucosyl transferase of platelets. Nature, 264, 670-672.

Meyer, F.A., and Frojmovic, M.M., 1979. Characteristics of the major platelet membrane site used in binding to collagen. Thrombos.Res., 15, 755-767.

Meyer, F.A., and Weisman, Z., 1978. Adhesion of platelets to collagen. The nature of the binding site from competitive inhibition studies. Thrombos.Res., 12, 431-446.

Meyer, F.A., and Weisman, Z., 1979. Platelet interaction with fibers and collagen-induced platelet aggregation. Thrombos.Haemostas., 42, 230 (Abstract).

Meyer, F.A., and Weisman, Z., 1980. Collagen-induced platelet aggregation. Dependence on triple helical structure and fiber diameter. Submitted for publication.

Meyer, F.A., Weisman, Z., and Frojmovic, M.M., 1979. Platelet adhesion to collagen is inhibited by 5'-adenosine diphosphate but unaffected by cell shape. Thrombos.Haemos., 42, 162 (Abstract).

Meyer, F.A., Weisman, Z., and Frojmovic, M.M., 1980. Platelet adhesion to collagen is inhibited by 5'-adenosine disphosphate but unaffected by cell shape. Submitted for publication.

Michaeli, D., and Orloff, K.G., 1976. Molecular considerations of platelet adhesion. Prog.Haemostasis Thromb. 3, 29-59.

Muggli, R., 1978. Collagen-induced platelet aggregation. Native collagen quaternary structure is not an essential structural requirement. Thrombos.Res., 13, 829-843.

Muggli, R., and Baumgartner, H.R., 1973. Collagen induced platelet aggregation: requirement for tropocollagen multimers. Thrombos. Res., 3, 715-728.

Nachman, R.L. and Ferris, B., 1972. Studies on the proteins of human platelet membranes. J.Biol.Chem., 247, 4468-4475.

Mustard, J.F., and Packham, M.A., 1977. Normal and abnormal haemostasis. Br.Med.Bull., 33, 187-192.

Nurden, A.T., Butcher, A.D., and Hawkey, C.M., 1977. Comparative studies on the glycoprotein composition of mammalian platelets. Comp.Biochem.Physiol., 56B, 407-413.

Nurden, A.T., and Caen, J.P., 1975. Specific roles for platelet surface glycoproteins in platelet function. Nature, 255, 720-722.

Ordinas, A., Hornebeck, W., Robert, L., and Caen, J.P., 1975. Interaction of platelets with purified macromolecules of the arterial wall. Path.Biol., 23 suppl., 44-48.

Packham, M.A., Evans, G., Glynn, M.F., and Mustard, J.F., 1969. The effect of plasma proteins on the interaction of platelets with glass surfaces. J.Lab.Clin.Med., 73, 686-697.

Phillips, D.R., 1972. Effect of trypsin on the exposed polypeptides and glycoproteins in the human platelet membrane. Biochemistry, 11, 4582-4588.

Puett, D., Wasserman, B.K., Ford, J.D., and Cunningham, L.W., 1973. Collagen-mediated platelet aggregation. Effects of collagen modification involving the protein and carbohydrate moieties. J.Clin.Invest., 52, 2495-2506.

Ruoslahti, E., and Engvall, E., 1978. Immunochemical and collagen binding properties of fibronectin. Ann.N.Y.Acad.Sci.U.S.A., 312, 178-191.

Santoro, S.A., and Cunningham, L.W., 1977. Collagen-mediated platelet aggregation. Evidence for multivalent interactions of intermediate specificity between collagen and platelets. J.Clin.Invest., 60, 1054-1060.

Santoro, S.A., and Cunningham, L.W., 1979. Fibronectin and the multiple interaction model for platelet-collagen adhesion. Proc.Natl.Acad.Sci.U.S.A., 76, 2644-2648.

Wang, C.L., Miyata, T., Weksler, B., Rubin, A.L., and Stenzel, K.H., 1978a. Collagen-induced platelet aggregation and release. I. Effects of side chain modifications and role of arginyl residues. Biochim.Biophys.Acta, 544, 555-567.

Wang, C.L., Miyata, T., Weksler, B., Rubin, A.L., and Stenzel, K.H., 1978b. Collagen-induced platelet aggregation and release. II. Critical size and structural requirements of collagen. Biochim. Biophys.Acta, 544, 568-577.

Wojtecka-Lukasik, E., Sopata, I., Wize, J., Skonieczna, M., Niedzwiecka-Namyslowska, I. and Kowalski, E., 1967. Adhesion of platelets to collagen devoid of telopeptides. Thromb.Diath. Haemorrh., 18, 76-79.

Yamada, K.M., Yamada, S.S., and Pastan, I., 1977. Quantitation of a transformation-sensitive adhesive cell surface glycoprotein. Decrease on several untransformed permanent cell lines. J.Cell Biol., 74, 649-654.

Zucker, M.B., Mosesson, M.W., Broekman, M.J., and Kaplan, K.L., 1979. Release of platelet fibronectin (cold-insoluble globulin) from alpha granules induced by thrombin or collagen; lack of requirement for plasma fibronectin in ADP-induced platelet aggregation. Blood, 54, 8-12.

THE ROLE OF CALCIUM IONS IN THE INDUCTION OF PLATELET ACTIVITIES

E.F. Lüscher, P. Massini, R. Käser-Glanzmann

Theodor Kocher Institute
University of Berne, Switzerland

ABSTRACT

Blood platelets can be stimulated into activity by a wide variety of chemically and functionally quite different agents. The end result is always the same and consists in aggregation, prostaglandin (PG) synthesis, the release reaction and manifestations of contractile and procoagulant activities, often preceded by shape change. This implies a common pathway and there is evidence, mainly from the work with ionophores that the crucial event is the intracellular availability of Ca^{2+} ions. Thus PG-synthesis depends on the cleavage of arachidonic acid from phospholipid by Ca^{2+}-activated phospholipase and contractile activity is mediated through Ca^{2+}-stimulated actomyosin, which also is involved in shape change. Less clear is the situation with respect to the release reaction, although there is no doubt that this is also mediated by Ca^{2+} ions.

Ca^{2+} ions are thought to be mobilized from different sites within the cell in response to a membrane-generated signal: from the stimulated membrane, from the dense tubular system (DTS), and perhaps also from mitochondria. Furthermore, the release-phase of activation is linked to an influx of Ca^{2+} ions from the outside. Increasingly, experimental evidence is becoming available for Ca^{2+}-release from the DTS, a structure known to actively accumulate Ca^{2+}. On the other hand, relatively little is as yet known with respect to the "second messenger(s)" responsible for the stimulation of the mediators which finally determine intracellular Ca^{2+}-release.

Extracellular Ca^{2+} also plays an essential role in controlling platelet activation. Whereas e.g. thrombin and collagen induce the platelets release reaction even in an EDTA-containing medium, other inducers such as ADP or adrenaline at low ($10^{-4}M$) Ca^{2+}-concentrations do so only as a consequence of Ca^{2+}-dependent aggregation; thus the inducers are not these agents per se, but rather the cell-cell contact. Furthermore, at physiological Ca^{2+} concentrations, release by these agents is greatly impaired even though aggregation takes place.

Preliminary evidence indicates that under these conditions thromboxane synthesis is also absent, implying that in a physiological suspension medium the plasma membrane of the platelet is unable to respond with a signal-producing configuration upon stimulation by ADP, adrenaline and other vasoactive amines.

INTRODUCTION

The inducers of platelet activation include an astonishing variety of agents. Even, if the list is restricted to those materials which play a role under physiological and pathological conditions, activating substances include thrombin, a proteolytic enzyme, macromolecular complexes such as collagen, IgG-containing immune complexes or aggregated IgG (cf. Pfueller and Lüscher, 1974) and low molecular weight substances such as adenosine diphosphate (ADP), thromboxane A_2, and vasoactive amines such as adrenaline, serotonin, and vasopressin. Nonetheless, the response of the platelet is always the same and is independent of the nature of the inducer, provided the concentration of the activator and the conditions in the suspension medium are adequate. In terms of manifestations of direct functional significance it can be summarized as follows: Aggregation, synthesis of prostaglandin (PG) and thromboxanes (TX), the release reaction, i.e. the specific secretion of substances from storage organelles and manifestations of contractile and procoagulant activities. Often, but not always, these events are preceded by fast morphological alterations termed shape change (cf. White 1974). It should also be noted that, depending upon the environment, some of these manifestations may proceed independent of the others; thus, thrombin and collagen will induce release also in the absence of aggregation, whereas other inducers depend on aggregation for release to occur. The relative uniformity of the platelet response to agents which must be expected to exert their influence over a variety of different receptors or mechanisms suggests that in every case one and the same essential effector system is enacted, which then determines the further course of events. Work on platelets as well as on other cells (for review see Bygrave 1978; Carafoli et al. (eds.), 1975) has provided ample evidence that this effector is the calcium ion. Since most of the known inducers of platelet activation are unable to penetrate into the cell, it must be assumed that they are capable of influencing the plasma membrane in such a way that a conformation capable of transmitting a signal to the interior of the platelet is created. The text of this message most likely reads: "Mobilize calcium ions". It is the purpose of this article to review briefly the consequences of the availability of Ca^{2+}ions in the cytoplasm, and the modes of their mobilization and removal. Furthermore, the effects of external calcium, which also influence platelet function to a considerable degree, will be briefly discussed.

THE CONSEQUENCES OF A RAISED CONCENTRATION OF CYTOPLASMIC CALCIUM

As in other cells the cytoplasmic Ca^{2+}-concentration of the resting platelet is in the neighborhood of $10^{-7}M$. Suitably ionophores such as A23187 or ionomycin (Gerrard et al. 1974; Massini and Lüscher 1974; Detwiler et al. 1978; Massini and Näf 1980) transport the cation across outer and inner membranes, resulting in the typical manifestations of platelet activation.
Contractile activity is based on the presence of considerable amounts of actomyosin in the platelets (cf. Cohen and Lüscher 1975; Lüscher 1976). Its most prominent manifestations are the spontaneous contraction of platelet aggregates and clot retraction. Actomyosin contraction is Ca^{2+}-mediated and its onset upon stimulation of the platelets therefore is convincing evidence for the appearance in the cytoplasm of concentrations of the cation of $10^{-6}M$ and higher.

Prostaglandin- and thromboxane synthesis is dependent upon the availability of arachidonic acid, which is cleaved from phospholipids by the action of phospholipase A_2, an enzyme which requires Ca^{2+} for activity and hence is activated in platelets by the ionophore A23187 (Pickett et al. 1977). As will be discussed later, cyclic adenosine-3',5'-monophosphate (cAMP) accelerates the removal of Ca^{2+} ions from the cytoplasm and accordingly decreases phospholipase activity (Bills et al. 1978; Rittenhouse-Simmons and Deykin 1978) and accordingly PG-synthesis (Minkes et al. 1977).

The release reaction is also produced by the addition of ionophore (Feinman and Detwiler 1974; Massini and Lüscher 1974). However, it is more difficult to establish a clear-cut link between Ca^{2+} ions and a process which obviously must involve the fusion of the organelle- and plasma membrane. Thromboxane A_2 is an efficient inducer of the release reaction; however, thrombin will still induce release under conditions of blocked PG-synthesis (Vargaftig 1977). This points to the existence of an alternative release-inducing agent, which in turn depends for its production on Ca^{2+} and phospholipase since release by thrombin is blocked by inhibitors of this enzyme (Vargaftig 1977). Recently, such an agent, derived from IgE-sensitized basophils has been described and its structure appears to be established as a 1-O-alkyl-2-acetyl-sn-glyceryl-3-phosphorylcholine (Demopoulous et al. (1979). This material, which is active as a release-inducer in pg amounts has been termed platelet activating factor (PAF) and is also produced by the stimulated platelets themselves (Chignard et al. 1979). It is difficult to define the relationship of PAF to the release mechanism but this substance as well as TX must be considered as being directly or indirectly involved in the release process.

The participation of the cytoskeleton in the release reaction has also been postulated for different types of cells (cf. e.g. Malaisse et al. 1975); however, in the platelet the contractile system can be inactivated without an effect on the secretory process (Kirkpatrick et al. 1979).

In conclusion, there can be no doubt that Ca^{2+} ions are essential for release to occur; however, it is also obvious that the cation essentially functions as a cofactor in the establishment of conditions which allow the production of the agent (or agents) which in fact bring about the release reaction. TXA_2 and/or PAF, both depending on Ca^{2+} for their production, are candidates for such a role, perhaps as parts of a more complex system.

Shape change is the early and fast transformation of the disk-shaped, resting platelet into a "spiny sphere", i.e. a spherical structure carrying long, filiform pseudopodia (Born 1970; White 1974). The disk-shaped platelet is characterized by a marginal bundle of microtubules, the persistence of which is incompatible with the transformation to a sphere with the same volume. Thus, shape change involves the decay of the microtubules and a second process which is responsible for pseudopode formation. Recent work has shown that the disks are first converted to spheres and that only these latter structures form spiny spheres (Rothen et al. 1980). Interestingly enough, the rate constants of the two steps (i.e. the formation of spheres and the transformation of the latter to "spiny spheres") are the same (Dubler et al. 1980). This might be interpreted to mean that shape change is due to the contraction of the submembranous network of actomyosin filaments, leading first to the rounding up of the cell and later, by a "pressure-flow" effect, to pseudopode formation. Similar mechanisms have been proposed for other, and particularly motile cells (Stocken 1977). Thus, shape change again is due to the availability of Ca^{2+} ions which lead to the depolymerization of the microtubules (Weisenberg 1972) and to actomyosin contraction.

WHERE DO THE CALCIUM IONS COME FROM ?

Different from e.g. the mastocyte which depends for secretion on the influx of external Ca^{2+}, the platelet can be activated by thrombin or collagen in an EDTA-containing medium. This means that Ca^{2+} ions can be mobilized

from internal stores. It is generally assumed that this
corresponds to a sequential reaction, first involving
the liberation of membrane-bound calcium, followed by
the mobilization from specific organelles, followed,
under physiological conditions by the influx from the
outside (Massini et al. 1978).

The mobilization of membrane-bound calcium is supported
by experimental evidence. By the use of the calcium-
specific fluorophore chlortetracyclin, Le Breton et al.
(1976) could demonstrate that concomitant with shape
change, calcium is lost from a membrane-bound form. How
this loss, which is the result of a stimulation-receptor
combination on the platelet surface, is achieved,
is not yet known. Some authors have drawn attention to
the fact that the degradation and resynthesis of inositol phosphatides is a very early event in stimulated
cells, including platelets, and is furthermore linked
to Ca^{2+} mobilization (for review see Mitchell 1975). It
is of particular interest that this response is observed
after stimulation with thrombin, collagen or ADP (in the
presence of fibrinogen), but not with ionophores (cf.
Kaulen 1978). This might indeed be interpreted to mean
that it is a causative and not a secondary event in Ca^{2+}-
mobilization.

Release of calcium from the dense tubular system (DTS).
The DTS is the equivalent to the sarcoplasmic reticulum
of muscle (cf. White 1972); it is a canalicular system
with a pronounced capacity for Ca^{2+} accumulation. It
forms a branched network, mainly underneath the plasma
membrane, but also extending into the interior of the
cell (Werner, 1980). Here again the question arises how
Ca^{2+} release from these structures is effected.
    Interestingly enough, the DTS is the site of pro-
staglandin synthesis (Käser-Glanzmann et al. 1978;
Gerrard et al. 1978 a,b), and the conclusion that the
platelet-activating PG's, in particular TXA_2 were directly involved in Ca^{2+}-release from the DTS appeared logical enough (cf. Gerrard et al. 1978a). However, later
work showed that TX-synthesis is not required; isolated
Ca^{2+}-accumulating vesicles release the cation under the
influence of the PG-endoperoxides PGG_2 and PGH_2 (Gerrard
et al. 1978b). Thus, the linkage of PG-synthesis and Ca^{2+}
mobilization appears clearly established. Again the
question remains what agent or mechanism takes over
under conditions of blocked PG-endoperoxide synthesis;
as mentioned earlier, thrombin or collagen will also
under these conditions induce the release reaction, which
obviously depends on the availability of larger amounts
of Ca^{2+}. Perhaps the results of experiments on the effects
of PAF on the DTS will shed light on this problem.
    Since the mobilization of membrane-bound Ca^{2+}
appears to be a very early event, it would appear logical

to assume that the cation thus made available would act as a "second messenger" responsible for the induction of the release of more Ca^{2+} from the DTS. It remains a fact, though, that the "early Ca^{2+}", responsible for shape change does not invariably lead to a progression of platelet activation: shape change, when induced by ADP remains an isolated phenomenon, unless it is followed by aggregation, which then triggers subsequent events, obviously by a mechanism which is more efficient in terms of Ca^{2+}-mobilization. It is as yet unclear whether this is due to quantitative or qualitative differences.

Calcium release from mitochondria. Mitochondria are known to accumulate considerable amounts of Ca^{2+} and in vitro conditions are known under which they also release the cation (cf. Carafoli et al. 1975). Most of these conditions, however, are such that their realization under in vivo conditions within the frame of a fast reaction appears rather unlikely (Scharf, 1980). At present it must rather be assumed that mitochondria play an important role in the removal of Ca^{2+} ions, but that they have only a minimal effect in triggering the fast events which characterize platelet activation.

Influx of Ca^{2+} ions from the outside. In the course of platelet activation, an influx of Ca^{2+} through the plasma membrane takes place. However, independent of the inducer used, this invariably coincides with the release reaction. This means that external Ca^{2+} plays at best a minor role in the events which trigger platelet activities (Massini and Lüscher 1976).
 The fact that the plasma membrane becomes Ca^{2+}-permeable in the course of activation, raises the question as to the persistence of this state. Thrombin-activated platelets which have undergone the release reaction can indeed return to the normal, resting state and can again be activated, although not by thrombin (Reimers et al. 1976). Clot retraction is a time consuming process and can be reversibly interrupted by the addition of EDTA to the external medium (Cohen and de Vries 1973). Thus, Ca^{2+} gates in the membrane appear to persist over much longer time than in other cells. It is as yet unknown, when and under what conditions resealing, which is a prerequisit for the reestablishment of the activable state, occurs.

Dense bodies (DB) are the storage site for biogenic amines and adenine nucleotides and at the same time the most important Ca^{2+}-reservoir of the platelet (Skaer et al. 1976). It is generally accepted that the contents of the DB are exclusively released to the outside and that there is no exchange of Ca^{2+} with the cytoplasm through the organelle membrane.

THE REMOVAL OF CALCIUM IONS FROM THE CYTOPLASM

It has been mentioned before that the DTS as well as the mitochondria are efficiently accumulating Ca^{2+} ions. The DTS is of particular interest, since cAMP is a powerful stimulator of the calcium pump (Käser-Glanzmann et al. 1977; cf. also Haslam in these Proceedings), thus explaining the activation-inhibiting effect of all agents which raise cAMP-levels by stimulating the adenylate cyclase. Therefore, all events leading to platelet stimulation via Ca^{2+}-release must be looked at on the background of the equilibrium between release of the cation and its removal.

At present it is not yet known whether platelets, in addition to subcellular Ca^{2+}-sequestrating structures, also have a plasma membrane-localized "extrusion pump", removing the cation to the outside. The solution of this problem depends on the development of more efficient methods for the separation of internal membrane systems from inside-out vesicles of plasma membrane origin.

THE ROLE OF EXTERNAL CALCIUM

The platelet activating activity of inducers such as ADP and the vasoactive amines depends on the presence of Ca^{2+} ions in the suspension medium. It is now established that the concentration of the cation is critical for the response of the platelet.
In a citrated platelet-rich plasma (about 10^{-4} M Ca^{2+}), ADP will induce shape change, aggregation and release. However, release is not the consequence of the direct effect of the nucleotide on the platelet but of aggregation, i.e. cell-cell contact, which in turn is dependent on external Ca^{2+}. It is noteworthy that this release reaction is blocked by inhibitors of PG synthesis (Mustard et al. 1975), which must be interpreted to mean that cell-cell contact has no effect equivalent to the one exerted by thrombin, collagen or immune complexes. Obviously, under these conditions the PAF is unable to compensate for deficient TX-synthesis.
The effect of ADP on platelets in a physiological suspension medium (1 mM Ca^{2+}) is strikingly different: aggregation proceeds normally; however, a drastically reduced release reaction is observed (Mustard et al. 1975); the same is true when adrenaline instead of ADP acts as the inducer (Massini 1976). Furthermore, there is evidence that also PG-synthesis is impaired (Massini 1980). All this implies that under these all-important conditions, those materials which are released from storage organelles are inactive as release inducers, obviously because intracellular processes requiring higher Ca^{2+} concentrations are not enacted. The conclusion is reached

that under these circumstances the plasma membrane is unable to assume the essential, signal-producing conformation.

It is of interest to note that such platelets are by no means unresponsive. Thus, the fibrinogen receptor, which is liberated in response to ADP exhibits optimal binding capacity in 1 mM Ca^{2+} (Marguerie et al. 1980). It seems reasonable to set fibrinogen binding by platelets in parallel to their "stickiness"; hence, "stickiness" is not directly related to the activating capacity of a membrane alteration.

In this context it is also noteworthy that shape change can be induced by ADP even in the presence of EDTA (Born 1970). This again demonstrates that ADP, independent of external Ca^{2+} exerts an action on the platelet membrane; however, again the crucial response, leading to PG-synthesis and release is missing.

CONCLUSION

It is obvious that intracellular Ca^{2+} ions play a decisive role in platelet activation. Their appearance in the cytoplasm is responsible for the onset of all manifestations which, besides adhesion, must be considered essential for platelet function in hemostasis and thrombosis. It is equally evident, though, that very important steps in the mobilization and function of Ca^{2+} are still poorly understood. The major problem consists certainly in the elucidation of the response of the plasma membrane to external stimuli, in particular in the differentiation between the minor and major signal-producing alterations. On the other hand, the nature and mode of action of the second messenger(s) which most likely include TX and PAF warrants also every attention. It is to be expected that the platelet will again serve as an easily accessible model for a series of reactions of very general importance for cell stimulation.

REFERENCES

Bills, T.K., Smith, J.B. and Silver, M.J., 1978. Intracellular regulation of the metabolism of arachidonic acid in human platelets. Thrombos. Haemostas. 40, 219-223.

Born, G.V.R.,1970. Observations on the change in shape of blood platelets brought about by adenosine diphosphate. J. Physiol., Lond. 209, 487-511.

Bygrave, F.L., 1978. Calcium movements in cells. Trends Biochem. Sci. 3, 175-178.

Carafoli, E., Clementi, F., Drabikowski, W. and Margreth, A. eds., 1975. Calcium transport in contraction and secretion. (North Holland, Amsterdam, Oxford).

Carafoli, E., Malmström, K., Capano, M., Sigel, E., and Crompton, M., 1975. Mitochondria and the regulation of cell calcium. in: <u>Calcium Transport in Contraction and Secretion</u>. E. Carafóli et al. eds. (North Holland, Amsterdam, Oxford) p. 53-64.

Chignard, M., le Couedic, J.P., Tence, M., Vargaftig, B.B. and Benveniste, J., 1979. The role of platelet-activating factor in platelet aggregation. <u>Nature, Lond</u>. 279, 799-800.

Cohen, I., and de Vries, A., 1973. Platelet contractile regulation in an isometric system. <u>Nature, Lond</u>. 246, 36-37.

Cohen, I., and Lüscher, E.F., 1975. The blood platelet contractile system. <u>Haemostasis</u> 4, 125-243.

Demopoulos, C.A., Pinkard, R.N., and Hanahan, D.J., 1979. Platelet activating factor. Evidence for 1-O-alkyl-2-acetyl-sn-glyceryl-3-phosphorylcholine as the active component (A new class of lipid chemical mediators). <u>J. Biol. Chem</u>. 254, 9355-9358.

Detwiler, T.C., Charo, I.F., and Feinman, R.D., 1978. Evidence that calcium regulates platelet function. <u>Thrombos. Haemostas</u>. 40, 207-211.

Dubler, D., Deranleau, D.A., Rothen, C., and Lüscher, E.F., 1980. Computer simulation of the shape change induced in human blood platelets by adenosine diphosphate. Submitted for publication.

Feinman, R.D. and Detwiler, F.C., 1974. Platelet secretion induced by divalent cation ionophore. <u>Nature, Lond</u>. 249, 172-173.

Gerrard, J.M., White, J.G., and Rao, G.H.R., 1974. Effects of the ionophore A23187 on blood platelets. 2. Influence on ultrastructure. <u>Amer. J. Pathol</u>. 77, 151-166.

Gerrard, J.M., White, J.G., and Peterson, D.A., 1978a. The platelet dense tubular system: its relationship to prostaglandin synthesis and calcium flux. <u>Thrombos. Haemostas</u>. 40, 224-231.

Gerrard, J.M., Butler, A.M., Graff, G., Stoddard, S.F., and White, J.G., 1978b. Prostaglandin endoperoxides promote calcium release from a platelet membrane preparation. <u>Prostaglandins Med</u>. 1, 373-385.

Haslam, R.J., 1980. in: <u>Platelets: Cellular Response Mechanisms and Their Biological Significane</u>. A. Rotman, ed., In press.

Käser-Glanzmann, R.,George,J.N., Jakábová, M., and Lüscher, E.F., 1977. Stimulation of calcium uptake into platelet membrane vesicles by adenosine 3',5'-cyclic monophosphate and protein kinase. <u>Biochim. Biophys. Acta</u> 466, 429-440.

Käser-Glanzmann, R., Jakábová, M., George, J.N., and Lüscher, E.F., 1978. Further characterization of calcium accumulating vesicles from human blood platelets. <u>Biochim. Biophys. Acta</u> 512, 1-12.

Kaulen, H.D., 1978. Dissociation of calcium-ionophore release and phospholipid reaction in human platelets. Thrombos. Res. 13, 577-582.

Kirkpatrick, J.P., McIntire,L.V.,Moake, J.L., and Cimo, P.L., 1979. Differential effects of cytochalasin B on platelet release, aggregation and contractibility: Evidence against a contractile mechanism for the release of platelet granular contents. Thrombos. Haemostas. 42, 1483-1489.

Le Breton, G.C., Dinerstein, R.J., Roth, L.J., and Feinberg, H., 1976. Direct evidence for intracellular divalent cation redistribution associated with platelet shape change. Biochem. biophys. Res. Comm. 71, 362-370.

Lüscher, E.F., 1976. Microfilaments in blood platelets. In: Molecular Basis of Motility; 26th Colloquium Mosbach 1975; L. Heilmeyer, J.C. Rüegg, Th. Wieland, ed. p. 175-185 (Springer, Berlin, Heidelberg, New York).

Marguerie, G.A., Edgington, T.S., and Plow, E.F., 1980. Interaction of fibrinogen with its platelet receptor as part of a multistep reaction in ADP-induced platelet aggregation. J. biol. Chem. 255, 154-161.

Malaisse, W.J., Herchuelz, A., Levy, J., Somers, G., Devis, G., Ravazzola, M., Malaisse-Lagae, F., and Orci, L., 1975. Insulin release and the movement of calcium in pancreatic islets. in: Calcium Transport Contraction and Secretion. E. Carafoli et al., eds. (North Holland, Amsterdam, Oxford) p. 211-226.

Massini, P., and Lüscher, E.F., 1974. Some effects of ionophores for divalent cations on blood platelets - comparison with the effects of thrombin. Biochim. Biophys. Acta 372, 109-121.

Massini, P., and Lüscher, E.F., 1976. On the significance of the influx of calcium ions into stimulated human blood platelets. Biochim. Biophys. Acta 436, 652-663.

Massini, P., 1976. The role of calcium in the stimulation of platelets. In: Platelets and Thrombosis. D.C.B. Mills, ed. (Academic Press, New York) p. 33-43.

Massini, P., Käser-Glanzmann, R., and Lüscher, E.F., 1978. Movement of calcium ions and their role in the activation of platelets. Thrombos. Haemostas. 40, 212-218.

Massini, P., and Näf, U., 1980. Ca^{2+}-ionophores and the activation of human blood platelets: The effects of ionomycin, beauvericin, lysocellin, virginiamycins, lasalocid-derivatives and McN4308. Biochim. Biophys. Acta (in press).

Massini, P., 1980. Personal communication.

Minkes, M., Stanford, N., Y.Chi, M.M., Roth, A.R., Needleman, P., and Majerus, P.W., 1977. Cyclic adenosine 3',5'-monophosphate inhibits the availability of arachidonate to prostaglandin synthetase in human platelet suspensions. J. clin. Invest. 59, 449-454.

Mitchell, R.H., 1975. Inositol phospholipids and cell surface receptor function. Biochim. Biophys. Acta 415, 81-147.

Mustard, J.F., Perry, D.W., Kinlough-Rathbone, R.L., and Packham, M.A., 1975. Factors responsible for ADP-induced release of platelet constituents. Am. J. Physiol. 228, 1757-1765.

Pfueller, S.L., and Lüscher, E.F., 1972. The effects of immune complexes on blood platelets and their relationship to complement activation. Immunochemistry 9, 1151-1165.

Pickett, W.C., Jesse, R.L., and Cohen, P., 1977. Initiation of phospholipase A_2-activity in human platelets by the calcium ionophore A23187. Biochim. Biophys. Acta 486, 209-213.

Reimers, H.J., Kinlough-Rathbone, R.L., Cazenave, J.P., Senyi, A.F., Hirsh, J., Packham, M.A., and Mustard, J.F., 1976. In vitro and in vivo functions of thrombin-treated platelets. Thrombos. Haemostas. 35, 151-166.

Rittenhouse-Simmons, S., and Deykin, D., 1978. The activation by Ca^{2+} of platelet phospholipase A_2: Effects of dibutyryl cyclic adenosine monophosphate and 8-(N,N-diethylamino)-octyl-3,4,5-ni-methoxybenzoate. Biochim. Biophys. Acta 543, 409-422.

Rothen, C., Deranleau, D.A., Dubler, D., and Lüscher, E.F., 1980. Evidence for a spherical intermediate in the platelet shape change reaction. Submitted for publication.

Scharf, R., 1980. personal communication.

Skaer, R.J., Peters, P.D., and Emmines, J.P., 1976. Platelet dense bodies: A quantitative microprobe analysis. J. Cell Sci. 20, 441-457.

Stockem, W.J., 1977. Basic mechanisms of movement: Pseudopodia, filopodia, axopodia, etc. Proc. 5th. Int. Congr. Protozool., p. 131-139.

Vargaftig, B.B., 1977. Carrageenan and thrombin trigger prostaglandin synthetase-independent aggregation of rabbit platelets: inhibition by phospholipase A_2 inhibitors. J. Pharm. Pharmac. 29, 222-228.

Weisenberg, R., 1972. Microtubule formation in vitro in solutions containing low calcium concentrations. Science 177, 1104-1105.

Werner, G., and Morgenstern, E., 1980. Three-dimensional reconstruction of human platelets using serial sections. Europ. J. Cell Biol. 20, 276-282.

White, J.G., 1972. Interaction of membrane systems in blood platelets. Amer. J. Path. 66, 295-372.

White, J.G., 1974. Shape change. In: Platelets, Thrombosis and Inhibitors. P. Didisheim, I. Shimamoto, H. Yamazaki, eds. p. 159-171 (Schattauer, Stuttgart, New York).

Platelet Membrane Structure and Receptors

Activation of the platelets takes place through their surfaces. The general structure of the platelet membrane, its composition and accessibility, and particularly its lipid and glycoprotein components, are considered to be important both individually and in their interaction with each other. There are obviously a number of receptors on the platelet membrane, some highly specific and others perhaps for less so. In these chapters the nature of the thrombin receptor, and the ADP and collagen receptors, are considered in particular, as is the interaction with fibrinogen and serotonin.

The platelet plasma membrane is morphologically indistinguishable from that of other cells, but it performs many cellular reactions which are unique to the platelet. Is surface material (mainly, glycoproteins) lost from platelets during activation and are new proteins thus exposed on the surface? Does actin, the main contractile protein of platelet, transverse the membrane during activation? Is there receptor aggregation and reorientation during thrombin activation? What is the nature of thrombin-platelet interaction? Is it an enzyme-substrate type of reaction or is it analogous to a hormone-receptor reaction? Which membrane proteins cause platelet aggregation? How can one monitor possible changes in membrane proteins during platelet activation? The proper assessment of how platelets function and how their response can be controlled depends on the answers to these and related questions.

MEMBRANE ALTERATIONS CAUSED BY PLATELET
AGGREGATION AND SECRETION

James N. George, Roger M. Lyons, and
Rebecca K. Morgan

Division of Hematology, Department of Medicine
University of Texas Health Science Center at
San Antonio, and the Veterans Administration
Hospital, San Antonio, Texas 78284

ABSTRACT

The effect of aggregation and secretion on membrane proteins was studied in washed human platelets by quantitative polyacrylamide gel electrophoresis (SDS-PAGE) analysis of platelets labeled with (^{125}I)-diazotized diiodosulfanilic acid (DD^{125}ISA). Reversible aggregation without secretion was stimulated by adenosine diphosphate (ADP) and secretion without aggregation was stimulated by thrombin in the presence of EDTA. No loss of platelet surface glycoproteins occurred during reversible ADP-induced platelet aggregation and no new proteins became exposed on the platelet surface following ADP aggregation. Thrombin-induced platelet secretion also caused no loss of platelet surface glycoproteins. However following platelet secretion, two new proteins were labeled by DD^{125}ISA: (1) actin and (2) the 149,000 mol wt glycoprotein (termed GP-G) which is contained in platelet granules and secreted in response to thrombin. The identity of DD^{125}ISA-labeled actin was confirmed by four criteria: (1) co-migration with actin in three different SDS-PAGE systems, (2) elution from a particulate fraction in low ionic strength buffer, (3) co-migration with actin in isoelectric focusing, and (4) binding to DNase I. The identity of actin and its appearance on the platelet surface after thrombin-induced secretion was also demonstrated by the greater binding of an anti-actin antibody to thrombin-treated platelets, detected with ^{125}I-Staphylococcal protein A.

INTRODUCTION

During involvement in hemostasis and thrombosis, blood platelets transform from discs to spheres with long pseudopods, aggregate with adjacent platelets, secrete their granule contents into the surrounding environment, accelerate plasma coagulation, and finally bind the developing fibrin strands and provide the power for clot retraction. To understand the platelet membrane changes associated with these events, we studied membrane surface proteins during two separable platelet activities: aggregation and secretion. Our study asked two questions: (1) is surface glycoprotein material lost from platelets during these reactions? (2) are new proteins exposed on the platelet surface following these reactions?

METHODS

The detailed methods for these experiments have been previously described (George, 1978a; George, Lyons, and Morgan, 1980).

RESULTS

In the first part of this study, four basic experiments were performed: (1) stimulation of $DD^{125}ISA$-labeled platelets with ADP, (2) labeling of platelets with $DD^{125}ISA$ after ADP stimulation, (3) stimulation of $DD^{125}ISA$-labeled platelets with thrombin, and (4) labeling of platelets with $DD^{125}ISA$ after thrombin stimulation. In each experiment platelets were analyzed by quantitative SDS-PAGE (George, 1978a). Figure 1 shows the analysis of $DD^{125}ISA$-labeled normal whole platelets by SDS-PAGE. GP-G is the major glycoprotein of platelet granules and is secreted during the platelet release reaction.

Effect of ADP-induced platelet aggregation on platelet membrane proteins. No significant loss of surface glycoproteins occurred during the reversible aggregation unaccompanied by platelet secretion caused by ADP stimulation of $DD^{125}ISA$-labeled platelets, as quantified by PAS (periodic acid-Schiff) staining and $DD^{125}ISA$ labeling (Table 1). Also no change in the pattern of radioisotope labeling was observed when $DD^{125}ISA$ was reacted with platelets which had previously undergone aggregation and disaggregation (Table 2). Specifically no new $DD^{125}ISA$-labeled peaks were present in the gel slices containing GP-G and actin.

Effect of thrombin-induced platelet secretion on platelet membrane proteins. Platelet secretion of GP-G occurred in each thrombin experiment and there was no difference in secretion between platelets labeled with $DD^{125}ISA$ before or after thrombin stimulation. we have previously shown that GP-G secretion correlates with secretion of ^{14}C-serotonin (George, 1978a). No loss of surface membrane glycoproteins occurred during the platelet secretion caused by thrombin stimulation of $DD^{125}ISA$-labeled platelets, as quantified by PAS staining and $DD^{125}ISA$ labeling (Table 3). When platelets were labeled with $DD^{125}ISA$ following thrombin stimulation there was no change in the labeling of the membrane glycoproteins but GP-G and actin bound significantly more $DD^{125}ISA$ (Table 4, Fig. 2). The new 149,000 mol wt $DD^{125}ISA$-labeled peak observed after thrombin-induced secretion was identified as GP-G on the basis of its exact and consistent co-migration with the GP-G PAS band. We considered the possibility that the change of $DD^{125}ISA$ labeling after thrombin stimulation might be due to lysis of a small fraction of platelets rather than exposure of new proteins on the membrane surface. This possibility was ruled out in two separate ways. First, the amount of platelet lysis was directly assessed by ^{51}Cr release during each of the steps of thrombin treatment and subsequent $DD^{125}ISA$ labeling.

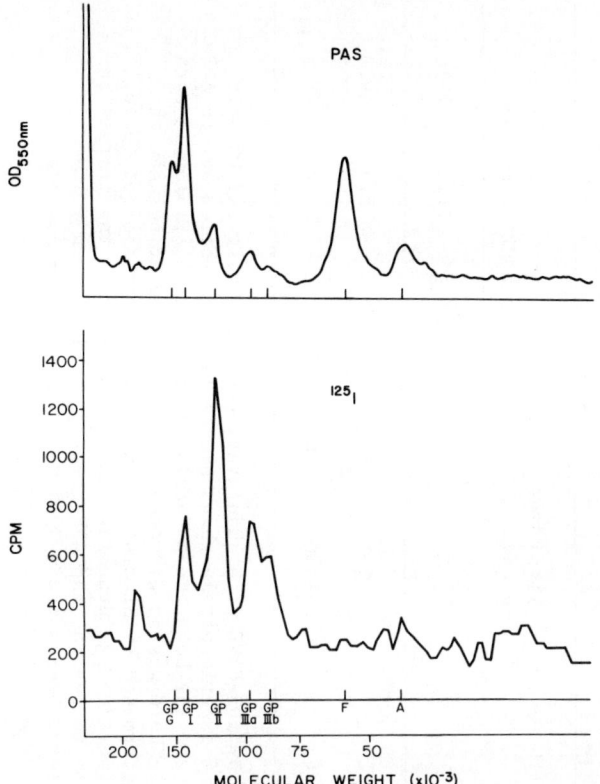

Fig. 1. SDS-PAGE analysis of normal whole platelets labeled with $DD^{125}ISA$. 200 μgm of DTT-reduced protein plus 5 μgm of fetuin were applied to the gel. The densitometry scan of the PAS reaction is shown in the top panel. The band labeled A (for actin) does not stain pink for carbohydrate by the PAS reaction but is seen on the gel as an opague white band and is detected by densitometry. The platelet glycoproteins are described by the nomenclature we have previously presented (George, 1978a): GP-G (mol wt 149,000), GP-I (mol wt 140,000), GP-II (mol wt 120,000), GP-IIIa (mol wt 98,000), and GP-IIIb (mol wt 88,000). The added fetuin is labeled as F. The gel is cut into 1 mm slices, after scanning the PAS reaction, for determination of $DD^{125}ISA$ radioactivity (bottom panel). A gel marking technique allows precise correlation of stained bands with radioactive peaks. Note the absence of $DD^{125}ISA$ labeling of GP-G and actin.

Table 1. Effect of ADP-Induced Aggregation on Platelet Membrane Glycoproteins

	PAS units			Total GP cpm	DDI^{125}ISA cpm				
						Percent distribution			
	I	II	IIIa	IIIb		I	II	IIIa	IIIb
ADP	1.06	.46	.39	.22	1561	16.6	40.1	23.3	19.9
Control	1.10	.47	.40	.26	1436	16.5	40.2	23.0	19.9

Data for the analysis of glycoproteins by SDS-PAGE with quantitative PAS staining and DDI^{125}ISA labeling represent the mean values for 6 experiments in which platelets were labeled before ADP treatment. Two to four gels were analyzed for both the ADP-treated and control samples in each experiment. No GP-G release occurred. There was no difference in any parameter between the ADP-treated and control platelets as determined by Student's t test for paired samples ($p > 0.1$). These data represent PAS units and cpm per 200 μgm protein. In two experiments the protein per platelet was determined and was the same in control and ADP-treated samples (mean values: control = 2.33×10^{-9} mg protein/platelet, ADP-treated = 2.29×10^{-9} mg protein/platelet).

Table 2. Effect of ADP-Induced Aggregation on Exposure of Platelet Membrane Proteins to DD^{125}ISA

	Membrane GP						
	Total Membrane GP (cpm)	Percent distribution				Actin (% membrane GP cpm)	GP-G (% membrane GP cpm)
		I	II	IIIa	IIIb		
ADP	2894	16.9	33.8	25.6	23.7	5.7 ± 0.4 (SE)	3.3 ± 1.3 (SE)
Control	2560	17.5	33.2	27.6	21.9	5.9 ± 0.6	3.1 ± 1.2

The data are the mean values for 4 experiments in which platelets were labeled with DD^{125}ISA after ADP aggregation and disaggregation. Three or four gels were analyzed for both the ADP-treated and control samples in each experiment. No GP-G release occurred. There was no difference in any parameter between the ADP-treated and control platelets (p> 0.5).

Table 3. Effect of Thrombin-Induced Secretion on Platelet Membrane Glycoproteins

	PAS units			Total GP cpm	$DD^{125}ISA$ Percent distribution		
	I	II	IIIa	IIIb		I	II	IIIa	IIIb
Thrombin	1.07	.39	.35	.25	2980	17.6	32.9	25.9	22.9
Control	1.08	.36	.35	.25	2709	17.6	33.0	25.0	23.5

Data for analysis of glycoproteins by SDS-PAGE with quantitative PAS staining and $DD^{125}ISA$ labeling represent the mean values for 9 experiments in which platelets were labeled before thrombin treatment. Two to four gels were analyzed for both the thrombin-treated and control samples in each experiment. Release of GP-G occurred in each experiment (13-73%, mean 45%). There was no difference in any parameter between the thrombin-treated and control platelets, as determined by Student's t test for paired samples ($p > 0.1$). These data represent PAS units and cpm per 200 μgm protein. In eight experiments the protein per platelet was not different in control and thrombin-treated samples (mean values: control = 2.67 ± 0.86 (SD) x 10^{-9} mg protein/platelet; thrombin-treated = 2.29 ± 0.86 (SD) x 10^{-9} mg protein/platelet; $p > 0.2$).

Table 4. Effect of Thrombin-Induced Secretion on Exposure of Platelet Membrane Proteins to DD^{125}ISA

	Membrane GP					Actin (% membrane GP cpm)	GP-G (% membrane GP cpm)
	Total Membrane GP	Percent distribution					
		I	II	IIIa	IIIb		
Thrombin	3427	19.2	34.3	25.7	20.9	12.6 $\pm$ 1.5 (SE)	10.0 $\pm$ 0.4 (SE)
Control	4120	17.6	34.1	25.7	22.7	6.3 $\pm$ 0.7	3.8 $\pm$ 0.3

The data are the mean values for seven experiments in which platelets were labeled with DD^{125}ISA after thrombin-induced secretion without aggregation (thrombin, 2 U/ml in the presence of 4 mM EDTA). Three to four gels were analyzed for both the thrombin-treated and control samples in each experiment. Release of GP-G occurred in each experiment (41-84%, mean = 66%). After thrombin treatment, DD^{125}ISA cpm were significantly greater on actin and GP-G as determined by Student's t test for paired samples (p <0.001). The total membrane GP cpm and the percent distribution of the cpm among the individual GP were the same in the thrombin-treated and control platelets (p >0.3).

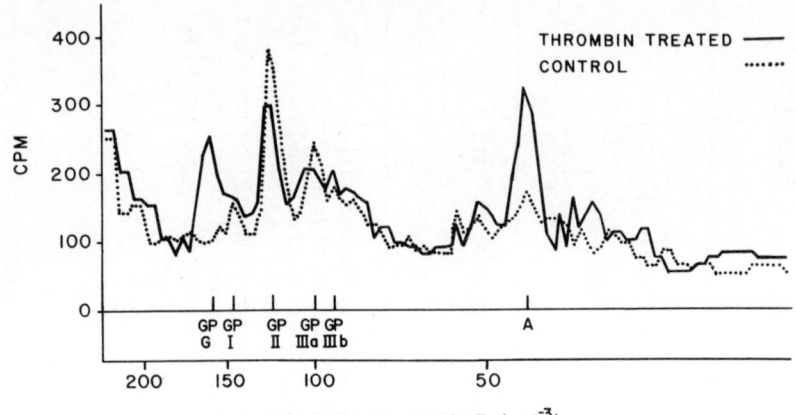

Fig. 2. Effect of thrombin on the surface exposure of platelet membrane proteins to $DD^{125}ISA$. Platelets were treated with thrombin in the presence of EDTA to stimulate secretion without aggregation, washed, labeled with $DD^{125}ISA$, and then analyzed by SDS-PAGE. Thrombin was omitted from the control sample. Gels were stained by PAS, the GP and actin bands were marked by ink, and then the gels were sliced for determination of radioactivity. The gels slices containing ink marks are shown by the marks on the abscissa. (Reprinted from George, Lyons, and Morgan, 1980, <u>Journal of Clinical Investigation</u>, with permission.)

^{51}Cr release was not different in thrombin-treated and control platelets (Table 5). Second, the $DD^{125}ISA$ labeling pattern of sonicated platelets was compared to that of thrombin-treated platelets. After lysis by sonication an actin-region protein was the most prominent peak, however none of the other major $DD^{125}ISA$ peaks of lysed platelets coincided with proteins which were labeled after thrombin. We calculated that many of the $DD^{125}ISA$ peaks seen in the platelet sonicate would have been readily apparent if the labeling of actin after thrombin stimulation was the result of cell lysis.

<u>Identification of actin on the platelet surface following thrombin-induced secretion</u>. The identity of the 40,000 mol wt $DD^{125}ISA$-labeled protein appearing on the platelet surface following thrombin-induced secretion as actin was confirmed by four experiments: (1) the $DD^{125}ISA$ peak co-migrated with actin in three different SDS-PAGE systems, (2) the $DD^{125}ISA$ peak was associated with a particulate fraction and was eluted in a low ionic strength buffer previously demonstrated to preferentially solubilize actin from membranes, (3) the isoelectric point of this $DD^{125}ISA$ peak was identical to actin, and (4) the $DD^{125}ISA$-labeled protein bound to DNase I and was eluted by 3 M guanidine (George, Lyons, and Morgan, 1980). Further

TABLE 5. Platelet Lysis During Thrombin-Induced Secretion and Subsequent $DD^{125}ISA$ Labeling.

Step in Experiment	Percent Platelet Lysis	
	Thrombin	Control
After thrombin treatment	2.0 ± 0.3	1.8 ± 0.4
After $DD^{125}ISA$ labeling	7.0 ± 1.9	5.1 ± 0.9
After final post-label wash	4.0 ± 1.0	3.9 ± 0.7

Data are the mean values ± SD for four experiments which were performed exactly as the experiments presented in Table 4. Fifty ml of blood were drawn, platelets were isolated and labeled with ^{51}Cr. Then the platelets were washed twice, treated with thrombin, then washed again. Platelet lysis was calculated by the percent release of ^{51}Cr in the supernatant wash fluid (Step 1). Then platelets were labeled with $DD^{125}ISA$, diluted, centrifuged, and ^{51}Cr release again determined (Step 2). Platelets were washed once more prior to SDS-PAGE analysis (Step 3). There was no difference between the thrombin-treated and control platelets at any step (p >0.1).

identification of actin on the surface of activated platelets was established by the binding of an anti-actin antibody (kindly provided by Dr. Giulio Gabbiani, Geneva, Switzerland) to thrombin-treated or control platelets and then quantitating the bound antibody with ^{125}I-Staphylococcal protein A (Zeltzer and Seeger, 1977). Table 6 demonstrates that significantly more anti-actin antibody was bound to thrombin-treated platelets than to control platelets. In contrast, the binding of non-immune IgG and a rabbit anti-platelet antibody was the same in both thrombin-treated and control platelets.

DISCUSSION

Because a variety of platelet functions change during activation, we studied the membrane protein changes in conditions which allow independent assessment of two major platelet reactions: aggregation and secretion.

Effect of aggregation on platelet membrane proteins. We demonstrated no loss of platelet surface glycoproteins during reversible ADP-induced platelet aggregation without secretion. Also we demonstrated no change in the $DD^{125}ISA$ labeling of membrane GP and no exposure of new proteins on the membrane surface following reversible aggregation. These data demonstrate the excellent reproducibility of the method of quantitative SDS-PAGE analysis of platelet membrane glycoproteins. These results with human platelets in vitro are analogous to our in vivo studies of circulating rabbit platelets double-labeled with $DD^{125}ISA$ for surface glycoproteins (George, Lewis, and Sears, 1976) and ^{51}Cr for internal cytoplasm. When these rabbits were given

TABLE 6. Effect of thrombin-induced secretion on the platelet binding of anti-actin (AAA) and anti-platelet (APA) antibodies

	AAA	APA
	(cpm of platelet-bound ^{125}I-SPA)	
Thrombin-treated platelets	8260	8370
Control platelets	3690	8127
	<0.025	>0.25

The data are the mean values for 6 experiments. Statistical comparisons were made by Student's t test for paired samples. Platelet-bound antibody was quantified by the subsequent binding of ^{125}I-SPA. As a control, the ^{125}I-SPA cpm bound to platelets reacted with nonimmune IgG were substracted from each sample. Nonimmune IgG bound equally to thrombin-treated and control platelets ($p > 0.7$). (Adapted from George, Lyons, and Morgan, 1980, Journal of Clinical Investigation, with permission.)

intravenous ADP, two-thirds of their platelets were removed from the circulation in less than one minute but all returned to the circulation by three minutes. There was no loss of platelet surface glycoproteins during this reversible ADP-induced sequestration (Fig. 3) (George, 1978b). Therefore platelets may be able to resume their normal function in the circulation after transient aggregation.

Effect of secretion on platelet membrane proteins. Our studies demonstrated no loss of platelet surface glycoproteins during thrombin-induced secretion (without aggregation). Although there was no change in DD^{125}ISA labeling of the membrane GP after thrombin-induced secretion, two new proteins were labeled: actin and the major granule glycoprotein (GP-G). The appearance of new proteins on the platelet surface following secretion is consistent with previous observations of the appearance of factor V activity (Miletich, Majerus, and Majerus, 1978; Osterud, Rapaport, and Lavine, 1977), lentil phytohemagglutinin binding sites (Faegler, Tillack, Chaplin, and Majerus, 1974), and lectin activity (Gartner, Williams, Minion, and Phillips, 1978) on the platelet membrane surface following thrombin treatment.

GP-G was initially considered to be a membrane protein because it remained with the platelet particulate fraction after a sonication procedure which completely solubilized a lyzosomal enzyme, β-glucuronidase (Baenziger, Brodie, and Majerus, 1972). Subsequently GP-G has been demonstrated to be a secreted granule protein (Hagen, Olsen, and Solum, 1976; Lawler, Slayter, and Coligan, 1978). The appearance of GP-G on the platelet surface may be due to adsorption of secreted GP-G onto the membrane.

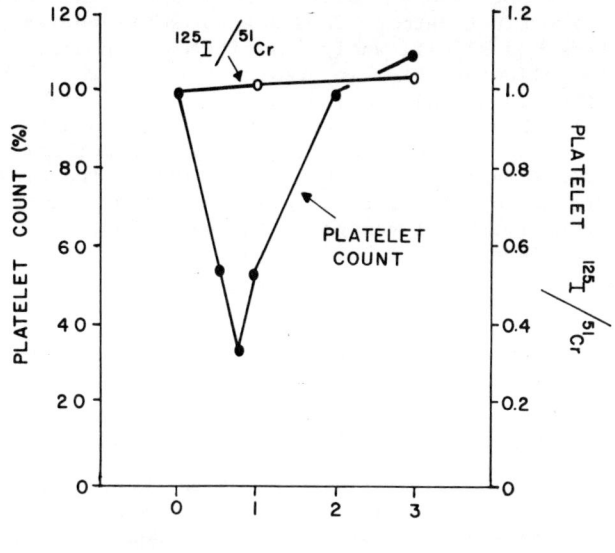

Fig. 3. Rabbit platelets were labeled simultaneously with ^{51}Cr and $DD^{125}ISA$ and infused into recipient rabbits. ADP (5 mg/kg) was given as a rapid infusion (<1 second) in 0.2 ml of saline. Platelet counts and samples for radioactivity were obtained before the infusion and assigned the values of 100%, for the platelet count, and 1.0, for the ratio of platelet $DD^{125}ISA$/platelet^{51}Cr. The data represent the average of experiments with two rabbits.

Actin is a membrane-associated protein in many cells with postulated functions in the regulation of cell shape and cell motility. The intimate association of actin filaments and platelet surface membranes has been demonstrated both morphologically (Zucker-Franklin, 1970) and biochemically (Taylor, Williams, and Crawford, 1976). Two previous studies with immunofluorescent techniques have suggested the appearance of actin on the surface of human platelets during activation (Bouvier et al, 1977; Diggle et al, 1979).

Alpha-actinin functions as the membrane attachment site for actin microfilaments in the tips of intestinal microvilli (Craig and Pardo, 1979). Evidence has been presented that platelet membrane GP IIIa may be α-actinin (Gerrard et al, 1979). Since this glycoprotein may span the plasma membrane (Phillips and Agin, 1974), it could function to anchor actin to the membrane and mediate the exposure of actin on the platelet surface. Therefore we studied the platelets from five patients from separate kindreds with Glanzmann's thrombasthenia which are deficient in GP IIIa and α-actinin (Gerrard et al, 1979). Our preliminary data (George and Morgan, 1980, plus observations on three more patients) demonstrated that these platelets released GP-G normally in response to thrombin and following thrombin treatment GP-G was normally labeled by $DD^{125}ISA$. However there was significantly less increase in actin labeling by $DD^{125}ISA$ following thrombin treatment in the thrombasthenic platelets than in normals. Also there was no increased binding of anti-actin antibodies to thrombasthenic platelets after thrombin treatment. These data are consistent with a hypothesis that membrane GP IIIa (α-actinin) may bind actin within the plasma membrane and that during thrombin-induced platelet activation GP IIIa may undergo a conformational change to expose actin to the external environment. Once exposed on the platelet surface, actin could provide a receptor site for polymerizing fibrin (Laki and Muszbek, 1974) in the process of clot retraction. The diminished or absent clot retraction in Glanzmann's thrombasthenia may be related to the diminished actin exposure on the surface of thrombasthenic platelets after thrombin treatment.

ACKNOWLEDGMENTS

The authors thank Mrs. Williadene Rampt for her expert assistance. This research was supported by a National Institutes of Health Grant HL 19996, a Grant-in-Aid from the American Heart Association with funds contributed in part by the Texas Affiliate, and the Research Service, Audie L. Murphy Veterans Administration Hospital, San Antonio, Texas

REFERENCES

Baenziger, N.L., Brodie, G.N., and Majerus, P.W., 1972. Isolation and properties of a thrombin-sensitive protein of human platelets. J. Biol. Chem., 247:2723-2731.

Bouvier, C.A., Gabbiani, G., Ryan, G.B., Badonnel, M-C., Majno, G., and Lüscher, E.F., 1977. Binding of anti-actin autoantibodies to platelets. Thromb. Haemost., 37:321-328.

Craig, S.W., and Pardo, J.V., 1979. Alpha-actinin localization in the junctional complex of intestinal epithelial cells. J. Cell Biol., 80:203-210.

Diggle, T.A., Toh, B.H., Firkin, B.G., and Pfueller, S.L., 1979. Human platelet actin: surface expression after platelet activation. Thromb. Haemost., 42:799-802.

Feagler, J.R., Tillack, T.W., Chaplin, D.D., and Majerus, P.W., 1974. The effects of thrombin on phytohemagglutinin receptor sites in human platelets. J. Cell Biol., 60:541-553.

Gartner, T.K., Williams, D.C., Minion, F.C., and Phillips, D.R., 1978. Thrombin-induced platelet aggregation is mediated by a platelet plasma membrane-bound lectin. Science, 200:1281-1283.

George, J.N., Lewis, P.C., and Sears, D.A., 1976. Studies on platelet plasma membranes. II. Characterization of surface proteins of rabbit platelets in vitro and during circulation in vivo using diazotized (^{125}I)-diiodosulfanilic acid as a label. J. Lab. Clin. Med., 88:247-260.

George, J.N., 1978a. Studies on platelet plasma membranes. IV. Quantitative analysis of platelet membrane glycoproteins by (^{125}I)-diazotized diiodosulfanilic acid labeling and SDS-polyacrylamide gel electrophoresis. J. Lab. Clin. Med., 92:430-446.

George, J.N., 1978b. Platelet behavior and aging in the circulation, in The Blood Platelet in Transfusion Therapy (Eds. Greenwalt and Jamieson), pp 39-64, Alan R. Liss, Inc., New York.

George, J.N., and Morgan, R.K., 1979. Actin exposure on the surface of normal platelets and thrombasthenic platelets following thrombin-induced secretion: mediated by platelet membrane α-actinin. Thromb. Haemost., 42:68 (Abst.).

George, J.N., Lyons, R.M., and Morgan, R.K., 1980. Membrane changes associated with platelet activation: exposure of actin on the platelet surface following thrombin-induced secretion. J. Clin. Invest., in press.

Gerrard, J.M., Schollmeyer, J.F., Phillips, D.R., and White, J.G., 1979. α-actinin deficiency in thrombasthenia: possible identity of α-actinin as glycoprotein III. Am. J. Path., 94:509-528.

Hagen, L., Olsen, T., and Solum, N.O., 1976. Studies on subcellular fractions of human platelets by the lactoperoxidase-iodination technique. Biochim. Biophys. Acta, 455:214-225.

Laki, K., and Muszbek, L., 1974. On the interaction of F actin and fibrin. Biochim. Biophys. Acta, 371:519-525.

Lawler, J.W., Slayter, H.S., and Coligan, J.E., 1978. Isolation and characterization of a high molecular weight glycoprotein from human blood platelets. J. Biol. Chem., 253:8609-8616.

Miletich, J.P., Majerus, D.W., and Majerus, P.W., 1978. Patients with congenital factor V deficiency have decreased factor Xa binding sites on their platelets. J. Clin. Invest., 56:924-936.

Osterud, B., Rapaport, S.I., and Lavine, K.K., 1977. Factor V activity of platelets, evidence for an activated factor V molecule and for a platelet activator. Blood, 49:819-834.

Phillips, D.R., and Agin, P.P., 1974. Thrombin substrates and the proteolytic site of thrombin action on human platelet plasma membranes. Biochim. Biophys. Acta, 352:218-227.

Taylor, D.G., Williams, V.M., and Crawford, N., 1976. Platelet membrane actin: solubility and binding studies with ^{125}I-labeled actin. Biochem. Soc. Trans., 4:156-160.

Zeltzer, P.M., and Seeger, R.C., 1977. Microassay using radioiodinated protein A from Staphylococcus aureus for antibodies bound to cell surface antigens of adherent tumor cells. J. Immunol. Methods, 17:163-175.

Zucker-Franklin, D., 1970. The submembranous fibrils of human platelets. J. Cell Biol., 47:293-299.

LIPID-PROTEIN INTERACTION IN ACTIVATED PLATELET MEMBRANE

Gila Fleischer,[a] Ilana Nathan,[a] Avinoam Livne,[b]
Alexander Dvilansky[a] and Abraham H. Parola[c]

[a]Department of Haematology, Soroka Medical Centre,
[b]Department of Biology, and [c]Department of Chemistry,
Ben Gurion University of the Negev, Beer-Sheva, Israel.

ABSTRACT

Attempts were made to correlate early events of platelet activation with the dynamic behaviour of the membrane lipids and proteins. Measurements of shape change, serotonin secretion as well as aggregation were conducted simultaneously along with fluorescence polarization studies of membrane components. Two fluorescent probes, N-carboxymethylisatoic anhydride, which binds to membrane glycoproteins, and 1,6-diphenyl-1,3,5-hexatriene, a lipophilic label, have been used to follow membrane microenvironmental changes. Activation of human platelets by thrombin resulted in a simultaneous increase in values of fluorescence polarization (P) of both probes during the stages of shape change and secretion, which further increased during platelet aggregation. The similar pattern of changes in P for both probes indicate the interdependence of lipids and proteins in the activated platelet membrane. The elevated "microviscosity" may be mediated primarily by clustering of membrane proteins, possibly controlled by the cytoskeleton and reflected by the mobility of aqueously exposed glycoproteins. Alternatively, the membrane lipids may play the primary role in passively modulating the observed dynamic behaviour of the membrane glycoproteins.

INTRODUCTION

The dynamic nature of biological membranes has recently been shown to play a major role in a variety of physiological processes (Nicolson, 1976a; Shinitzky and Henkart, 1979). There is growing evidence (Wallach et al., 1975) in various cell systems on the non-randomized, controlled and interdependent motions of various membranal components which mediate cell division, growth (Nicholau et al., 1978) and transformation (Parola and Souroujon, 1979; Parola et al., 1979; Rosenthal et al., 1978; Fuchs et al., 1975), transport (Van Dijck et al., 1975), phagocytosis (Berlin and Fera, 1977), capping and agglutination (Nicolson, 1976a, b), adhesion and aggregation (Nicolson, 1973). Membrane lipids may, in part, regulate protein diffusion (Ediddin, 1974) and association (Grant and McConnell, 1974), cell antigenicity (Shinitzky and Souroujon, 1979; Lewis and McConnell, 1978; Rubenstein et al., 1979; Borochov and Shinitzky, 1976), the activity of membrane bound enzymes (Coleman, 1973; Linden et al., 1973) and membrane fusion (Papahadjopoulous et al., 1974). This chapter deals with the dynamic nature of the platelet membrane in association with the activation of the blood platelet (Nathan et al., 1979). Interestingly, the dynamic changes of membrane proteins and lipids during the course of activation appear to be interdependent (Nathan et al., 1980).

Two major concepts have recently been advanced in attempts to explain the dynamic interdependence of membranal proteins and lipids. One relates membrane protein motion to the cytoskeletal manifold, subjecting the cell surface to a strict and coordinated cytoplasmic control (Nicolson, 1976b). The other is the passive modulation of protein mobility (Shinitzky and Barenholtz, 1978; Shinitzky, 1979) whereby lipid-lipid (Shattil and Cooper, 1976) and lipid-protein (Wallach et al., 1975) interactions selectively control the vertical motion of membrane proteins, resulting in differential exposure and reactivity of these reactive membranal components.

Blood platelets present an attractive experimental system to study lipid-protein interaction due to the unique physiological role played by blood platelets, in which the plasma membrane is directly involved e.g. shape change, release and aggregation. In addition, the platelet may serve as an easily obtainable and controllable model system for a number of biological tissues, e.g. the smooth muscles (Booyse and Rafelson, 1971) and the nervous systems (Sneddon, 1973; de Gaetano, 1978). While the detailed molecular mechanism of platelet aggregation is not clear (Weiss, 1975), it is known that platelet activation is associated with major changes in membrane lipids and proteins. Most profound are the exposure of platelet factor 3 activity (Hardisty and Hutton, 1966), hydrolysis and mobilization of archidonic acid (Rittenhouse-Simons and Deykin, 1977; Deykin, 1976) leading to prostaglandin synthesis (Smith and Silver, 1976), an increased turnover of phospholipids (Deykin, 1976), and phosphorylation of lipids (Kaulen and Gross, 1976), an increased exposure of sialic acid (Wu and Ku, 1979), of glycoproteins (George et al., 1978; Nurden and Caen, 1978) and of receptors to lectins (Gartner et al., 1978). Dynamical alterations in the organization of the cytoskeletal system, concomitant with platelet activation, were reported as well (Marcus, 1969).

The assessment of dynamic changes in platelets may be crucial not only for the better understanding of platelet activation, but also in reference to platelet dysfunction (Cooper, 1977) in thrombotic disorders (Harker and Slichter, 1972), hyper betalipoproteinemia (Shattil and Cooper, 1978) and atherosclerosis (Ross and Glomset, 1976).

Membrane dynamic changes during platelet activation. The use of biologically inert fluorescent probes for cell membranes is instrumental in gaining valuable information on aspects of membrane structures such as the nature of the microenvironment of the labelled sites and freedom of rotation of the labelling reagents (Radda and Vanderkooi, 1972). In the present work we embarked upon the study of intact, fluorescently labelled platelets. Two fluorescent probes have been employed. The polar N-carboxy-methyl isatoic anhydride (NCMIA) which binds covalently to plasma membrane glycoproteins containing free-NH_2 group (Nathan et al., 1980) and 1,6-diphenyl-1,3,5-hexatriene (DPH), a lipophilic noncovalent label (Nathan et al., 1979). Following these two labels, enabled the study of the dynamic changes associated with platelet membrane lipids and proteins, during the course of platelet activation. The methods and experimental details are presented in the respective studies.

Platelets treated by these two labels retained most of their physiological integrity, as evident by the absence of excess leakage of lactate dehydrogenase (a cytoplasmic enzyme) and of ^{14}C-serotonin (a dense body marker). Labelled platelet activation and aggregation by thrombin proceeded normally. Shape change induced by thrombin and by ADP was unaltered with DPH-labelled platelets; NCMIA labelled platelets which responded normally to activation and aggregation by thrombin, failed to exhibit characteristic shape change pattern.

Platelet aggregation, induced by thrombin, was monitored by the decrease in the 600 nm scattering intensity, due to platelet clumping and is shown in Fig.1. Aggregation was accompanied by a 14% increase in DPH fluorescence intensity.

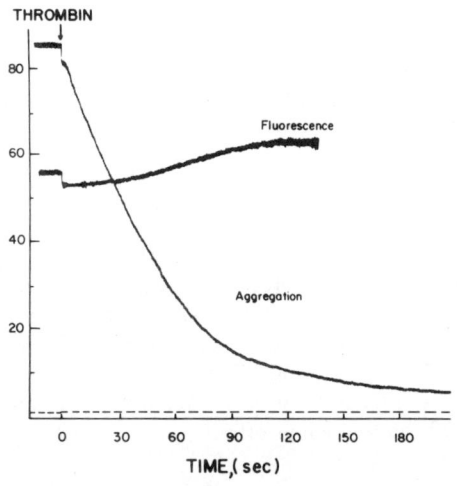

Fig. 1. Changes in fluorescence during thrombin-induced aggregation of DPH-labelled platelets. Fluorescence determined at 360 nm of excitation/429 nm of emission and aggregation followed at 600 nm of excitation/600 nm of emission. Identical course of aggregation was obtained with unlabelled platelets. The scatter contribution of unlabelled platelets at 360 nm of excitation/429 nm of emission is shown as a dashed line.

NCMIA-labelled platelets similarly showed a 9% increase in fluorescence intensity. This increase in fluorescence is directly linked to the process of platelet aggregation since no change in fluorescence was evident when thrombin was added to platelets without the continuous mixing required for aggregation. Moreover, the increase in emission intensity is apparently unrelated to early events of platelet activation or to alteration in individual platelets, since no clear change in intensity was detected when individual platelet secreted or changed shape. Thus, the increased fluorescence emission may be attributed to the formation of hydrophobic enclaves within the dense aggregate.

In order to evaluate the microenvironmental changes of these probes in the platelet membrane it is valuable to compare the changes in the probes fluorescence intensity with their sensitivity to model solvents of varying dielectric constants. DPH fluorescence intensity is sixty fold more sensitive to solvent effect (benzene vs water) than NCMIA is. It is thus concluded that the relative increase in fluorescence emission of DPH-labelled platelets is much smaller than that for NCMIA labelled platelet. This may indicate a smaller change in the already hydrophobic microenvironment of the lipophilic DPH in the individual platelet as compared with the aqueously exposed glycoproteins. We may envisage that upon aggregation the glycoproteins are caught in the newly formed hydrophobic enclaves within the dense aggregate.

The course of aggregation of platelets activated by thrombin and the changes in fluorescence polarization (P) associated with aggregation are shown in Fig. 2. Aggregation was clearly accompanied by an increase in P of both NCMIA and DPH labelled platelets, representing a decreased rotational freedom of the probes in their respective microenvironment.

When activated by thrombin in the presence of EDTA, labelled platelets rapidly changed shape and secreted their intragranular content but did not aggregate. Fig. 3 shows that under these conditions thrombin caused an increase in P in both NCMIA and DPH labelled platelets. Fig. 4 shows the effect of ADP upon DPH-labelled platelets. Under these conditions, only platelet shape change takes place, but neither secretion nor aggregation occur. The fast initial increase in fluorescence polarization exhibits a magnitude and kinetics similar to that observed in Fig. 3, yet the ADP effect is characterized with a secondary decline in P values, apparently related to the known reversibility of the ADP shape change effect.

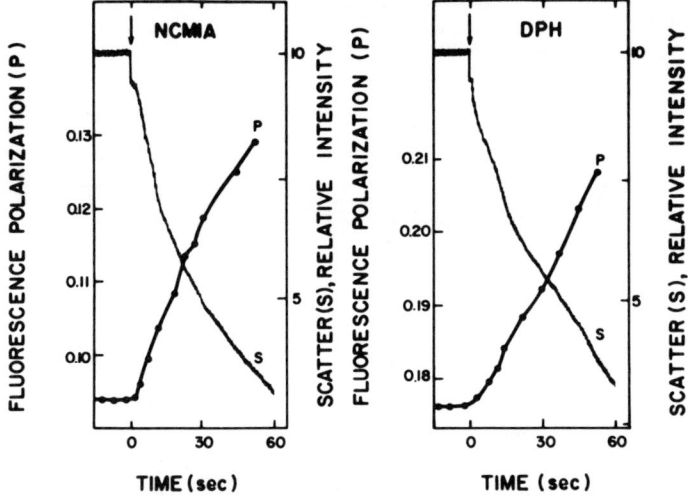

Fig. 2. Rotational dynamics of NCMIA-labelled and DPH-labelled platelets during aggregation induced by thrombin. Measurements carried out on 3 ml platelet suspension, $3 \pm 0.5 \times 10^8$ platelets/ml. Aggregation was induced by 1 u/ml thrombin added at zero time (arrow). Excitation and emission slits were 4 nm for scatter and 4 and 20 nm for P measurements respectively. With excitation at 345 and 350 nm fluorescence emission was followed at 425 and 430 nm for NCMIA and DPH respectively. A 390 nm cut off filter was used. P was calculated according to Rosenthal et al. (1978) and scatter (S) was followed at 600 nm.

These studies taught us some useful lessons.

A. It is essential to eliminate excess labelling reagent, since the free label may mask the effects of the bound label. This may account, at least in part, for the absence of any change in fluorescence observed by other workers (Horne et al., 1975).

B. The change in turbidity of platelet suspensions is the basis for their clinical tests. Yet, scatter contribution to the fluorescence studies should be minimized (Mely-Goubert et al., 1979). While primary scattering can be reduced to minimum by proper labelling and filtration conditions, secondary scattering (Teale, 1969; Lentz et al., 1979) effects could not be excluded totally and present an inherent limitation. Thus, since secondary scattering reduces the observed fluorescence polarization values, it is conceivable that changes in scatter associated with aggregation may present an additional contribution to the observed increase in fluorescence polarization. It is, therefore, of interest that P values do increase even during shape change when only minor change in turbidity occurs. Time resolved fluorescence spectroscopy

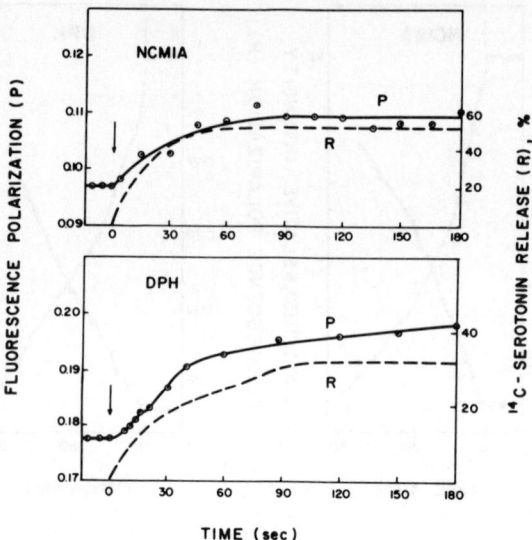

Fig. 3. The effect of thrombin, in the presence of 5 mM EDTA, on the rotational dynamics and on serotonin release of NCMIA-labelled and DPH-labelled platelets. Thrombin 1 u/ml was added at zero time (arrow). The procedure for P measurement detailed in Fig. 2 was followed. Release of ^{14}C-serotonin, is represented by the dashed curve.

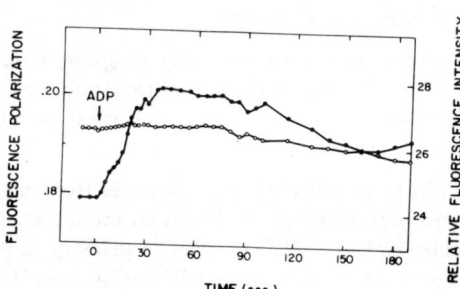

Fig. 4. The effect of ADP (5 µM) on fluorescence polarization (●) and intensity (O) of DPH-labelled platelets.

studies will further assist in overcoming primary scatter contribution. We now undertake detailed studies of secondary scatter contribution to further evaluate its contribution in our studies.

C. In assigning the increased polarization associated with platelet aggregation to decreased rotational freedom of the probe, it must be ascertained that increased P is not due to decrease in the probe's lifetime. In the present study this is evident from the increase in fluorescence intensity during aggregation. Furthermore, in using a probe which binds non-covalently such as DPH, it is imperative to ascertain that no redistribution of the probe takes place between the platelet and the medium during the activation process. We have indeed verified that such redistribution did not occur (Nathan et al.,1979).

D. The similar response to both ADP and thrombin in the presence of EDTA, indicates that increase in P in the activated platelet indeed reflects alterations during shape change (and release) rather than a specific interaction with either of the inducers. While changes in P values do indicate variation in the dynamic characteristics of the probes immediate environment, the exact nature of these dynamic effects cannot be verified by the averaging steady-state procedure, and require additional time-resolved fluorescence studies (Parola et al., 1979).

INTERPRETATION OF THE DYNAMIC CHANGES

It is of interest to examine functional implications for the dynamic changes observed during platelet activation on the basis of mechanisms already proposed.

Non-activated platelets. P values obtained with DPH indicate that phospholipids in the discoid platelet are characterized with a state of relatively high fluidity. This fluid state apparently allows the rapid lateral movement of receptors in the membrane and their random distribution (Nicolson, 1973). NCMIA signals that the aqueously exposed membrane glycoproteins have a relatively high rotational freedom in the unactivated platelet.

The observed depolarization in nanosecond time-scale of NCMIA labelled platelets could arise from an independent motion of the bound probe and from segmental motion of the labelled protein. Cherry and associates (1975,1977) pointed out that rotational correlation times for membrane proteins are much slower than those of proteins in aqueous solution (Weber, 1952). Both fluorescent lectin (Shinitzky et al., 1973) and NCMIA labelled plasma membrane glycoproteins in respective cell systems and exhibited rotational timescale corresponding to aqueous solution of proteins. Depolarization of fluorescently labelled glycoproteins could arise from the fast rotation of the aqueously exposed portion of the glycoproteins, presumably around the protein axis which is normal to the plane of the membrane (Cherry et al., 1977).

Activated platelets. As activation is initiated and platelets change shape, P of NCMIA-labelled platelets is elevated. This elevation may be interpreted as a decrease in the rotational mobility of membrane glycoproteins. The restriction in the protein motion may be caused by mechanisms, such as aggregation of membrane receptor proteins (Nicolson, 1973) and reduced rotation controlled by the cytoskeleton (Nicolson, 1976b). The concomitant elevation in membrane lipid microviscosity reflects an overall increase in lipid packing and in lipid-lipid interaction. Such alterations could cause a vertical motion of membrane proteins as described for several systems (Shinitzky and Souroujon, 1979; Borochov and Shinitzky, 1976).

The processes in platelets leading to the release reaction involve the activation of phospholipase A and the generation of lysolecithin. Lysolecithin, in turn, is known to fluidify membrane lipids (Lucy, 1970) and is likely to lead to a mosaic of regions of higher fluidity. Furthermore, the release process involves fusion of the granule membranes with membranes of the intracellular cannalicular system (White, 1970). The regions of fusions probably exhibit localized and transient increase in fluidity, undetected by us, since only an overall change in microviscosity was recorded. An analogous situation has been proposed for the process of phagocytosis, where an overall increase in microviscosity coincided with higher lipid fluidity of selective sites, associated with lateral phase transition (Berlin and Fera, 1977).

Concerning the aggregating platelets, increase in P reflects two types of alterations: changes corresponding to individual activated platelets (Fig. 3) and changes due to linkages among these platelets. Apparently the linkages between the pseudopod membranes further decrease the rotational freedom of the probe molecules. Reduced secondary scattering in aggregating platelets may add to the observed increase in P. The functional significance of membrane microviscosity in platelet activation, is evident from studies of the sensitivity of platelets to inducers. The sensitivity of platelets to aggregation by epinephrine and ADP was enhanced in platelets in which lipid microviscosity was elevated by incorporated cholesterol (Shattil and Cooper, 1976; Shattil et al., 1978).

The kinetics of changes in P of NCMIA and DPH-labelled systems are very similar. This similarity may indicate the interdependence of the lipids and proteins in the course of changes during activation. The nature of this interdependence of the major membrane components is still unclear.

REFERENCES

Berlin, R.D., and Fera, J.P., 1977. Changes in membrane microviscosity associated with phagocytosis: effects of colchicine. Proc. Natl. Acad. Sci. U.S.A. 74, 1072-1076.

Booyse, F.M., and Ratelson, M.E., 1971. Human platelet contractile proteins: location, properties and function. Ser. Hematol., 4, 152-174.

Borochov, H., and Shinitzky, M., 1976. Vertical displacement of membrane proteins mediated by changes in microviscosity. Proc. Nat. Acad. Sci. U.S.A. 73, 4526-4530.

Cherry, R.J., 1975. Protein mobility in membranes. FEBS Lett. 55, 1-7.

Cherry, R.J., Heyn, M.P., and Oesterhelt, D., 1977. Rotational diffusion and excision coupling of bacteriorhodopsin in the cell membrane of Halobacterium halobium. FEBS. Lett. 78, 25-30.

Coleman, R., 1973. Membrane-bound enzymes and membrane ultrastructure. Biochem. Biophys. Acta., 300, 1-30.

Cooper, R.A., 1977. Abnormalities of cell membrane fluidity in the pathogenesis of disease. N. Engl. J. Med. 297, 371-377.

Deykin, D., 1976. Platelet lipids and platelet function, in Platelets in Biology and Pathology (Eds. Gordon, J.L.) pp 111-119. North-Holland, Amsterdam.

Ediddin, M., 1974. Rotational and translational diffusion in membranes. Annu. Rev. Biophys. Bioeng. 3, 179-201.

Fuchs, P., Parola, A., Robbins, P.W., and Blout, E.R., 1975. Fluorescence polarization and viscosities of membrane lipids of 3T3 cells. Proc. Natl. Acad. Sci. (U.S.A.) 72, 3351-3354.

de Gaetano, G., 1978. Blood platelets as a pharmacological model of serotoninergic synaptosomes, in Platelets: A multidisciplinary approach. (Ed. de Gaetano, G.), pp 373-384. Raven, New York.

Gartner, T.K., Williams, D.C., Minion, F.C., and Phillips, D.R., 1978. Thrombin-induced platelet aggregation is mediated by a platelet plasma membrane-bound lectin. Science, 200, 1281-1283.

George, J.N., Lewis, P.C., Morgan, R.K., 1978. Studies on platelet plasma membranes. III. Membrane glycoprotein loss from circulating platelets in rabbits: Inhibition by aspirin-dipyridamole and acceleration by thrombin. J. Lab. Clin. Med. 91, 301-306.

Grant C.W.M., and McConnell, H.M., 1974. Glycophoria in lipid bilayers. Proc. Nat. Acad. Sci. U.S.A. 71, 4653-4657.

Hardisty, R.M., and Hutton, R.A., 1966. Platelet aggregation and the ability of platelet Factor 3. Br. J. Haematol. 12, 764-776.

Harker, L.A., and Slicter, S.J., 1972. Platelet and fibrinogen consumption in man. N. Engl. J. Med. 287, 999-1005.

Horne, W.C., Guilmette, K.M., and Simons, E.R., 1975. Fluorescent labeling of human platelets. Blood, 46, 751-759.

Kaulen, H.D., and Gross, R., 1976. Metabolic properties of human platelet membranes. II. Thrombin-induced phosphorylation of membrane, lipids and demonstration of phosphorylating enzymes in the platelet membrane. Thromb. Haemostasis, 35, 364-376.

Lenz, B.R., Moore, B.M., and Barrow, D.A., 1979. Effect of membrane suspension turbidity on DPH fluorescence anisotropy. Biophys. J., 25, 164a.

Lewis, J.T., and McConnell, H.M., 1978. Model lipid bilayer membranes as targets for antibody-dependent, cellular and complement mediated immune attack. Ann. N.Y. Acad. Sci. 308, 124-238.

Linden, C.D., Wright, K.L., McConnell, H.M., and Fox, C.F., 1973. Lateral phase separations in membrane lipids and the mechanism of sugar transport in Escherichia Coli. Proc. Nat. Acad. Sci. U.S.A., 70, 2271-2275.

Lucy, J.A., 1970. The fusion of biological membranes. Nature (London) 227, 815-817.

Marcus, A.J., 1969. Platelet function (First of three parts). N. Eng. J. Med. 280, 1213-1220.

Mely-Goubert, B., Calvo, F., and Rosenfeld, C.I., 1979. Study of platelet membrane proteins through fluorescence polarization of diphenyl hexatriene. Biomedicine, 31, 155-156.

Nathan, I., Fleischer, G., Livne, A., Dvilansky, A., and Parola, A.H., 1979. Membrane microenvironmental changes during activation of human blood platelets by thrombin. J. Biol. Chem. 254, 9822-9828.

Nathan, I., Fleischer, G., Dvilansky, A., Livne, A., Parola, A.H., 1980. Membrane dynamic alterations associated with activation of human platelets by thrombin. Biochim. Biophys. Acta. in press.

Nicholau, C., Hildenbrand, K., Reimann, A., Johnson, S.M., Vaheri, A., and Friis, R.R., 1978. Membrane lipid dynamics and density dependent growth control in normal and transformed avian cells. Exp. Cell. Res., 113, 63-73.

Nicolson, G.L., 1973. The relationship of a fluid membrane structure to cell agglutination and surface topography. Ser. Haematol. 6, 275-291.

Nicolson, G.L., 1976a. Trans-membrane control of the receptors on normal and tumor cells. I. Cytoplasmatic influence over cell surface components. Biochim. Biophys. Acta. 457, 57-108.

Nicolson, G.L., 1976b. Trans-membrane control of the receptors on normal and tumor cells. I. Cytoplasmatic influence over cell surface components. Biochim. Biophys. Acta., 458, 1-72.

Nurden, A.T., Caen, J.P., 1978. Annotation. Membrane glycoproteins and human platelet function. Br. J. Haematol. 38, 155-160.

Papahadjopoulous, D., Poste, G., Shaeffer, B.E., and Vail, W.J., 1974. Membrane fusion and molecular segregation in phospholipid vesicles. Biochim. Biophys. Acta, 352, 10-28.

Parola, A.H., and Souroujon, M., 1979. Membrane dynamic alteration associated with the tumorigenicity of polyoma-transformed and revertant hamster cells. Int. J. Cancer, 24, 800-805.

Parola, A.H., Robbins, P.W. and Blout, E.R., 1979. Membrane dynamic alterations associated with viral transformation and reversion. Decay of fluorescence emission and anisotropy studies of 3T3 cells. Exp. Cell. Res. 118, 205-214.

Radda, G.K., and Vanderkooi, J., 1972. Can fluorescence probes tell us anything about membranes? Biochim. Biophys. Acta, 265, 509-549.

Rittenhouse-Simons, S., and Deykin, D., 1977. The mobilization of arachidonic acid in platelets exposed to thrombin or ionophore A23187. J. Clin. Invest. 60, 495-498.

Rosenthal, S.L., Parola, A.H., Blout, E.R., and Davidson, R.L., 1978. Membrane alterations associated with "transformation" by BUdR in BUdR-dependent cells. Fluorescence polarization studies with a lipid probe. Exp. Cell. Res. 112, 419-429.

Ross, R., and Glomset, J., 1976. The pathogenesis of atherosclerosis. N. Eng. J. Med. 295, 369-377, 420-425, 1976.

Rubenstein, J.L.R., Smith, B.A., and McConnell, H.M., 1979. Lateral diffusion in binary mixtures of cholesterol and phosphatidylcholines. Proc. Natl. Acad. Sci. U.S.A., 76, 15-18.

Shattil, S.J., and Cooper, R.A., 1976. Membrane microviscosity and human platelet function. Biochemistry, 15, 4832-4837.

Shattil, S.J., and Cooper, R.A., 1978. Role of membrane lipid composition, organization and fluidity in human platelet function, in Progress in Hemostasis and thrombosis, 4: 59-86. (Ed. Spaet T.H.) Grune and Stratton, New York.

Shinitzky, M., Inbar, M., and Sachs, L., 1973. Rotational diffusion of lectins bound to the surface membrane of normal lymphocytes. FEBS. Lett., 34, 247-250.

Shinitzky, M., and Barenholz, Y., 1978. Fluidity parameters of lipid regions determined by fluorescence polarization. Biochim. Biophys. Acta, 515, 367-394.

Shinitzky, M., and Henkart, P., 1979. Fluidity of cell membranes: Current concepts and trends. Int. Rev. Cytol., 60, 121-147.

Shinitzky, M., and Souroujon, M., 1979. Passive modulation of blood-group antigens. Proc. Natl. Acad. Sci. U.S.A., 76, 1-3.

Shinitzky, M., 1979. The concept of passive modulation of membrane response, in Physical chemical aspects of cell surface events and cellular regulation (Eds. Blumentnol R.S. delisi, Co) pp. 173-181, Elsevier, North Holland, Amsterdam.

Smith, J.B., Silver, M.J., 1976. Prostaglandin synthesis by platelets and its biological significance in Platelets in Biology and Pathology (Ed. Gordon, J.L.), pp. 331-352, North Holland, Amsterdam.

Sneddon, J.M., 1973. Blood platelets as a mode for monoamine containing neurons, in Progress in Neurobiology (Eds. Kerkut, G.A. and Phillis, J.W.) Vol. 1, pp. 151-198, Pergamon, New York.

Teale, F.W.J., 1969. Fluorescence depolarization by light-scattering in turbid solutions. Photochem. and Photobiol. 10, 363-374.

Van Dijck, P.W.M., Ververgaet, P.H.J. Th., Verkleij, A.J., Van-Deenen, L.L.M. and de Gier, J., 1975. Influence of Ca^{++} and Mg^{++} on the thermotropic behaviour and permeability properties of liposomes prepared from dimyristoyl phosphatidylglycerol and mixtures of dimyristoyl phosphatidylglycerol and dimyristoyl phosphatidylcholine. Biochim. Biophys. Acta 406, 465-478.

Wallach, D.F.H., Bieri, V., Verma, S.P., and Schmidt-Ulrich, R., 1975. Modes of lipid-protein interactions in biomembranes. Ann. N.Y. Acad. Sci., 264, 142-160.

Weber, G., 1952. Polarization of the fluorescence of macromolecules. 1. Theory and experimental methods. Biochem. J., 51, 145-167.

Weiss, H.J., 1975. Platelet physiology and abnormalities of platelet function. N. Engl. J. Med., 293, 531-541, 580-588.

White, J.G., 1970. A search for the platelet secretory pathway using electron dense tracers. Amer. J. Pathol., 58, 31-49.

Wu, K.K., and Ku, C.S.L., 1979. Effect of platelet activation on the platelet surface sialic acid. Thromb. Res., 14, 697-704.

LABELLING AND SEPARATION OF PLATELET MEMBRANE PROTEINS

A. Rotman

Department of Membrane Research
The Weizmann Institute of Science
Rehovot, Israel

ABSTRACT

Specific reagents for membrane glycoproteins were synthesized and used to label the platelet membrane. One of these reagents, 3,5-diiodo-L-tyrosine hydrazide (DITH) is a very polar reagent and under suitable conditions is relatively impermeant. The other reagent for glycoprotein labelling, 2,4-dinitrophenyl-β-alanine hydrazide, is more hydrophobic but can be recognized by anti DNP antibodies and thus was used as a probe that enabled the isolation of membrane glycoproteins. Another reagent used was diiodo arsanilic acid diazonium salt (DIAA). This proved to be impermeant and a good probe for quantitative isolation of the labelled membrane proteins using anti-arsanilic acid antibodies. The use of iodonaphtyl azide (INA) to label platelet membrane proteins from within the lipid core is also described.

INTRODUCTION

The central role played by the protein components of membranes has been recognized, but progress in the isolation of these proteins, particularly integral ones, has been slow. Knowledge of the stereochemical and structural arrangement of membrane proteins is of the utmost importance to the understanding of their functions and for their isolation. One of the methods for identifying membrane proteins and their relative location in the membrane is covalent labelling.

The advantage of this labelling is the fact that the proteins are labelled in the intact cell i.e. in their natural environment and conformation. Usually the labelled proteins are identified by SDS gel electrophoresis. There are two principal methods of labelling cell membranes, the chemical method and the enzymatic method. The chemical method is usually accomplished by the interaction of a relatively small molecule with specific or nonspecific membrane macromolecules. Among these reagents one can mention the diazodiiodosulfanilic acid (George et al. 1980, George et al. 1978, George, 1978), sodium borohydride (Andersson and Gahmberg, 1978, Bunting et al. 1978), 4,4'-Diisothiocyano stilbene disulphonate (Cabantchik and Rothstein 1972), and the photoaffinity labelling reagents Iodonaphtyl azide (Bercovici and Gitler, 1978, and

N-(4-azido-2nitrophenyl)-2 aminoethyl sulphonate, Staros and Richards, 1974, Marchesi et al. 1969). The enzymatic labelling methods usually involve interaction of the added enzyme with the membrane proteins and this interaction enables the incorporation of the radioactive label e.g. iodine. Labelling of platelet membrane proteins using the lactoperoxidase method was carried out by Nachman et al. (1973), Phillips and Agin (1973), Phillips (1972), Tanner et al. (1974), Gates et al. (1975), Hagen et al. (1976), Phillips and Agin (1974), Phillips and Agin (1977a). Another enzyme catalyzed reaction is the galactose oxidase tritiation which is based on the oxidation of terminal galactose residues on glycoproteins (Gahmberg and Hakomori (1973), Steck and Dawson (1974), followed by reduction.

Specific labelling allows one to determine the existence and location of various proteins and glycoproteins on the cell membrane. Thus, these labelling procedures revealed the presence of the major glycoproteins on platelet membrane and were very useful in the determination of thos glycoproteins missing in some platelet disorder diseases (Phillips and Agin (1977 b), Phillips et al. (1975)).

RESULTS

a. <u>Labelling of Platelet Membrane Glycoproteins</u>. The general approach is to generate aldehyde groups on the membrane glycoproteins and then either to reduce the aldehyde with $[^3H]$-NaBH$_4$ or to react it with radioactive hydrazide. In both cases a relatively minor modification leads to a very efficient radioactive labelling of the glycoprotein. This method is based on the fact that sialic acid, present on most glycoproteins of the platelet membrane can be oxidized quite selectively with sodium periodate to form the aldehyde (Van Lenten and Ashwell, 1971).
We used this principle to specifically label glycoprotein I and glycoprotein III on the platelet membrane and to isolate other glycoproteins. The periodate ovidation and subsequent reactions of the   is shown in Fig. 1. Periodic acid will cleave the bond between two vicinal hydroxyl groups on the side chain of the sialic acid of a glycoprotein. The aldehyde formed can be either reduced with tritiated sodium borohydride or react with a hydrazide derivative. The Schiff base formed as a result of the interaction between the aldehyde and the hydrazide is stabilized by reduction with sodium cyanoborohydride resulting in a labelled glycoprotein modified in the sialic acid moiety.

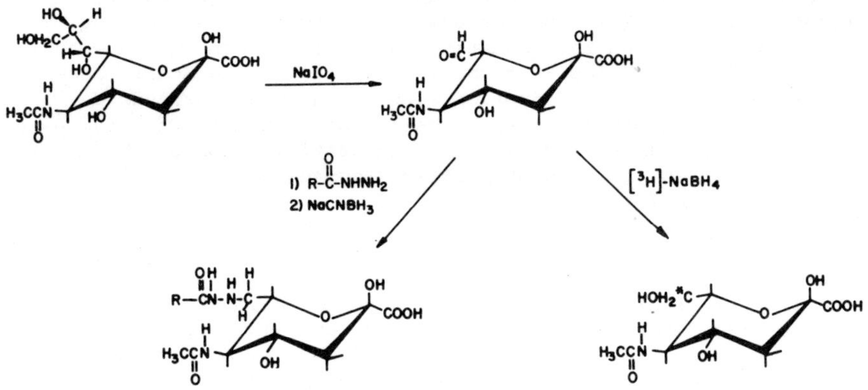

Fig. 1. Periodate oxidation of sialic acid and treatment of the aldehyde formed with [^{3}H]-NaBH$_4$ or with hydrazide.

1. <u>Sodium Borohydride</u>. When washed human platelets were treated with sodium periodate in the concentration range of 0.1 mM-20 mM and then reduced with [^{3}H]-sodium borohydride, a selective labelling was obtained in glycoprotein III (Rotman, Linder and Pribluda, 1980). No difference in the labelling pattern was observed when the periodate concentration was increased. The only change observed was the intensity of the labelling. When the aldehyde was treated with the hydrazide derivative a different pattern of labelling was obtained.

2. <u>3,5-diiodo-L-tyrosine hydrazide (DITH) (Fig. 2)</u>.

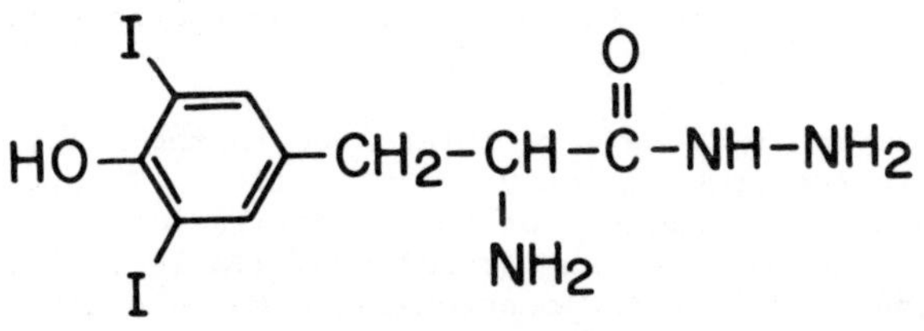

Fig. 2. 3,5 Diiodo-L-Tyrosine hydrazide.

This compound was prepared by esterification of diiodo tyrosine and conversion of the methyl ester to the hydrazide by treatment with hydrazine hydrate. The advantage of this reagent lies in the fact that it is easy to prepare with radioactive iodine (according to the method of Helmkamp and Sears, 1970) and that it is fairly polar and thus will label mainly external glycoproteins. Using this reagent we were able to specifically label glycoprotein I on platelets membrane. This labelling was done by treatment of washed platelets with 0.1 mM sodium periodate at room temperature over 15 min at pH = 7.2 and then reacting the platelet suspension with the radioactive 3,5-diiodo-L-tyrosine hydrazide. The Schiff base formed was stabilized by reduction with sodium cyanoborohydride The fact that glycoprotein I was labelled specifically has tremendous importance, taking into account the participation of this glycoprotein in the process of platelet aggregation.

b. <u>Labelling of Proteins from within the Lipid Bilayer</u>. One of the most important questions in membrane biochemistry is that of the relative location of an integral protein with relation to the lipid bilayer. Thus, the question of receptor exposure might be related to the interaction of the membrane proteins with the phospholipids to the bilayer (Fleisher et al.(In these proceedings), Jamieson et al. (In these proceedings)). Among the most promising reagents for the study of proteins that transverse the membrane is the Iodonaphtyl azide (INA) (Bercovici and Gitler 1978). This is a site-directed photoactivated labelling reagent which labels membrane proteins that span the membrane. The mechanism of labelling with this reagent is shown in Fig. 3.

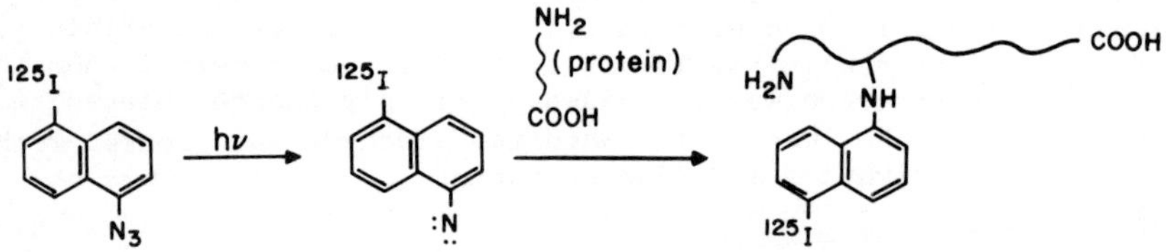

Fig. 3. The structure of Iodonaphtyl azide, its photochemical conversion to the nitrene and the insertion to protein.

In this part of the study we were interested in the relative location of actin in resting and activated platelets. Thus, platelets were treated with trace amounts of the highly radioactive INA, divided into 4 equal samples and irradiated, (Table 1). The samples were analyzed by two dimensional SDS gel electrophoresis and autoradiography. Results are shown in Table 1.

TABLE 1. Labelling of platelets with INA.

Sample	Conditions	Labelling of actin
1	Control, non aggregated	traces
2	aggregated by 1 u/ml thrombin	traces
3	aggregated by 10 µM ADP in the presence of fibrinogen	traces
4	treated with 0.1% triton X-100	very high

In other experiments we have shown that there is no specific binding of ^{125}I-DNAse to human platelets and there is no change in the binding during activation.

c. <u>Isolation of Platelet Membrane Proteins</u>. The other kine of labelling reagents is that enabling separation of the labelled proteins. The platelets are labelled with a reagent containing a haptenic group. These groups are chosen so that antibodies against them are easily prepared. Thus, when these antibodies are coupled to sepharose one can separate the labelled proteins on affinity column containing the antibodies. The general rationale of this method is shown in Fig. 4.

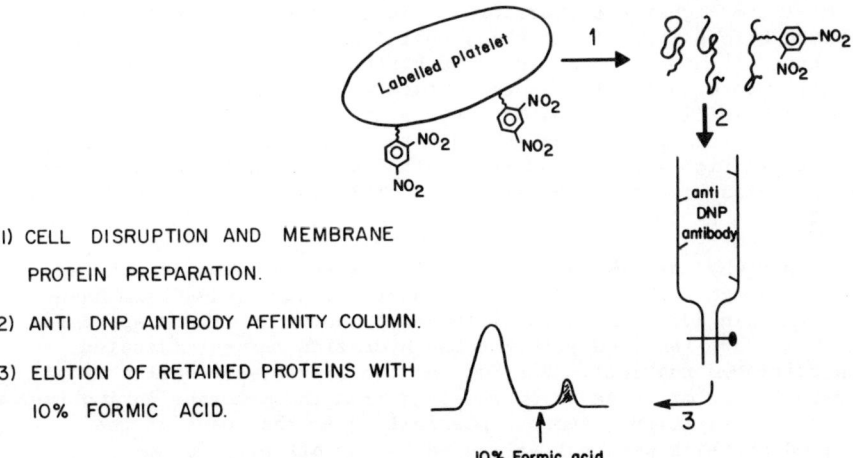

1) CELL DISRUPTION AND MEMBRANE PROTEIN PREPARATION.
2) ANTI DNP ANTIBODY AFFINITY COLUMN.
3) ELUTION OF RETAINED PROTEINS WITH 10% FORMIC ACID.

Fig. 4. The isolation of DNP-labelled glycoproteins from platelet membrane by the use of affinity chromatography. The same method was used to isolate membrane proteins labelled with Diazodiiodo arsanilic acid.

In this contribution we describe two such labelling reagents. One, 2,4-dinitro phenyl-β-alanine hydrazide (Fig. 5a) is designed to label glycoproteins and is recognized by anti DNP antibodies. The other, Diazo diiodoarsanalic acid (Fig. 5b) is designed to label outside-oriented proteins and is recognized by anti-arsanilic acid antibodies. Both antibodies are easy to prepare and purify.

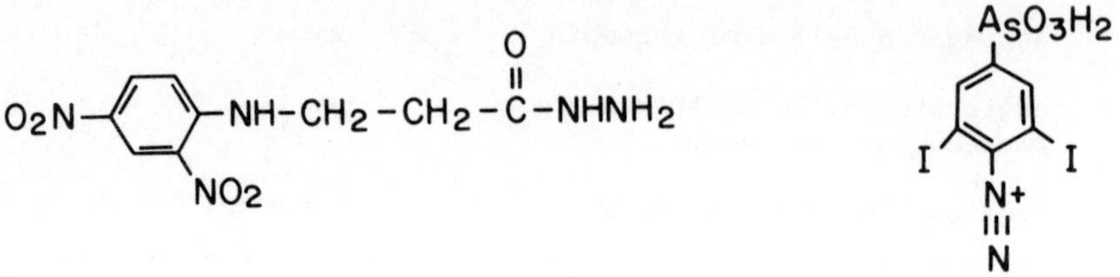

Fig. 5. 2,4-dinitrophenyl-β-alanine hydrazide (a)
Diazo diiodoarsanilic acid (b)

1. **Isolation of glycoproteins labelled with 2,4-dinitrophenyl-β-alanine hydrazide**: The mechanism of labelling with this reagent is shown in Fig. 1 (R=2,4-dinitrophenyl-β-alanyl), namely interaction of the hydrazide group with aldehyde formed from periodate oxidation of sialic acid-containing glycoproteins. As this compound is less polar than DITH, the chances that it will cross the membrane into the cell are higher and therefore it is necessary to isolate the membrane before identifying the labelled glycoproteins. The main advantage of this compound is the fact that its covalent binding to the glycoproteins enabled us to isolate at least part of these glycoproteins by affinity chromatography using anti-DNP antibodies attached to sepharose beads (the general scheme of this isolation is shown in Fig. 4). Using this method we were able to isolate 3 main proteins having molecular weight of 130,000, 100,000 and 80,000.

The reason why not all the glycoproteins were isolated is not yet clear. In other studies (Rotman, Linder, Kaplan , 1980) we have shown that in addition to these three glycoproteins there are a few more which are labelled with the DNP hydrazide reagent (studied with tritiated reagent). Part of the labelled glycoproteins might be cytoplasmic or those being released from the membrane during the membrane preparation. Another possibility is that part of the labelled proteins were not attracted by the affinity column.

2. **Isolation of outside exposed proteins.** Use of Diazodiiodoarsanilic acid (Fig. 5b). This reagent is quite similar to the diazodiiodo sulfanilic acid used by George (1976). The preparation of the reagent from the commercial available arsanilic acid is very easy. When tested on erythrocytes the compound proved to

be impermeant. Thus, incubation of 10^{-4} M ^{125}I-diiodo arsanilic acid diazonium salt with human erythrocytes at 4° for 10' results in only 5% labelling of hemoglobin used as an intracellular marker (Rotman, Linder and Kaplan, 1980). The mode of reaction of this reagent with protein is shown in Fig. 6.

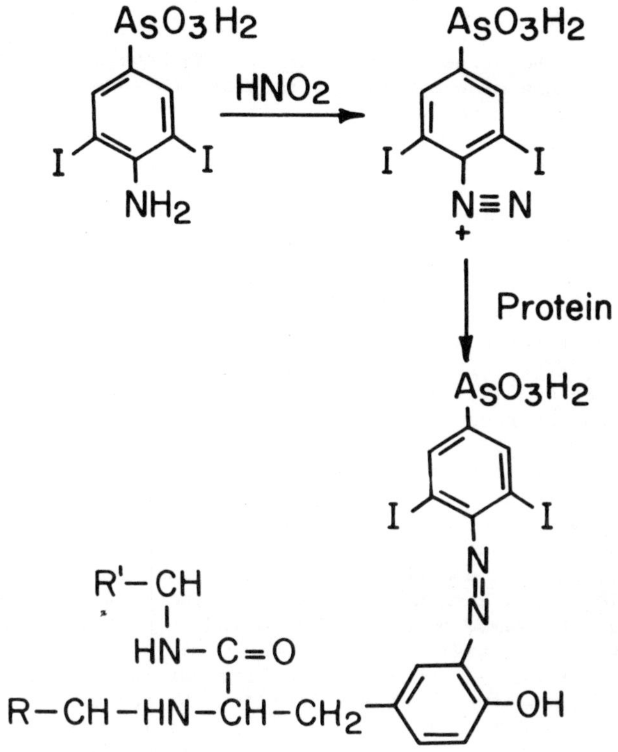

Fig. 6. Preparation of Diazodiiodoarsanilic acid from diiodoarsanilic acid and reaction of the diazonium ion with tyrosin group of a protein. R, R'=polypeptide chain.

When platelets were incubated with this reagent the main labelling appeared to be associated with an 85,000 daltons protein. The main advantage of the arsanilic acid reagent is the fact that it is a good immunogen and thus could be used to isolate the labelled proteins by affinity chromatography. Using a similar procedure to the one described in section 1, we were able to isolate the labelled protein on affinity chromatography using anti arsanilic acid antibodies attached to sepharose. As we know that diazo diiodoarsanilic acid does not penetrate into the cell it is logical to assume that this protein is exposed to the outer side of the membrane. The labelling pattern of platelets treated with diazodiiodoarsanilic acid is completely different from that obtained by George (1976) who used the reagent diazodiiodosulfanilic acid. The reason for this difference in labelling pattern is not clear to us in view of the similar nature of these reagents. One of the possible reasons might be a difference in the charge of these reagents, but this question has not been investigated by us.

DISCUSSION

a. <u>Labelling of Membrane Glycoproteins</u>. We have described the preparation and use of a few simple reagents to label and identify platelets membrane components. In addition we have described the preparation of other reagents which enabled us to isolate the labelled macromolecules by affinity chromatography. These methods are applicable in principle to other cell systems although they were used by us only in the platelet system. Comparing our reagents with those known in the literature, we conclude that the diiodo tyrosine hydrazide is a very efficient and promising reagent. Higher specific activity can be obtained with this reagent than by use of tritriated sodium borohydride. In addition, the relatively high polarity of the hydrazide prevents it from penetrating easily into the cell, a property which makes it a very appealing reagent. Thus, Rifkin et al. (1972) labelled the external glycoproteins of influenza virus by reducing the Schiff's base formed by pyridoxal phosphate with tritiated sodium borohydride but they obtained some labelling of internal proteins, a rather high background and some 6% non-specific reduction. However, under proper conditions Hunt and Brown (1974) and Roberts and Yuan (1974) obtained good results with pyridoxal in tissue culture cells. Comparison of the labelling pattern obtained with sodium borohydride to that with diiodo-tyrosine hydrazide shows a marked difference although in both cases the precursor was the same: oxidized (by periodate) sialic acid, 3,5-Diiodo-L-tyrosine hydrazide reacted mainly with the aldehyde groups formed on glycoprotein I while sodium borohydride reduced mainly the aldehydes formed on glycoprotein III. The reason for these differences in labelling is not yet clear. It is possible that the difference in labelling is a result of the electrical and charge environment of the oxidized glycoporteins. While sodium $[^3H]$-borohydride reduction proceeds through a hydride ion $[^3H^-]$, i.e. a negative species, the interaction of the oxidized glycoprotein with 3,5-Diiodo-L-tyrosine hydrazide is via the positive charge hydrazide group. Therefore, it is possible that the immediate environment of glycoprotein III is less negative than that of glycoprotein I. This difference in electrical charge of the two glycoproteins might result from the presence of high concentration of sialic acid on glycoprotein I (Nurden and Caen, 1975).

The disadvantage of the hydrazide derivatives as compared to the other reagents especially the photoaffinity ones is the fact that pretreatment of platelets with periodate is reported to affect their properties (Cazenave et al. 1976). Thus, sodium periodate in the concentration range of 1-10 mM caused aggregation of stirred washed rabbit platelets which was not followed by the release reaction. Rabbit platelets treated with the same concentrations of periodate

(1-10 mM)without stirring did not undergo aggregation. Under these conditions the platelets kept their discoid shape but lost their ability to aggregate in response to ADP, collagen, thrombin and arachidonic acid. (Cazenave et al. 1976). Therefore it is obvious that the periodate oxidation changed some of the biological properties of the platelets, eventually as a result of glycoprotein modification. Another disadvantage is the relatively slow reaction of the hydrazide as compared to the photoaffinity labelling reagents. Usually, in order to obtain a reasonable labelling (enough to be detected on SDS gel electrophoresis for example) one has to incubate periodate treated platelets with the diiodotyrosine hydrazide over a period of at least 10 min. This is a long period of time when compared to the shape change process which is over within seconds or the aggregation which is finished within 2-3 min. Therefore, it might be very difficult to follow possible changes in the exposure of membrane glycoproteins during the aggregation process with this reagent. However, one can use it to map the exposure of glycoproteins before and after aggregation.

The photoactivated labelling reagents have the advantage of rapid activition and efficient labelling can be achieved during 1-2 min. Therefore, it is possible to follow the aggregation process and even the shape change by using the appropriate photoaffinity labelling reagent. The reagent that we used (Iodonaphtyl azide) is actually a site-directed photolabelling reagent. It is not specific to any receptor or group of macromolecules except to those which reside in the lipid bilayer of the membrane. We used the Iodonaphtyl azide as a probe which will enable us to answer the very basic question: Does actin penetrate the lipid bilayer in resting platelets and does actin transverse the membrane and become exposed outside the cell as a result of activation? Reports by George (In these Proceedings) indicate that actin is exposed on the outer side of the activated platelet. Our results cast some doubt as to the presence of actin in the lipid bilayer. Therefore, if actin is exposed to a small extent at the surface of the cell it might be that traces of the protein are released during the activation process.

b. **Isolation of Platelet Membrane Proteins**. A few methods were reported in the last few years concerning the use of affinity chromatography in the isolation of platelet membrane components. These methods were based mainly on the use of sepharose-bound lectin and involved the step by membrane solubilization (Clemetson et al. 1977, Nachman et al. 1977, Bowles and Rotman 1978). Unlike the method described here the earlier reports made use of soluble membrane preparations and did not label specific membrane proteins in order to separate them.

Using the principle described here, namely, labelling of the intact platelet with a reagent containing an haptenic group followed by isolation of the labelled proteins on antibodies affinity columns, one has many options. By choosing the appropriate labelling reagent and the haptenic group it is possible in principle to label many kinds of membrane macromolecules. In this paper we describe two such reagents. One of them is based on the haptenic group dinitrophenyl (DNP) and is specific for glycoproteins (due to the hydrazide moiety). The other is based on the haptenic group arsanilic acid and is designed to label outside oriented proteins.

ACKNOWLEDGEMENT

The generous financial support of the Gatsby Foundation (London, England) is highly appreciated.

REFERENCES

Anderson, L.C., and Gahmberg, C.G., 1978. Surface glycoproteins of human white blood cells. Analysis by surface labelling. Blood, 52, 57-62.

Bercovici, T., and Gitler, C., 1978. 5-[^{125}I] Iodonaphtyl Azide, a reagent to determine the penetration of proteins into the lipid bilayer of biological membrane. Biochemistry, 17, 1484-1489.

Bowles, D.J., and Rotman, A., 1978. Agglutination activity association with a glycoprotein extract of human platelet plasma membranes. Possible involvement in platelet aggregation. FEBS Lett.,90, 283-285.

Bunting, R.W., Peerschke, E.I., and Zucker, M.B., 1978. Human platelet sialic acid content and tritium incorporation after ADP-induced shape change and aggregation. Blood,52, 643-653.

Cabantchik,Z.I., and Rothstein, A., 1972. The nature of the membrane sites controlling anion permeability of human red blood cells as determined by studies with disulfonic stilbene derivatives. J.Memb.Biol., 10, 311-330.

Cazenave, J.P., Reimers, H.J., Kinlough-Rathbone, R.L., Packham, M.A., Mustard, J.F., 1976. Effect of sodium periodate on platelet functions. J.Lab.Invest., 34, 471-481.

Clemetson, K.J., Pfueller, S.L., Lüscher, E.F., and Jenkins, C.S.P., 1977. Isolation of the membrane glycoproteins of human blood platelets by lectin affinity chromatography. Biochim.Biophys. Acta, 464, 493-508.

Fleisher, G., Nathan, I., Livne, A., Dvilansky, A., and Parola, A.H., Lipid-protein interaction in activated platelet membrane. In press.

Gahmberg, C.G., and Hakomori, S.I., 1973. External labelling of cell surface galactose and galactosamine in glycolipid and glycoprotein of human erythrocytes. J.Biol.Chem., 248, 4311-4317.

Gates, R.E., Phillips, D.R., Morrison, M., 1975. The distinguishing characteristics of the plasma membrane are its exposed proteins. Biochem.J., 147, 373-376.

George, J.N., Potterf, R.D., Lewis, P.C., and Sears, D.A., 1976. Studies on platelet plasme membrane I. Characterization of surface proteins of human platelets labelled with diazotized (^{125}I)-diiodosulfanilic acid. J.Lab.Clin.Med.,88, 232-246.

George, J.N., 1978. Studies on platelet plasme membranes. IV. Quantitative analysis of platelet membrane glycoproteins by ^{125}I-diazotized diiodosulfanilic acid labelling and SDS polyacrylamide gel electrophoresis. J.Lab.Clin.Med., 92, 430-446.

George, J.N., Lyons, R.M., and Morgan, R.K., 1980. Membrane alterations caused by platelet aggregation and secretion. In press.

Hagen, I., Olsen, T., Solum, N.O., 1976. Studies on subcellular fractions of human platelets by the lactoperoxidase-iodination technique. Biochim.Biophys.Acta, 455, 214-225.

Hunt, R.C., and Brown, J.C., 1974. Surface glycoproteins of mouse L cells. Biochemistry, 13, 22-28.

Jamieson, G.A., Jung, S.M., Ordinas, A., and Marcum, J.M., The influence of receptor mobility and association on the high affinity binding of thrombin to platelets. In press.

Marchesi, V.T., Steers, E. Jr., Tillack, T.W., and Marches, S.L., 1969. Some properties of spectrin - a fibrous protein isolated from red cell membranes, in Red Cell Membrane Structure and Function (Eds. G.A. Jamieson and T.J. Greenwalt) pp 117-130. J.B. Lippincott Co., Philadelphia.

Nachman, R.L., Hubbard, A., and Ferris, B., 1973. Iodination of human platelet membrane, studies on the major surface glycoproteins. J.Biol.Chem., 248, 2928-2936.

Nachman, R.L., Tarasov, E., Weksler, B.B., and Ferris, B., 1977. Wheat germ agglutinin affinity chromatography of human platelet glycoproteins. Thromb.Res. 12, 91-104.

Nurden, A.T., and Caen, J.P., 1975. Specific roles for platelet surface glycoproteins in platelet function. Nature, 255, 720-722.

Phillips, D.R., 1972. Effect of trypsin on the exposed polypeptides and glycoproteins in the human platelet membrane. Biochemistry, 11, 4582-4588.

Phillips, D.R., and Agin, P.P., 1973. Thrombin-induced alterations in the surface structure of the human platelet plasma membrane. Ser.Haematol., 6, 292-310.

Phillips, D.R., and Agin, P.P., 1974. Thrombin substrates and the proteolytic site of thrombin action on human platelet plasma membranes. Biochim.Biophys.Acta, 352, 218-227.

Phillips, D.R., Jenkins, C.S.P., Lüscher, E.F., and Larrieu, M.J., 1975. Molecular differences of exposed surface proteins on thrombasthenic platelet plasma membranes. Nature, 257, 599-600.

Phillips, D.R., and Agin, P.P., 1977a. Platelet plasma membrane glycoproteins. Identification of a proteolytic substrate for thrombin. Biochem.Biophys.Res.Commun., 75, 940-947.

Phillips, D.R., Agin, P.P., 1977b. Platelet membrane defects in Glanzmann's thrombasthenia: Evidence for decreased amounts of two major glycoproteins. J.Clin.Invest., 60, 535-545.

Rifkin, D.B., Compans, R.W., and Reich, E., 1972. A specific labelling procedure for proteins on the outer surface of membranes. J.Biol.Chem., 247, 6432-6437.

Roberts, R.M., and Yuan, B.O., 1974. Chemical modification of the plasma membrane polypeptides of cultured mammalian cells as an aid to studying protein turnover. Biochemistry, 13, 4846-4855.

Rotman, A., Linder, S., and Kaplan, M., 1980. Isolation of platelet plasma proteins by affinity chromatography. Submitted.

Rotman, A., Linder, S., and Pribluda, V., 1980. Specific labelling of platelet membrane glycoproteins. Submitted.

Staros, J.V., and Richards, F.M., 1974. Photochemical labelling of the surface proteins of human erythrocytes. Biochemistry, 13, 2720-2726.

Steck, T.L., and Dawson, G., 1974. Topographical distribution of complex carbohydrates in the erythrocytes membrane. J.Biol. Chem., 249, 2135-2142.

Tanner, M.J.A., Boxer, D.H., Cumming, J.,and Verrier-Jones, J., 1974. A set of surface proteins common to the circulating human platelet and lymphocyte. Biochem.J. 141, 909-911.

Van Lenten, L., and Ashwell, G., 1971. Studies on the chemical and enzymatic modification of glycoproteins. A general method for the tritiation of sialic acid-containing glycoproteins. J.Biol.Chem., 246, 1889-1894.

PLATELET GLYCOPROTEINS IN RELATION TO HUMAN PLATELET FUNCTION

A.T. Nurden, D. Dupuis, D. Pidard, T. Kunicki and J.P. Caen
Unité 150 INSERM, Hôpital Lariboisière, Paris 10, France

ABSTRACT

Glanzmann's thrombasthenia, the Gray platelet syndrome and the Bernard-Soulier syndrome are congenital platelet disorders associated with defined abnormalities of platelet function. Molecular deficiencies of different platelet glycoproteins are characteristic for each disorder and suggest specific roles for glycoproteins in different aspects of platelet function.

INTRODUCTION

When platelets aggregate a stimulus received at a receptor within the platelet plasma membrane sets in motion a chain of events which results in the formation of bonds between adjacent cells. Recent ultrastructural studies have defined the types of contact located within platelet aggregates (Skaer et al, 1979). Areas of tight contact were apparent, as were 50 nm intercellular spaces spanned by bridges linked to attachment points extending from the outer surface of the plasma membrane. Cell contact interactions in mammalian cell systems are often mediated by membrane glycoproteins (Nicolson, 1976) and glycoproteins have been shown to be major components of the normal human platelet surface (George et al 1979). Evidence supporting a possible role for membrane glycoproteins in platelet surface contact interactions has come from studies performed on platelets isolated from patients with congenital or acquired disorders of platelet function.

GLANZMANN'S THROMBASTHENIA

A disease with an autosomal recessive inheritance, thrombasthenia (GT) is characterised by the absence of platelet aggregation in response to ADP and all physiologic aggregation-inducing agents (see Hardisty, 1977). As discussed elsewhere (Nurden and Caen, 1979) the basic defect appears to lie in the inability of GT platelets to form the platelet-platelet linking bonds which conclude the aggregation mechanism. The platelets of the majority of patients are also unable to support clot retraction (Caen et al 1966). However, platelets of the occasional patient, termed type II thrombasthenia by Caen (1972), support at least 50 % of the normal clot retraction although the platelet aggregation defect remains unchanged.
Abnormalities in the membrane glycoprotein (GP) composition of GT platelets were first described by Nurden and Caen (1974) who noted a

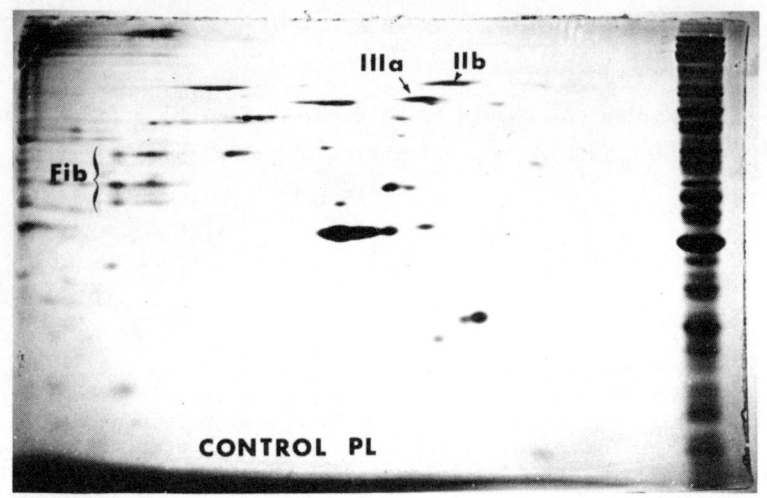
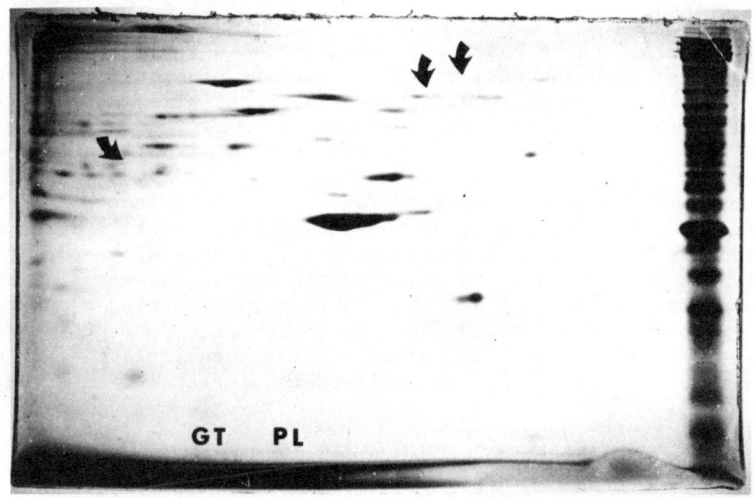

Fig. 1. Two-dimensional electrophoresis of normal human and GT platelets. Washed platelet suspensions were solubilised by 2 % SDS in the presence of 5 mM N-ethyl maleimide. Prior to the first dimension separation by isoelectric focusing (IF) the samples (200 ug protein) were made 9M with urea and triton X-100 added to give a 4 : 1 ratio with respect to the SDS. IF was then performed as described by Ames and Nikaido (1976). Following IF, the gels were incubated with 2 % SDS and 5 % 2-mercaptoethanol, placed onto 8-12 % exponential gradient slab gels and SDS-PAGE performed according to Laemmli (1971). Protein was detected with coomassie blue R 250.

severely reduced carbohydrate staining intensity of the GP II band, and a lower than normal staining intensity of the GP III band following SDS-polyacrylamide gel electrophoresis (SDS-PAGE). These, and subsequent studies performed on the platelets of a large number of patients in several laboratories have been reviewed elsewhere (Nurden and Caen, 1979). Our current studies suggest that GT platelets are either missing, or have severely reduced amounts, of membrane glycoproteins IIb and IIIa. This finding is illustrated in Figures 1 and 2. In Figure 1 a two-dimensional polyacrylamide gel electrophoresis procedure has been used to separate these glycoproteins from other polypeptides of similar size or charge. GP IIb migrates with a pI of 4.8-5.1 and apparent M.wt. of 135.000, IIIa with a p_I of 5.0 - 5.3 and apparent M. wt. of 116,000. The coomassie blue stained spots corresponding to IIb and IIIa are missing from the gel performed using platelets isolated from the GT patient. Autoradiographic analysis of gels performed using platelets whose surface proteins had been labelled with ^{125}I by the lactoperoxidase-catalysed procedure confirmed the apparent absence of IIb and IIIa from the platelets of this patient.

Figure 2 illustrates the analysis of ^{125}I-labelled GT and normal human platelets by crossed immunoelectrophoresis (CIE) using a polyspecific rabbit antiserum prepared against normal human platelets. A major ^{125}I-labelled precipitate, termed band 16 by Hagen et al (1980), is severely diminished in intensity in the GT platelet profile. The other major ^{125}I-labelled precipitates were present in their normal positions and were of normal intensity. Platelets from 9 GT patients have now been analysed by CIE in our laboratory, the results obtained for 3 patients as reported by Hagen et al (1980) and those studied subsequently all show either the absence of band 16 or its presence in severely reduced quantities (< 15 %). SDS-PAGE analysis of band 16 eluted from the agarose gel following either (i) its precipitation by the polyspecific rabbit antihuman platelet antibody preparation (Hagen et al, 1980) or (ii) a monospecific alloantibody, IgG L... (Kunicki and coworkers, manuscript in preparation) has shown the presence of GP IIb and IIIa in the precipitate.

The IgG L... is an alloantibody isolated from the serum of a GT patient which induced a "thrombasthenia-like" functional state on normal human platelets (Levy-Toledano et al, 1978). Kunicki and Aster (1978) have reported that a platelet-specific alloantigen (Pl^{A1}) is deleted in thrombasthenia and subsequently showed that the antigen is located on GP IIIa (Kunicki and Aster, 1979). Recently, van Leeuwen et al (1979) reported being able to inhibit platelet aggregation by an antibody with anti-Pl^{A1} specificity. Thus two antibodies both of which interact with membrane glycoprotein antigens missing or severely modified on GT platelets, inhibit aspects of human platelet function deficient in thrombasthenia, strongly suggesting that the glycoprotein defects are related to the platelet functional abnormalities.

Both SDS-PAGE and CIE have confirmed the low concentration of fibrinogen in GT platelets (see Figure 1) as previously reported by other authors. The amount of fibrinogen present in the platelets of different patients was variable (not detected in the platelets of 6 patients, and present in low to relatively normal concentrations in 3 patients). There was no quantitative relationship between the

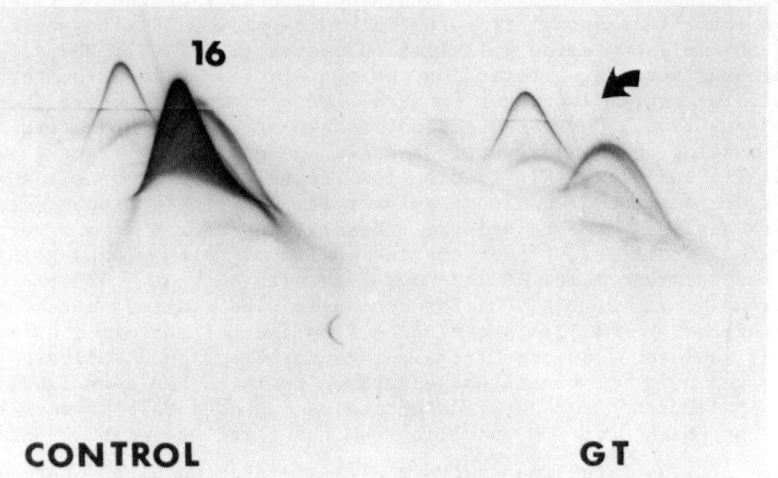

Fig. 2. Analysis of ^{125}I-labelled normal human and GT platelets (patient A.C.) by crossed immunoelectrophoresis (CIE). Washed platelet suspensions were labelled with ^{125}I by the lactoperoxidase-catalysed procedure (Phillips and Poh Agin, 1977). The platelets were solubilised in the presence of 1 % triton X-100 and CIE performed according to the procedures of Hagen et al (1980). The immunoglobulin fractions of a multispecific rabbit antiserum prepared against washed, normal human platelets was incorporated into the superior gel for the second dimension. Autoradiography of the dried, protein-stained plates, was performed using Kodak X-Omat MA film.

amount of fibrinogen present and the extent of the GP deletion, although those patients with detectable band 16 (GP IIb/IIIa) tended to be those with detectable platelet fibrinogen. These latter patients (Type II thrombasthenia) supported a modified clot retraction. The partial correction of clot retraction in thrombasthenia by the addition of Mg^{2+} (Caen et al, 1966) or by ristocetin and ATP (Chediak et al, 1978) distinguished the clot retraction abnormality from the aggregation defect, perhaps by partially correcting the binding of fibrin to the GT platelet surface.

GRAY PLATELET SYNDROME

An extremely rare platelet disorder, the Gray platelet syndrome has recently been shown by White (1979) to be due to a selective platelet ɑ-granule deficiency. We have studied the platelets of 2 such patients, a brother and sister where an ultrastructural examination has shown a specific absence of platelet ɑ-granules (Breton-Gorius and coworkers, unpublished studies). Analysis of the platelets isolated from both patients has shown the presence of distinct protein and glycoprotein deficiencies. These findings are illustrated in Figure 3.

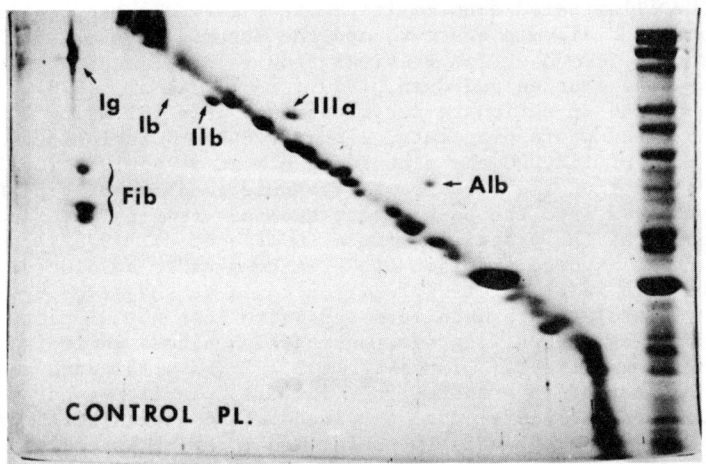

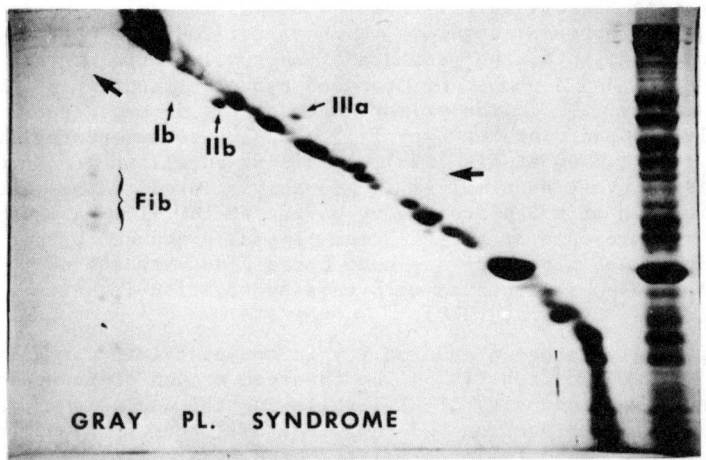

Fig. 3. Glycoprotein and protein defects in the Gray platelet syndrome. Washed normal human platelets and those isolated from a patient (H.B.) with a selective α-granule deficiency were solubilised by 2 % SDS in the presence of 5 mM N-ethyl maleimide. Two-dimensional SDS-PAGE was performed according to the procedure of Phillips and Poh Agin (1977). The first dimension was performed using 7 % (0.2 % bis) polyacrylamide gels, after electrophoresis the polypeptides were reduced by incubation with 5 % 2-mercaptoethanol. Second dimension electrophoresis was performed using 8-12 % exponential gradient slab gels. Proteins were detected with coomassie blue R 250.

Among the illustrated abnormalities are a markedly reduced platelet fibrinogen and albumin content, and the absence of a major platelet glycoprotein termed GP Ig. Previous studies on GP Ig have been reviewed elsewhere (Nurden and Caen, 1979 ; George et al, 1978). It is a prominent band on periodate-Schiff stained gels following SDS-PAGE of solubilised whole platelets, with a reduced (disulphide bond) apparent M.wt of 142,000 and a nonreduced M.wt of 450,000 (Lawler et al, 1978). During the release of α-granule constituents, part of GP Ig is released into the supernatant and part remains membrane bound and exposed at the platelet surface (George et al, 1978). The role of this surface exposed fraction of GP Ig remains to be elucidated. A possible role in platelet aggregation could be suggested by the fact the Gray platelets are much less sensitive than normal platelets to aggregation by several aggregation-inducing agents including thrombin, epinephrine and the Ca^{2+} ionophore A 23187 (Levy-Toledano and coworkers, manuscript in preparation). The Gray platelet syndrome is a relatively recent addition to the platelet congenital disorders and as such will be a potentially useful model during investigations into the role of α-granule proteins in platelet function.

BERNARD-SOULIER SYNDROME

Another platelet disorder with an autosomal recessive inheritance, the Bernard-Soulier (B-S) syndrome is characterised by a moderate to severe thrombocytopenia, the presence of unusually large platelets on blood smears and a number of proposed platelet function abnormalities (see Hardisty, 1977). The primary haemostatic defect appears to be a markedly reduced platelet capacity to adhere to subendothelium (Weiss et al, 1974 ; Caen et al, 1976). As discussed elsewhere (Nurden and Caen, 1979), this abnormality is probably related to the absence of agglutination of B-S platelets by bovine factor VIII_{VWF} or by ristocetin in the presence of normal human plasma. A reduced binding of thrombin to B-S platelets has been correlated with the decreased aggregation response observed with this aggregation-inducing agent (Jamieson and Okumura, 1978).

A specific glycoprotein abnormality in B-S platelets was first described by Nurden and Caen (1975) who observed a much decreased carbohydrate staining intensity of GP I following the analysis of isolated B-S platelet membranes on SDS-PAGE. Further studies on unfractionated platelets confirmed the abnormality (Caen et al 1976). These, and other studies on the glycoproteins and proteins of B-S platelets have been discussed previously (Nurden and Caen, 1979). We have recently been able to more accurately define the GP I defect using improved methods of platelet glycoprotein analysis. Four B-S patients have been examined. The platelets of each of these patients exhibited a specific abnormality on SDS-PAGE which, in terms of the glycoprotein nomenclature of Phillips and Poh Agin (1977) was an apparent absence of GP Ib, the major periodate-Schiff staining GP of normal human platelets (Nurden and Caen, 1979). The amount of radioactivity incorporated into GP Ib during lactoperoxidase catalysed ^{125}I-labelling of platelet surface proteins is small compared with that incorporated into other membrane glycoproteins, therefore a SDS-PAGE procedure giving a high resolution is required for its specific analysis. In our hands the

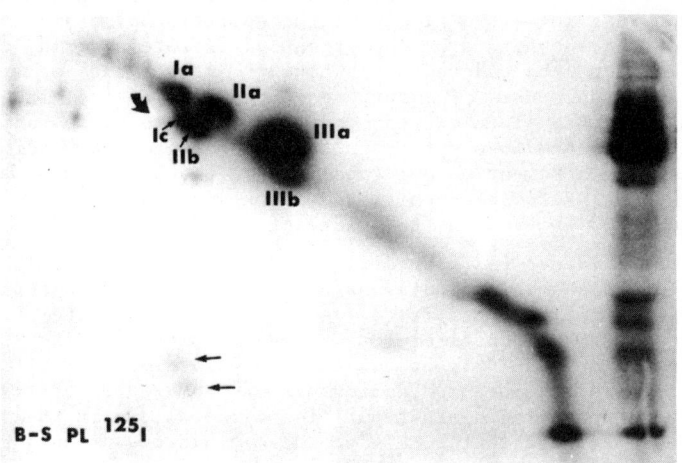

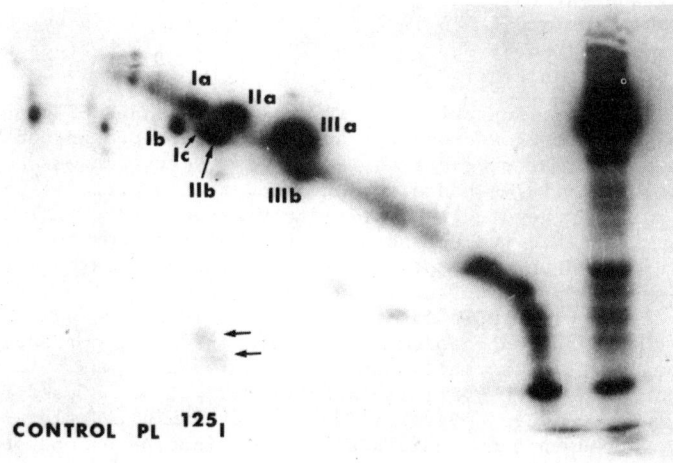

Fig. 4. Glycoprotein Ib defect in Bernard-Soulier platelets. Washed normal human and B-S platelets (patient N.V.) were labelled with ^{125}I by the lactoperoxidase-catalysed procedure (Phillips and Poh Agin, 1977). Two-dimensional SDS-PAGE was performed as described in the legend to Figure 3. Autoradiographic analysis of the dried polyacrylamide slab gels was performed using Kodak X-Omat MA film. The two horizontal arrows in the lower half of each gel mark the faint spots corresponding to the β-subunits of Ic and IIb (Phillips and Poh Agin, 1977).

two-dimensional nonreduced/reduced SDS-PAGE system of Phillips and Poh Agin (1977) most clearly separates Ib from the other membrane glycoproteins. This is a result of the splitting of a small M.wt polypeptide (β-subunit) from the parent glycoprotein during disulphide bond reduction, the reduced GP Ib having a faster rate of migration during electrophoresis. The surface composition of ^{125}I-labelled normal human and B-S platelets is compared in Figure 4. No radioactivity was located in the Ib position on the B-S platelet autoradiograph, note also the apparent normal labelling of the other major membrane glycoproteins. Periodate-Schiff and coomassie blue staining confirmed the absence of Ib from the B-S platelet gel.

Additional evidence for a specific glycoprotein abnormality in B-S platelets has been provided by Hagen et al (1980) who observed the absence of an immunoprecipitate (band 13) when B-S platelets were analysed by CIE. Glycocalicin or GP Is are names given to a solubilised fraction of "GP I" liberated from the platelet surface during platelet lysis (Okumura and Jamieson, 1976). Hagen et al (1980) used an antiserum prepared against purified glycocalicin in their CIE studies, and concluded that both glycocalicin and its precursor membrane glycoprotein were absent from the platelets of the two B-S patients examined. These, and our previous results (see Nurden and Caen, 1979) strongly suggest that the precursor of glycocalicin is GP Ib as defined by Phillips and Poh Agin (1977), a view supported by the SDS-PAGE analysis performed by George et al (1978) but a view recently challenged by Nachman et al (1979).

In another study, Kunicki et al (1978) showed that B-S platelets lacked the receptor for drug-dependent antibodies present on the platelets of all normal subjects tested. This observation was important as Moore et al (1978) had also suggested that a platelet surface Fc receptor for aggregated IgG was closely associated with the GP I complex. Our current studies indicate that the receptor for quinine- and quinidine-dependent antibodies is indeed associated with membrane GP Ib (Kunicki and coworkers, manuscript in preparation) but that this receptor differs from the Fc receptor described by Moore et al (1978). Other evidence to emphasise the possible importance of the GP I components in normal human platelet function was obtained using an alloantibody, IgG P..., isolated from a polytransfused B-S patient (see Nurden and Caen, 1979). This antibody inhibited platelet adhesion to subendothelium and platelet agglutination as induced by ristocetin in the presence of normal human plasma but did not inhibit ADP-induced platelet aggregation (Tobelem et al, 1976). It was, in fact, inducing a "Bernard-Soulier" type of reactivity onto normal human platelets.

ACQUIRED PLATELET GLYCOPROTEIN DISORDERS

So far we have described molecular deficiencies of glycoproteins in platelets of patients with rare congenital disorders of platelet function. It may be speculated that these deficiencies arise through a basic genetic defect manifested at an early stage in the synthesis of the glycoproteins or, as in the case of the Gray platelet-syndrome, in the incorporation of proteins into the platelet α-granules during platelet maturation. A modified platelet surface structure may also arise from the incorporation of glycoproteins into the membrane with incomplete or modified oligosaccharide chains, or by the subsequent degradation of glycoproteins after their incorporation in the platelet membrane. Such pathways may be the origin of certain acquired platelet GP disorders. Recently, the presence of a GP Ib abnormality in platelets isolated from Tn-syndrome donors was correlated with a platelet galactosyltransferase defect (Cartron and Nurden, 1979). It was suggested that subpopulations of platelets in these patients possessed GP Ib molecules deficient in sialic acid and subterminal galactose groupings leaving the Tn-antigen (terminal α-glycosidically linked N-acetyl-D-galactosamine residues) exposed. Markedly altered periodate-Schiff profiles have been noted following the analysis of platelets isolated from patients with myeloproliferative disorders (Bolin et al, 1977). It remains to be proved whether these acquired defects are related to specific alterations in different aspects of platelet function. However, Moore and Nachman (1979) have recently shown that marked changes in the accessibility of the platelet Fc receptor to aggregated IgG occur in patients with myeloproliferative disorders. Such a change would be expected if this receptor is associated with a GP I component (see earlier in the text). Furthermore, Greenberg et al (1979) have shown that GP modifications are often associated with a shortening in platelet survival time, a phenomenon often observed in patients with glycoprotein disorders (in particular those affecting GP I).

CONCLUSIONS

We have discussed the possible involvement of surface glycoproteins as mediators of different aspects of platelet function in terms of the evidence obtained from studies performed on platelets isolated from patients with congenital or acquired platelet disorders. Strong evidence suggests that different glycoproteins play specific roles in platelet function, but the precise mechanisms for the different pathways of platelet aggregation and adhesion remain to be elucidated. When platelets adhere to subendothelium it is the initial contact which arrests the platelet and this is followed by platelet activation and spreading (Sheppard and French, 1971). A role for GP I components during either the initial arrest of the platelet or during the formation of the cohesive bonds attaching the "spread" platelet to subendothelium could explain the adhesion defect in the B-S syndrome. During aggregation, platelets are activated by the aggregation-inducing agent with the result that cohesive forces are able to link one platelet surface with another. It has been known for a long time that both Ca^{2+} and fibrinogen are essential cofactors in the mechanism of platelet aggregation. After ADP-induced platelet activation, fibrinogen is able to bind to receptor sites newly exposed at the platelet surface, these receptors are resistant to digestion with chymotrypsin and are absent from the surface of GT platelets (Mustard et al, 1979). Binding of fibrinogen to a receptor located on (or associated with) a polypeptide region of GP IIb or IIIa may be an essential step in platelet aggregation. The fibrinogen may then be directly involved in the formation of the interplatelet bonds. Alternatively, fibrinogen and Ca^{2+} may be cofactors for the expression of a "lectin-like" activity at the platelet surface as proposed for thrombin-induced platelet aggregation by Gartner et al (1978). As shown by Skaer et al (1979), the protein bridges between aggregated platelets are relatively large, the release of the filamentous GP Ig from α-granules (see earlier in text) would make this an additional candidate for the lectin activity present at the platelet surface after platelet activation. The continuation of studies on platelets from patients with congenital or acquired glycoprotein defects may further contribute to the elucidation of the mechanisms underlying the different processes essential to the normal haemostatic functioning of the blood platelet.

REFERENCES

Ames, G.F., and Nikaido, K., 1976. Two-dimensional gel electrophoresis of membrane proteins. Biochemistry, 15, 616-623

Bolin, R.B., Okumura, T., and Jamieson, G.A., 1977. Changes in distribution of platelet membrane glycoproteins in patients with myeloproliferative disorders. American Journal of Haematology, 3, 63-71

Caen, J.P., 1972. Glanzmann's thrombasthenia. Clinics in Haematology, 1, 383-392

Caen, J.P., Castaldi, P.A., Leclerc, J.C., Inceman, S., Larrieu, M.J., Probst, M. and Bernard, J., 1966. Congenital bleeding disorders with long bleeding time and normal platelet count. I. Glanzmann's thrombasthenia (Report of fifteen patients). American Journal of Medicine, 41, 4-26

Caen, J.P., Nurden, A.T., Jeanneau, C., Michel, H., Tobelem, G., Levy-Toledano, S., Sultan, Y., Valensi, F., and Bernard, J., 1976. Bernard-Soulier syndrome : a new platelet glycoprotein abnormality. Its relationship with platelet adhesion to subendothelium and with the Factor VIII von Willebrand protein. Journal of Laboratory and Clinical Medicine, 87, 586-596

Cartron, J.P. and Nurden, A.T., 1979. Galactosyltransferase and membrane glycoprotein abnormality in human platelets from Tn-syndrome donors. Nature, 282, 621-623

Chediak, J., Lambert, E., and Maxey, B., 1978. Correction of clot retraction in thrombasthenia by ATP and ristocetin. Thrombosis Research, 12, 875-882

Gartner, T.K., Williams, D.C., Minion, F.C., and Phillips, D.R., 1978. Thrombin-induced platelet aggregation is mediated by a platelet plasma membrane-bound lectin. Science, 200, 1281-1283

George, J.N., Morgan, R.K., and Lewis, P.C., 1978. Studies on platelet plasma membranes. IV. Quantitative analysis of platelet membrane glycoproteins (^{125}I)-diazotised diiodosulfanilic acid labeling and SDS-polyacrylamide gel electrophoresis. Journal of Laboratory and Clinical Medicine, 92, 430-446

Greenberg, J.P., Packham, M.A., Guccione, M.A., Rand, M.L., Reimers, H.J., and Mustard, J.F., 1979. Survival of rabbit platelets treated in vitro with chymotrypsin, plasmin, trypsin, or neuraminidase. Blood, 53, 916-927

Hagen, I., Nurden, A.T., Bjerrum, O.J., Solum, N.O., and Caen, J.P., 1980. Immunochemical evidence for protein abnormalities in pla-

telets from patients with Glanzmann's thrombasthenia and the
Bernard-Soulier syndrome. Journal of Clinical Investigation, 65,
722-731

Hardisty, R.H., 1977. Disorders of platelet function. British Medical
Bulletin, 33, 207-212

Jamieson, G.A., and Okumura, T., 1978. Reduced thrombin binding and
aggregation in Bernard-Soulier platelets. Journal of Clinical
Investigation, 61, 861-864

Kunicki, T., Johnson, M.M., and Aster, R.H., 1978. Absence of the
platelet receptor for drug-dependent antibodies in the Bernard-
Soulier syndrome. Journal of Clinical Investigation, 62, 716-
719

Kunicki, T.J., and Aster, R.H., 1978. Deletion of the platelet-specific alloantigen Pl^{A1} from platelets in Glanzmann's thrombasthenia. Journal of Clinical Investigation, 61, 1225-1231

Kunicki, T.J., and Aster, R.H., 1979. Isolation and immunologic characterization of the human platelet alloantigen Pl^{A1}. Molecular
Immunology, 16, 353-360

Laemmli, U.K., 1970. Cleavage of structural proteins during the assembly of the head of bacteriophage T4. Nature, 227, 680-685

Lawler, J.W., Slayter, H.S., and Coligan, J.E., 1978. Isolation and
characterization of a high molecular weight glycoprotein from
human blood platelets. Journal of Biological Chemistry, 253,
8609-8616

Levy-Toledano, S., Tobelem, G., Legrand, C., Bredoux, R., Degos L.,
Nurden, A.T., and Caen, J.P., 1978. An acquired IgG antibody
occuring in a thrombasthenic patient : its effect on normal human platelet function. Blood, 51, 1065-1071

Moore, A., Ross, G.D., and Nachman, R.L., 1978. Interaction of platelet membrane receptors with von Willebrand factor, ristocetin,
and Fc region of immunoglobulin G. Journal of Clinical Investigation, 62, 1053-1060

Moore, A., and Nachman, R.L., 1979. Platelet Fc receptor : Increased
expression in myeloproliferative platelets. Blood, 54 supplement
1, 254 (abstract)

Mustard, J.F., Kinlough-Rathbone, R.L., Packham, M.A., Perry, D.W.,
Harfenist, E.J., and Pai, K.R.M., 1979. Comparison of fibrinogen association with normal and thrombasthenic platelets on exposure to ADP or chymotrypsin. Blood, 54, 987-993

Nachman, R.L., Kinoshita, T., and Ferris, B., 1979. Structural analysis of human platelet membrane glycoprotein I complex. Proceedings of the National Academy of Sciences, U.S.A., 76, 2952-2954

Nicolson, G.L., 1976. Transmembrane control of the receptors on normal and tumor cells. I. Cytoplasmic influence over cell surface
components. Biochimica et Biophysica Acta, 457, 57-108

Nurden, A.T., and Caen, J.P., 1974. An abnormal platelet glycoprotein
pattern in three cases of Glanzmann's thrombasthenia. British
Journal of Haematology, 28, 253-260

Nurden, A.T., and Caen, J.P., 1975. Specific roles for platelet surface glycoproteins in platelet function. Nature, 255, 720-722

Nurden, A.T., and Caen, J.P., 1979. The different glycoprotein abnormalities in thrombasthenic and Bernard-Soulier platelets. Seminars in Haematology, 16, 234-250

Okumura, T., and Jamieson, G.A., 1976. Platelet glycocalicin. I. Orientation of glycoproteins of the human platelet surface. Journal of Biological Chemistry 251, 5944-5949

Phillips, D.R., and Poh Agin, P., 1977. Platelet plasma membrane glycoproteins. Evidence for the presence of nonequivalent disulfide bonds using nonreduced-reduced two-dimensional gel electrophoresis. Journal of Biological Chemistry, 252, 2120-2126

Sheppard, B.L., and French, J.E., 1971. Platelet adhesion in the rabbit abdominal aorta following the removal of the endothelium : a scanning and transmission electron microscopical study. Proceedings of the Royal Society of London, 176, 427-432

Skaer, R.J., Emmines, J.P., and Skaer, H. le B., 1979. The fine structure of cell contacts in platelet aggregation. Journal of Ultrastructural Research, 69, 28-42

Tobelem, G., Levy-Toledano, S., Bredoux, R., Michel, H., Nurden, A., Caen, J.P., and Degos, L., 1976. New approach to determination of specific functions of platelet membrane sites. Nature, 263, 427-429

Van Leeuwen, E.F., Zonnevels, G.T.E., von Riesz, L.E., Jenkins, C.S.P., Van Mourik, J.A., von dem Borne, A.E.G. Kr., 1979. Absence of the complete platelet-specific alloantigens Zw (Pl^{A1}) on platelets in Glanzmann's thrombasthenia and the effect of anti-Zw^a antibody on platelet-function. Thrombosis and Haemostasis, 42, 422 (abstract)

Weiss, H.J., Tschopp, T.B., Baumgartner, H.R., Sussman, I.I., Johnson, M.M., and Egan, J.J., 1974. Decreased adhesion of giant (Bernard-Soulier) platelets to subendothelium-further implications on the role of the von Willebrand factor in hemostasis. American Journal of Medicine, 57, 920-925

White, J.G., 1979. Ultrastructural studies of the Gray platelet syndrome. American Journal of Pathology, 95, 445-462

PLATELET MEMBRANE GLYCOPROTEINS AS THROMBIN AND
AGGREGATION RECEPTORS

D.R. Phillips, L.K. Jennings, M.C. Berndt,
H.R. Prasanna, J.E.B. Fox and H.H. Edwards

Department of Biochemistry
St. Jude Children's Research Hospital,
Memphis, Tennessee 38101 U.S.A.

INTRODUCTION

Thrombin-induced platelet aggregation is the end result of a complex series of reactions. It is initiated by stimulus-platelet interaction and, after many biochemical and morphological events, culminates with the physical association of activated platelets. The initial stimulatory action appears to be an interaction of thrombin with a membrane surface component since thrombin does not enter platelets (Tollefsen, et al., 1974) and can activate platelets when covalently bound to agarose beads (Workman, et al., 1976). The catalytic activity of thrombin is required for activation to occur (Davey and Lüscher, 1967). We have recently identified a surface membrane glycoprotein that is directly hydrolyzed by thrombin (Phillips and Agin, 1977a), a reaction discussed below in greater detail. Although the nature of the transmembrane signal is not understood, recent studies have shown several intracellular changes that occur rapidly after thrombin-platelet interaction: i) the turnover of phosphatidyl inositol is increased (the "PI response", Michell, 1975). This involves the cleavage of phosphatidyl inositol to produce a diglyceride and inositol phosphate followed by the subsequent resynthesis of phosphatidyl inositol. In the presence of exogenously added [^{32}P]phosphate, radioactivity is rapidly incorporated into this phospholipid (Lloyd and Mustard, 1974). Recent evidence suggests that the liberated diglyceride may be the source of arachidonic acid required for platelet prostaglandin biosynthesis (Bell, et al., 1979); ii) the intracellular Ca^{++} concentration is increased (Lüscher and Massini, 1975); iii) two intracellular proteins show increased phosphorylation (Lyons, et al., 1975). One of these (P-20) is a light chain of myosin while the other is a polypeptide with an apparent molecular weight of 47,000 (P-47) (Daniel, et al., 1977; Haslam, et al., 1979). P-20 is phosphorylated by a myosin light chain kinase that is regulated by calmodulin and therefore activated by μM levels of calcium (Dabrowska, et al., 1978); iv) the cytoskeletal structures within platelets are altered, perhaps as a consequence of these changes in Ca^{++} and phosphorylation. Few actin filaments are observed in unstimulated platelets while many are observed in activated platelets, particularly in filopodia (Zucker-Franklin, et al., 1967; White, 1968). As will be discussed below, we have now quantitated the rate and extent of actin polymerization during thrombin activation.

The morphological changes that occur during thrombin-induced aggregation are extensive. The platelets change shape from discs to spheres with many filopodia extending out from the central mass of the platelet. The contents of three storage organelles, α-granules, dense bodies and lysosomes, are secreted to the outside of the platelet. Concomitant with these changes, the newly polymerized actin and associated proteins form an extensive cytoskeleton within the platelet. The membrane surface of the activated platelet has different properties as well. For example, the surface of the activated platelet has specific receptors that bind Factor Va, assisting in the Factor Xa-catalyzed hydrolysis of prothrombin to thrombin (Miletich, et al., 1977). Enhancement of other coagulation reactions has been observed as well. Of fundamental importance is the cohesive nature of the membrane surfaces of activated platelets so that platelets aggregate.

All of these above reactions are not prerequisites for aggregation: aggregation induced by γ-thrombin can precede dense body secretion (Huang and Detwiler, 1980); inhibition of arachidonic acid metabolism does not prevent aggregation induced by high α-thrombin concentrations (Kinlough-Rathbone, et al., 1977); aggregation can occur before the expression of thrombin-induced procoagulant activity. In our laboratory, we have concentrated on three problems directly related to the aggregation response. The first is the identity of the thrombin receptor. The second is the thrombin-induced intracellular changes in actin filament polymerization. The third is the identification of the membrane proteins which cause platelet aggregation, i.e., the aggregation sites.

THROMBIN RECEPTOR

Our working hypothesis for the identification of the thrombin receptor on human platelets is that interaction of thrombin with its receptor involves a hydrolytic event (Phillips and Agin, 1974; Phillips and Agin, 1977a). This hypothesis is based on several studies showing that the catalytic site of α-thrombin plays a crucial role in inducing the platelet response. For example, α-thrombin blocked with active-site directed inhibitors such as DFP, PMSF and TLCK does not stimulate platelets (Tollefsen, et al., 1974; Workman, et al., 1977; Ganguly, 1974; Davey and Lüscher, 1967). Further, a number of proteases such as trypsin (Davey and Lüscher, 1967), papain (Martin, et al., 1975) and thrombocytin (Niewiarowski, et al., 1979) whose cleavage specificities overlap with that of α-thrombin, activate platelets. Our approach, therefore, is to identify the protein(s) on the membrane surface that is hydrolyzed by thrombin and then to determine if this hydrolysis results in platelet activation.

The membrane glycoproteins on the surface of the platelets were labeled by sequential treatment of intact cells with either neuraminidase, galactose oxidase and [^{3}H]NaBH$_4$, or periodate and [^{3}H]NaBH$_4$. Of the more than 30 glycoproteins identified on the surface of human platelets, only one, glycoprotein V (M_r = 82,000) was hydrolyzed following the addition of α-thrombin (Phillips and Agin, 1977a). A new molecular species (M_r = 69,500) appeared in the supernatant after this proteolytic event. Glycoprotein V hydrolysis was the only observable catalytic event, even on treatment of labeled platelets with high thrombin concentrations (10 U/ml) for 15 min at 37°C. Hydrolysis of glycoprotein V appeared to be unique to proteolytic activation of platelets. Activation of platelets by nonproteolytic stimuli such as collagen, ADP/fibrinogen and the calcium ionophore, A23187, did not cause either the loss of glycoprotein V from the platelet membrane or the appearance of the new species in the supernatant. However, activation of platelets by other proteolytic stimuli did cause the hydrolysis of glycoprotein V. These proteases include some with broad specificity like trypsin, thermolysin, papain and bromelain that hydrolyzed many surface glycoproteins and others with high specificity like γ-thrombin, thrombocytin and α-clostripain that specifically hydrolyzed only glycoprotein V. Hydrolysis by these more specific proteases also produced the same hydrolytic fragment as that produced by α-thrombin. Hydrolysis of glycoprotein V did not occur when platelets were treated with catalytically inactive α-thrombin. Glycoprotein V can be classified a peripheral membrane protein since it is eluted from the plasma membrane by varying the ionic strength. We have recently purified glycoprotein V to apparent homogeneity. The purified glycoprotein is a thrombin substrate and on hydrolysis yields an apparently identical fragment to that observed on thrombin treatment of platelets. This finding indicates that hydrolysis of glycoprotein V during thrombin-induced platelet activation is a direct result of thrombin catalysis. The alternative possibility, that hydrolysis is a secondary event, resulting from activation of a membrane-bound or secreted protease, seems unlikely since secretion induced by other stimuli caused no hydrolysis of glycoprotein V. Glycoprotein V on intact platelets can be modified by reagents such as sodium periodate, neuraminidase and galactose oxidase indicating that it would also be accessible to extracellular proteases.

The available data indicate that hydrolysis of glycoprotein V is of physiological significance with respect to thrombin activation of platelets. Hydrolysis of this glycoprotein is observed at all α-thrombin concentrations above the threshold concentration required to elicit platelet aggregation. In addition, measurement of the rate of glycoprotein V hydrolysis shows that the hydrolytic event precedes aggregation. Further studies with the purified glycoprotein are designed to establish whether hydrolysis of this surface glycoprotein is the primary stimulus in platelet activation by thrombin.

ACTIN POLYMERIZATION DURING THROMBIN-INDUCED ACTIVATION

Although 15% or more of the total platelet protein is actin (Bettex-Galland and Lüscher, 1965), few actin filaments have been observed in unstimulated platelets. However, filopodia produced by activated platelets have extensive filaments (Zucker-Franklin, et al., 1967; White, 1968), suggesting an increase in the formation of actin filaments following platelet activation.

We have measured the amount of actin filaments in control and activated platelets by a method based on the observation of Bray and Thomas (1976) who showed that filamentous actin within non-muscle cells is resistant to Triton solubilization, while the unpolymerized actin is Triton soluble. Using this Triton extraction procedure, it is possible to solubilize most cellular structures except for the cytoskeletal structural elements. We have isolated platelet cytoskeletons by first treating platelet suspensions with 1% Triton X-100 containing 5 mM EGTA and then isolating the insoluble filamentous structures by centrifugation (Phillips, et al., 1980). Such cytoskeletons were composed of four proteins; actin, myosin, actin-binding protein and an as-yet-unidentified protein with an apparent molecular weight of 31,000. Thrombin-activated platelets (activated with thrombin in the presence of EDTA to prevent aggregation) showed a marked increase in the amount of these proteins in the Triton-insoluble filaments. The time course of new filament formation was extremely rapid. About 35% of the total platelet actin of unstimulated platelets was in the form of polymerized filaments, but within 15 s, this value increased to close to 60%. The other cytoskeletal proteins were also increased during this time interval. Electron micrographs of these cytoskeletal preparations revealed dramatic structural changes which coincided with the increased actin polymerization. The cytoskeletal structures of washed, unstimulated platelets consisted of randomly dispersed filaments with equivalent dimensions to actin filaments. However, when platelets were activated with thrombin for only 15 s, defined cytoskeletons of individual platelets were observed that had the appearance of hollow spheres approximately 2.1 µm in diameter. After platelets had been incubated with thrombin for 2 min and subsequently extracted with Triton, the cytoskeletons had condensed to structures with diameters of approximately 1.5 µm. Extraction of platelets at longer time intervals after activation (>5 min) revealed cytoskeletal structures that were not as tightly knit as those in the 2-min preparation, with filaments distributed throughout the structure. Thus, during thrombin-induced activation, actin rapidly polymerizes into filaments which are more structured than in unactivated platelets.

The question arises, does the increase in actin polymerization and subsequent structural reorganization have a role in platelet functions like secretion, aggregation and clot retraction? Measurement of the time course of 5-hydroxytryptamine (5-HT) secretion during thrombin-induced activation showed that the maximum rate of 5-HT secretion occurred approximately 15 s after thrombin addition; i.e., after most actin had already polymerized. Thus, actin polymerizes fast enough to be critical to the physiological response of the platelet. PGE_1 or PGI_2 inhibit both thrombin-induced platelet activation and actin polymerization, again consistent with a cause and effect relationship between these two reactions. Examination of the effects of other platelet stimuli on actin polymerization indicate that the effect of thrombin is not unique. Addition of adenosine diphosphate to an unstirred suspension of platelets in the absence of exogenous fibrinogen, conditions in which shape change but not aggregation can occur, also led to a rapid increase in actin polymerization. Thus, actin polymerization and/or structural reorganization may be necessary in some platelet functions.

Since filopodia produced by activated platelets often contain bundles of actin filaments, our finding of increased actin polymerization following thrombin activation may have direct bearing on the mechanism of platelet filopod formation. Pollard, et al. (1977) have considered two possibilities; either that the actin in filopodia of activated platelets comes from preformed filaments or that actin polymerization is necessary for filopodia formation. Previously it has been difficult to distinguish between these possibilities because of the uncertainties of actin filament quantitation by electron microscopy (Pollard, 1976). Our finding that actin is polymerized following thrombin activation suggests that actin filaments used for filopodia formation come from newly formed filaments. Nachmias, et al. (1977) made a similar conclusion by examining the effect of local anesthetics on actin polymerization. They showed that while lidocaine-treated platelets lacked filopodia and did not have recognizable filaments after Triton extraction, filopodia and filaments did form when the drug was removed, prompting these authors to suggest that filament assembly may also take place during normal activation of discoid platelets. The data, however, provide no information as to whether actin is added to filaments in filopodia or if filaments are formed in the central regions of the platelet and subsequently extended into filopodia. Both alternatives have been observed in the acrosome process of sperm, another reaction dependent upon the extrusion of actin filaments from a cell body (Tilney, 1975).

AGGREGATION SITES ON THE PLATELET MEMBRANE

The cytoskeletons of activated platelets, i.e., platelets activated with thrombin in the presence of EDTA to prevent aggregation, do not show any apparent relationship to each other - they are disperse in the Triton extraction medium. We have found, however, that when thrombin-aggregated platelets are extracted with Triton, the resulting cytoskeletal structures remain aggregated. This rather surprising observation has permitted the direct identification of platelet membrane aggregation sites. We asked, if the cytoskeletons of aggregated platelets remain aggregated, what is holding them together? Either the filamentous material in each structure is interacting directly with the filaments in an adjacent structure or the interaction is mediated by a membrane component(s). If a membrane component mediates this interaction, it might be associated with the cytoskeletons of aggregated platelets.

To detect any membrane surface proteins and glycoproteins in the cytoskeletal preparation, intact platelets were radiolabeled with ^{125}I by lactoperoxidase-catalyzed iodination (Phillips, 1972). We found that essentially none of the labeled membrane surface proteins and glycoproteins were retained either with the cytoskeletons from washed, control platelets or from thrombin-activated platelets. In contrast, when thrombin-aggregated platelets were Triton extracted, two glycoproteins, IIb and III, were selectively retained with the aggregated cytoskeletons. The selective retention of glycoproteins IIb and III with aggregated cytoskeletons appears to result from the macromolecular associations of these glycoproteins with adjacent platelets on the outer membrane surface and actin cables on the inner membrane surface.

Glycoproteins IIb and III are major membrane glycoproteins which appear to be noncovalently associated as an intramembranous complex (see Phillips, 1980, and refs. therein). Several other observations support the conclusion that glycoproteins IIb and III are aggregation sites on the membrane surface. First, glycoproteins IIb and III are deficient in the platelets of patients with Glanzmann's thrombasthenia (Phillips and Agin, 1977b). Although this deficiency is observed in the platelets from all patients yet examined, variable expression is observed as would be expected with a genetic disorder. The deficiency of glycoproteins IIb and III on thrombasthenic platelets appears to be related to the inability of these platelets to aggregate. Second, Fab´ fragments of an antibody with apparent specificity toward glycoprotein IIb inhibit aggregation of normal platelets (Degos, et al., 1975).

Although the glycoprotein IIb/III complex appears to be implicated as an aggregation site on the membrane, it is not known how these glycoproteins perform this function. Do these glycoproteins interact with complimentary molecules on adjoining membrane surfaces, or do they interact directly with other IIb and III molecules? Are these interactions mediated by polyvalent, extracellular molecules that bridge interacting cells? What is the role of carbohydrate in the function of the aggregation sites? Is the mobility or lateral position of the glycoprotein IIb/III complex affected by aggregation or by aggregating stimuli?

We have recently developed a membrane binding assay which should prove useful in addressing these questions. This assay measures the binding of radiolabeled platelet plasma membranes to control and thrombin-activated platelets by separating platelets from solution by rapid centrifugation through 27% sucrose and determining the amount of radioactive membranes associated with the platelets. Using this method, we have shown that purified membranes have functional aggregation sites and that thrombin-activated platelets have increased expression of aggregation receptors. Future work with this system is designed to delineate the structure/function relationships of specific membrane components, particularly the glycoprotein IIb/III complex, as aggregation sites.

REFERENCES

Bell, R.L., Kennerly, D.A., Stanford, N., and Majerus, P.W., 1979. Diglyceride lipase: a pathway for arachidonate release from human platelets. Proc. Natl. Acad. Sci. (US), 76, 3238-3241.

Bettex-Galland, M., and Lüscher, E.F., 1965. Thrombosthenin, the contractile protein from blood platelets and its relation to other contractile proteins, in Advances in Protein Chemistry (Ed. Anfinsen, et al.), vol. 20, pp 1-35. Academic Press.

Bray, D., and Thomas, C., 1976. Unpolymerized actin in fibroblasts and brain. J. Molec. Biol., 105, 527-544.

Dabrowska, R., Sherry, J.M.F., Aromatorio, D.K., and Hartshorne, D.J., 1978. Modulator protein as a component of the myosin light chain kinase from chicken gizzard. Biochemistry, 17, 253-258.

Daniel, J.L., Holmsen, H., and Adelstein, R.S., 1977. Thrombin-stimulated myosin phosphorylation in intact platelets and its possible involvement in secretion. Thromb. Haemostasis, 38, 984-989.

Davey, M.G., and Lüscher, E.F., 1967. Actions of thrombin and other coagulant and proteolytic enzymes on blood platelets. Nature (Lond.), 216, 857-858.

Degos, L, Dautigny, A., Brouet, J.C., Colombani, M., Ardaillous, N., Caen, J.P., and Colombani, J., 1975. A molecular defect in thrombastenic platelets. J. Clin. Invest., 56, 236-240.

Ganguly, P., 1974. Binding of thrombin to human platelets. Nature (Lond.), 247, 306-307.

Haslam, R.J., Lynham, J.A., and Fox, J.E.B., 1979. Effects of collagen, ionophore A23187 and prostaglandin E1 on the phosphorylation of specific proteins in blood platelets. Biochem. J., 178, 397-406.

Huang, E.M., and Detwiler, T.C., 1980. Reassessment of the evidence for the role of secreted ADP in biphasic platelet aggregation. Mechanism of inhibition by creatine phosphate plus creatine phosphokinase. J. Lab. Clin. Med., 95, 59-68.

Kinlough-Rathbone, R.L., Packham, M.A., Reimers, H.-J., Cazenave, J.-P., and Mustard, J.F., 1977. Mechanisms of platelet shape change, aggregation, and release induced by collagen, thrombin, or A23187. J. Lab. Clin. Med., 90, 707-719.

Lloyd, J.V., and Mustard, J.F., 1974. Changes in ^{32}P-content of phosphatidic acid and the phosphoinositides of rabbit platelets during aggregation induced by collagen or thrombin. Br. J. Haematol., 26, 243-253.

Lüscher, E.F., and Massini, P., 1975. Common pathways of membrane reactivity after stimulation of platelets by different agents. Biochemistry and Pharmacology of Platelets, Ciba Foundation Symposium 35, pp 5-21, Elsevier.

Lyons, R.M., Stanford, N., and Majerus, P.W., 1975. Thrombin-induced protein phosphorylation in human platelets. J. Clin. Invest., 56, 924-936.

Martin, B.M., Feinman, R.D., and Detwiler, T.C., 1975. Platelet stimulation by thrombin and other proteases. Biochemistry, 14, 1308-1314.

Michell, R.H., 1975. Inositol phospholipids and cell surface receptor function. Biochim. Biophys. Acta, 415, 81-147.

Miletich, J.P., Jackson, C.M., and Majerus, P.W., 1977. Interaction of coagulation Factor Xa with human platelets. Proc. Natl. Acad. Sci. (US), 74, 4033-4036.

Nachmias, V., Sullender, J., and Asch, A., 1977. Shape and cytoplasmic filaments in control and lidocaine-treated human platelets. Blood, 50, 39-53.

Niewiarowski, S., Kirby, E.P., Brudzynski, T.M., and Stocker, K., 1979. Thrombocytin, a serine protease from Bothrops atrox venom. 2. Interaction with platelets and plasma-clotting factors. Biochemistry, 18, 3570-3577.

Phillips, D.R., 1972. Effects of trypsin on the exposed polypeptides and glycoproteins in the human platelet membrane. Biochemistry, 11, 4582-4588.

Phillips, D.R., and Agin, P.P., 1974. Thrombin substrates and the proteolytic site of thrombin action on human platelet plasma membranes. Biochim. Biophys. Acta, 352, 218-227.

Phillips, D.R., and Agin, P.P., 1977a. Platelet plasma membrane glycoproteins. Identification of a proteolytic substrate for thrombin. Biochem. Biophys. Res. Commun., 75, 940-947.

Phillips, D.R., and Agin, P.P., 1977b. Platelet membrane defects in Glanzmann's thrombasthenia. Evidence for decreased amounts of two major glycoproteins. J. Clin. Invest., 60, 535-545.

Phillips, D.R., 1980. An evaluation of membrane glycoproteins in platelet adhesion and aggregation, in Progress in Hemostasis and Thrombosis (Ed. T.H. Spaet), vol. 5., in press. Grune and Stratton.

Phillips, D.R., Jennings, L.K., and Edwards, H.H., 1980. Identification of membrane proteins mediating the interaction of human platelets. J. Cell Biol., in press.

Pollard, T.D., 1976. The role of actin in the temperature-dependent gelation and contraction of extracts of Acanthamoeba. J. Cell Biol., 68, 579-601.

Pollard, T.D., Fujiwara, K., Handin, R., and Weiss, G., 1977. Contractile proteins in platelet activation and contraction. Ann. N.Y. Acad. Sci., 283, 218-236.

Tilney, L.G., 1975. Actin filaments in the acrosomal reaction of Limulus sperm. J. Cell Biol., 64, 289-310.

Tollefsen, D.M., Feagler, J.R., and Majerus, P.W., 1974. The binding of thrombin to the surface of human platelets. J. Biol. Chem., 249, 2646-2651.

White, J.G., 1968. Fine structural alterations induced in platelets by adenosine diphosphate. Blood, 31, 604-622.

Workman, E.F., White, G.C., II, and Lundblad, R.L., 1976. Platelet-thrombin interactions as assessed by affinity chromatography. Thromb. Res., 9, 491-503.

Workman, E.F., Jr., White, G.C., II, and Lundblad, R.L., 1977. Structure-function relationships in the interaction of α-thrombin with blood platelets. J. Biol. Chem., 252, 7118-7123.

Zucker-Franklin, D., Nachman, R.L., Marcus, A.J., 1967. Ultrastructure of thrombosthenin, the contractile protein of human blood platelets. Science, 157, 945-946.

THE PLATELET THROMBIN RECEPTOR

Thomas C. Detwiler and Sang William Tam

Department of Biochemistry,
S.U.N.Y. Downstate Medical Center
Brooklyn, New York 11203   U.S.A.

ABSTRACT

The activation of platelets by thrombin has the characteristics of an agonist-receptor equilibrium reaction. Neither the nature of the interaction of thrombin with its receptor nor the changes in the receptor that lead to generation of a signal are known. Two recent observations suggest possible approaches to the study of the receptor processing that generates the signal. First, bound thrombin becomes more slowly dissociable with time, suggesting a change in the nature of the thrombin-receptor complex; this transition is observed only with active thrombin. Second, pre-treatment of platelets with chymotrypsin results in a long lag before the platelet response to thrombin. While the rate of binding is not affected, hirudin can inhibit if added any time during the lag, suggesting that the chymotrypsin-sensitive step involves coupling of binding to signal generation.

INTRODUCTION

Thrombin is one of the most potent platelet agonists. It is difficult to quantitate this potency for platelets in plasma, which contains high concentrations of protease inhibitors as well as the potential for generating more thrombin, but with platelets suspended in buffer, maximum activation can be observed with thrombin concentrations of 2-4 nM, well below the concentration of thrombin required for appreciable fibrin formation ($K_m \simeq 1$ μM) (Fenton et al., 1979). Thrombin is also a powerful platelet agonist; for example, no other "physiological" platelet agonist (or combination of agonists) at any concentration can cause as much secretion or prostaglandin synthesis.

The mechanism of the thrombin-platelet interaction is an intriguing problem. While it is tempting to assume that thrombin catalyzes the hydrolysis of specific surface proteins, such a mechanism has not been proved, and there are several reasons to question a simple catalytic mechanism. We have suggested, instead, that the thrombin-platelet interaction is more nearly analogous to a hormone-receptor reaction than to an enzyme-substrate reaction. The basis of this suggestion is briefly outlined below, and recent explorations into the nature of the processing of the thrombin-receptor complex are described.

SUMMARY OF WORK LEADING TO CURRENT STUDIES.

Initial studies in our lab involved analyses of the kinetics of the thrombin-platelet reaction, monitoring secretion of either Ca^{2+} or ATP as the most readily quantifiable parameter of platelet activation (Detwiler and Feinman, 1973a,b). Two of the conclusions from these initial studies are important here. The first conclusion was that the reaction was fast. With a concentration of thrombin that gave half maximal secretion, the thrombin-dependent processes (those that were inhibited by hirudin) were complete within about 15 sec; with higher concentrations of thrombin this time was reduced to only a few seconds. This observation should be kept in mind when designing the interpreting studies of the thrombin-platelet reaction; only reactions that occur very quickly can be considered to cause platelet activation. This also might be considered the best evidence that platelet activation results from the action of thrombin on the surface, since it doesn't seem to allow time for internalization.

The second conclusion was that at low concentrations of thrombin the extent of platelet activation was a function of thrombin concentration but was independent of the time of incubation of platelets with thrombin. This was considered inconsistent with a simple enzyme-catalzyed mechanism, and it was suggested instead that platelet stimulation was the consequence of receptor occupancy, in analogy with hormone-receptor reactions. At the time, tight binding of thrombin to receptors, with essentially no turnover, was envisioned. Thus, it was considered that the dependence of the extent of activation on thrombin concentration was a reflection of the titration of receptors. It was, however, subsequently shown that bound thrombin was in rapid equilibrium with free thrombin, and that at the point of half maximal stimulation, at least 80% of the thrombin was not bound (Martin et al., 1976). With very low concentrations of thrombin, unbound[1] (and fully active) thrombin was in equilibrium with platelets that were only partially stimulated (but capable of full stimulation). Thus, stimulation of platelets by thrombin has the characteristics of agonist-receptor equilibrium processes, with the degree of stimulation a function of the number of receptors occupied, which is in turn a function of the concentration of thrombin and the association constant for formation of the thrombin-receptor complex (Martin, Feinman, and Detwiler, 1975).

[1] Although thrombin binds "tightly" relative to many familiar biological associating systems (i.e., K_D for the thrombin-platelet complex is estimated to be about 1 nM), the concentration of receptors is so low (e.g., for 2×10^8 platelets/ml, there would be about 0.1 n moles high affinity sites/L) that the amount of thrombin bound will always be a small fraction of total thrombin.

In apparent contradiction to the equilibrium aspect of the reaction, it has been demonstrated i) that platelet activation requires catalytically active thrombin, ii) that the reaction is influenced by competitive inhibitors and pH as predicted for a thrombin-catalyzed reaction, and iii) that protease specificity is consistent with hydrolysis of a peptide with a basic amino acid (Martin, Feinman and Detwiler, 1975). In an attempt to reconcile these apparent contradictions, a model was proposed (eq. 1) with aspects of an enzyme-

$$T + R \overset{K}{\rightleftharpoons} TR \underset{k_{-cat}}{\overset{k_{cat}}{\rightleftharpoons}} TR^o \qquad (1)$$

catalyzed reaction and a thrombin-receptor equilibrium reaction. This model indicates association between thrombin (T) and a platelet surface receptor (R) with an equilibrium constant K. The receptor can be modified by reaction with the catalytic site on thrombin to give a modified receptor complex (TR°), with the degree of stimulation determined by the number of TR°, or perhaps by the ratio TR°/R_{total}. The essential feature of this model is that the formation of TR° is reversible, so that the concentration of TR° is dependent on the concentration of thrombin by mass action relationships. Since no dissociation of TR° is shown, there is no turnover of thrombin; that is, thrombin doesn't leave a modified receptor and go on to modify another receptor until, with sufficient time, all receptors have been modified by even a very low concentration of thrombin. Thus, the model is consistent with the observations that the extent of stimulation depends on thrombin concentration but is independent of time of incubation.

Recent research on this problem has involved two general approaches. Based on the postulated mechanism of a thrombin-catalyzed hydrolysis of a surface protein, thrombin-induced changes in the composition of surface proteins have been analysed, and, following experimental approaches used for a variety of cell surface receptors, attempts have been made to characterize (number, binding affinity, etc.) and to isolate the platelet thrombin receptor.

Numerous studies (e.g., Tollefsen, Feagler and Majerus, 1974; Martin et al., 1976) of the binding of labeled thrombin to platelets have reached similar conclusions: thrombin binds with high affinity ($K_D \simeq 1$ nM) to 200-500 sites and with lower affinity ($K_D \simeq 1$ μM) to 2,000-20,000 sites, with either negative cooperativity or site heterogeneity. There has, however, been disagreement about the rates of association and dissociation. Most binding measuremnts have involved methods (filtration with washing of the filtrate) that would only measure bound thrombin that dissociated very slowly. Using these methods, most workers (e.g., Tollefsen, Feagler and Majerus, 1974) also observed slow binding, with equilibrium established only after 15-30 min. Since, as discussed above, only very rapid binding could be considered to cause platelet activation, we measured binding after centrifugation of platelets through a non-aqueous fluid, permitting quick separation of platelets and bound thrombin from free thrombin without any re-equilibration during separation (Martin et al., 1976). We found that association was fast, with equilibration quicker than the limits of the measurement, which we estimate to be 5-15 sec.

As with any studies of agonist action, it is difficult to determine the extent to which measured thrombin binding is related to its action. Two types of evidence suggest that at least the high affinity binding is significant. The significance of binding is suggested by the fact that as binding affinity is modified by changes in the ionic composition of the medium, platelet stimulation is a function of the amount of thrombin bound, not the total concentration of thrombin (Shuman and Majerus, 1975). The high affinity sites are indicated by the fact that their K_D is equal to the concentration required for half maximal stimulation (Martin et al., 1976). On the other hand, it has been reported that while inhibited thrombin binds the same as active thrombin and displaces active thrombin from its binding sites, it does not act as a competitive inhibitor for platelet stimulation by active thrombin (Tollefsen, Feagler and Majerus, 1974). Thus, the role of measured binding in platelet stimulation must be viewed with skepticism.

PRELIMINARY STUDIES OF RECEPTOR PROCESSING

Some modification, or processing, of the receptor during or after formation of the thrombin-receptor complex is an implicit requirement for generation of a biological signal. The processing could involve hydrolysis of a peptide bond, formation of a covalent bond, a change in conformation, some combination of these, or any of numerous other changes in a receptor that could cause transfer of information to another membrane or cytoplasmic component. We have recently observed two phenomena that may offer a means of analyzing this processing of the thrombin-receptor complex.

<u>Dissociation rates decrease with time of incubation</u>. We have been concerned with the rates of association and dissociation of thrombin-platelet complexes for several years, and we previously reported that part of the bound thrombin became only slowly dissociable after incubation for 30 min, an observation made by measuring the amount of bound thrombin at intervals after dilution of a mixture of thrombin and platelets (Detwiler and Wasiewski, 1977). Since large dilutions are necessary to get substantial dissociation, this is a rather awkward assay. It has been observed that hirudin, a high affinity thrombin inhibitor, completely blocks saturable (specific) binding but has no effect on non-saturable (non-specific) binding (Ganguly and Sonnichsen, 1976; Tam and Detwiler, 1978). We observed that when hirudin was added to a platelet suspension after thrombin, the thrombin bound to saturable sites dissociated quickly (Tam, Fenton and Detwiler, 1979). Thus, addition of hirudin permitted a simple way to follow the dissociation of thrombin-receptor complexes.

The effect of addition of hirudin to a thrombin-platelet mixture is shown in Fig. 1. As previously reported (Martin et al., 1976), the amount of bound thrombin was essentially constant after 5 or 10 sec of its addition, consistent with the known rapid platelet activation by thrombin. When hirudin was added 5 sec after thrombin, all of the saturable binding was dissociated within about 15 sec. But if

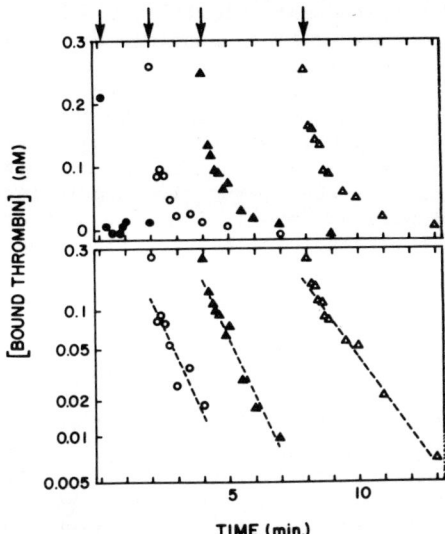

Fig. 1. Hirudin-induced dissociation of thrombin from platelets. Platelets were incubated with 4 nM ^{125}I-thrombin before adding 5 units/ml of hirudin after either 5 sec, 2, 4 or 8 min (arrows). Bound thrombin represents only saturable binding (total bound minus bound in the presence of an excess of unlabeled thrombin).

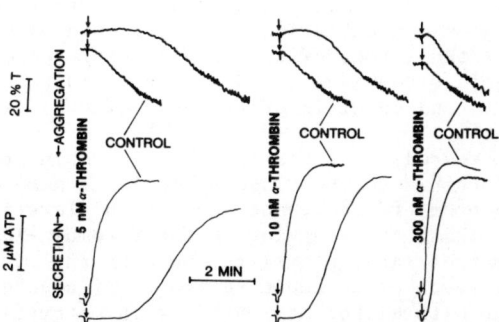

Fig. 2. Thrombin-induced aggregation and secretion by control platelets and by platelets pre-treated with 1 μM chymotrypsin for 10 min. Aggregation and secretion were measured as described by Charo, Feinman and Detwiler, 1977.

hirudin was not added until 2 min after thrombin, about 30% of the bound thrombin dissociated more slowly; the slowly dissociable component increased to about 80% of saturable binding by 8 min. Thus, while the total amount of bound thrombin did not change over the 8 min period, there was a change in the nature of the binding from dissociation too rapid to measure to dissociation with a first order rate constant of about 10^{-2} sec^{-1}. This change to a more slowly dissociable form was not observed with inhibited thrombin. It is thus possible that the slowly dissociable form represents a physiologically significant processing of the thrombin-receptor complex. On the other hand, the change is considerably slower than the actual platelet activation, so it is possible that the more slowly dissociable state is a <u>consequence</u>, not a <u>cause</u> of platelet activation by thrombin.

<u>Binding of thrombin is coupled to signal generation by a chymotrypsin-sensitive mechanism</u>. Since chymotrypsin was known to catalyze rather extensive hydrolysis of platelet surface proteins but not to stimulate platelets or to block stimulation by subsequent addition of thrombin (Martin and Detwiler, unpublished observations), we explored the possibility that it could be a useful probe of surface proteins involved in thrombin receptor function. Preliminary experiments revealed that chymotrypsin treatment of platelets caused them to respond to subsequent addition of thrombin with an uncharacteristic long lag (Fig. 2). This effect, which could largely be overcome by very high concentrations of thrombin, was observed only with stimulation by thrombin; it was not observed with ADP, epinephrine, collagen or the ionophore A23187, and it was observed to only a very slight extent with stimulation by trypsin or γ-thrombin (Tam, Fenton and Detwiler, 1980).

The dramatic increase in the lag of thrombin-induced responses was observed with short incubations with low concentrations of chymotrypsin. The maximum lag was observed after a 2 min incubation of platelets with 1 μM chymotrypsin, and only after longer incubations with much higher concentrations (e.g., 10 min with 50 μM) was inhibition of the extent of thrombin-induced responses seen. Thus, the long lag in thrombin-induced responses must have resulted from rather limited and specific proteolysis of the platelet surface.

The observed responses of platelets to thrombin presumably follow binding of thrombin to the platelet surface, some change in a thrombin receptor/effector, and changes in platelet regulatory messengers. Thus, the long lag in the thrombin-induced responses by chymotrypsin-treated platelets could be the result of modifications at the level of thrombin action or of subsequent steps. We observed that with either untreated or chymotrypsin-treated platelets, addition of hirudin at any time prior to the beginning of secretion caused essentially complete inhibition, whereas addition after the beginning of secretion had little effect. We conclude that the long lag observed with chymotrypsin-treated platelets involves the action of thrombin, not subsequent steps. We were not able to detect differences in the rate of binding or in the number or affinities of high affinity binding sites. While interpretation of binding studies is complicated by uncertainty whether the measured binding is directly related to platelet activation, the binding studies together with the hirudin experiments described above suggest that chymotrypsin modifies a step between the initial interaction of thrombin with platelets (the binding step) and the generation of the signal.

We consider it significant that chymotrypsin treatment has little effect on the platelet response to γ-thrombin or trypsin, and that the pattern of the chymotrypsin-treated platelet response to α-thrombin is similar to that of untreated platelets to γ-thrombin or trypsin. It appears that chymotrypsin-treated platelets have lost the advantage normally conferred to α-thrombin due, presumably, to a specific recognition site involved in high affinity binding. While this high affinity binding is not essential for reaction with the signal generating site, it appears to greatly facilitate the reaction. Chymotrypsin appears to disconnect the binding and signal generating aspects of the thrombin receptor.

Conclusions. Without purification of the thrombin receptor, a formidable task because there is apparently so little of it and because there is presently no assay for it except in intact platelets, the mechanism by which thrombin modifies the receptor to generate the biological signal can be studied only indirectly. Two approaches to these studies are described. Measurement of dissociation of bound thrombin by hirudin revealed a thrombin-induced modification of the receptor, either directly or through a change in environment accompanying platelet activation. Limited proteolysis of the platelet surface appears to partially uncouple the initial thrombin-platelet binding from the subsequent processing of the receptor (or effector) that leads to signal generation.

REFERENCES

Charo, I.F., Feinman, R.D., and Detwiler, T.C., 1977. Interrelations of Platelet Aggregation and Secretion. J. Clin. Invest., 60, 866-873.
Detwiler, T.C., and Feinman, R.D., 1973a. Kinetics of the thrombin-induced release of Ca(II) by platelets. Biochemistry, 12, 282-289.
Detwiler, T.C., and Feinman, R.D., 1973b. Kinetics of the thrombin-induced release of ATP by platelets. Comparison with release of calcium. Biochemistry, 12, 2462-2467.
Detwiler, T.C., and Wasiewski, W.W., 1977. The equilibrium reaction of thrombin with platelets, in Chemistry and Biology of Thrombin (Eds. Lundblad, Fenton and Mann), pp. 465-478, Ann Arbor Science, Ann Arbor.
Fenton, J.W. II, Landis, B.H., Walz, D.A., Bing, D.H., Feinman, R.D., Zabinski, M.P., Sonder, S.A., Berliner, L.J., and Finalyson, J.S., 1979. Human thrombin: preparative evaluation, structural properites and enzymic specificity, in The Chemistry and Physiology of the Human Plasma Proteins (ed. Bing) pp. 151-183, Pergamon Press, New York.
Ganguly, P., and Sonnichsen, W.J., 1976. Binding of thrombin to

human platelts and its possible significance. Brit. J. Haematol., 34, 291-301.

Martin, B.M., Feinman, R.D., and Detwiler, T.C., 1975. Platelet stimulation by thrombin and other proteases. Biochemistry, 14, 1308-1314.

Martin, B.M., Wasiewski, W.W., Fenton, J.W. II, and Detwiler, T.C., 1976. Equilibrium binding of thrombin to platelets. Biochemistry, 15, 4886-4893.

Shuman, M.A., and Majerus, P.W., 1975. The perturbation of thrombin binding to human platelets by anions. J. Clin. Invest. 56, 945-950.

Tam, S.W., and Detwiler, T.C., 1978. Binding of thrombin to platelet membranes. Biochim. Biophys. Acta, 543, 194-201.

Tam, S.W., Fenton, J.W.II, and Detwiler, T.C., 1979. Dissociation of thrombin from platelets by hirudin. Evidence for receptor processing. J. Biol. Chem., 254, 8723-8725.

Tam, S.W., Fenton, J.W.II, and Detwiler, T.C., 1980. Platelet thrombin receptors. Binding of α-thrombin is coupled to signal generation by a chymotrypsin-sensitive mechanism. J. Biol. Chem., in press.

Tollefsen, D.M., Feagler, J.R., and Majerus, P.W. 1974. The binding of thrombin to the surface of human platelets. J. Biol. Chem. 249, 2646-2651.

THE INFLUENCE OF RECEPTOR MOBILITY AND ASSOCIATION ON THE HIGH AFFINITY BINDING OF THROMBIN TO PLATELETS[*]

G. A. Jamieson, Stephanie M. Jung,
Antonio Ordinas and J. Michael Marcum
American Red Cross Blood Services
Bethesda, Maryland 20014 USA

INTRODUCTION

The binding of thrombin to platelets exhibits complex kinetics suggestive of two types of binding site or of negative cooperatively within a single molecular class of receptors (Tollefsen, 1974; Martin et al., 1975).

We have considered that the latter situation might arise from the ability of receptors to interact with one another in the plane of the platelet membrane and have utilized two different approaches to study this. In the first, we have studied the effect of modifying the membrane microviscosity of platelets on the binding of thrombin and, in the second, we have utilized lectins and chemical crosslinking agents to maintain glycoprotein receptors in close proximity to each other.

RESULTS

<u>Liposome Studies</u>. Platelets were modified in their membrane composition with respect to cholesterol and phospholipid by incubation with appropriate liposomes (Shattil et al., 1975) and their ability to bind thrombin was studied using a centrifugal technique (Chuang et al., 1977). Under these conditions, the cholesterol:phospholipid ratios found were in accord with published values as shown in Table I. Platelets that had been enriched in cholesterol by incubation with cholesterol-rich liposomes showed an increase in their ability to bind thrombin in the high affinity range from 3000 sites to 8600 sites while in those depleted of cholesterol, by incubation with phospholipid-rich liposomes, the number of sites was decreased to 1700 sites per platelet. Platelets which had been incubated with liposomes containing normal cholesterol:phospholipid ratios were used as controls and showed normal binding of thrombin (3000 sites/platelet). In each case it was the number of available high affinity sites that was changed while the affinity at those sites remained constant ($Kd \sim 1nM$).

---

[*]Contribution No. 490 from the American Red Cross Blood Services Laboratories.

TABLE I. High Affinity Binding to Cholesterol-Modified Platelets

	Chol:PL	nH	Kd (nM)
Enriched	1.06	8700	0.8
Normal	0.62	3000	1.0
Depleted	0.45	1700	1.0

Chemical Crosslinking. We have previously shown that platelets fixed with formaldehyde retain the ability to bind thrombin with high affinity (Okumura et al., 1978) and that the number of high affinity sites (3000) and the affinity at those sites (Kd 3 nM) is similar to that in control, washed platelets. In extension of this work we have examined the effect of glutaraldehyde, a more vigorous protein fixative and crosslinking agent. Platelets treated with glutaraldehyde showed a striking increase in the ability to bind thrombin (Table II). The number of high affinity binding sites found in the glutaraldehyde-fixed fixed platelets (34,000) was similar to the total number of high and low affinity sites found in normal washed platelets while the affinity was essentially unchanged (Kd 2 nM). In fact, low affinity sites could not be detected in the glutaraldehyde-fixed platelets.

TABLE II. High Affinity Binding to Fixed Platelets

	nH	Kd
Control	6000	1.7
Formaldehyde	4500	1.6
Glutaraldehyde	34000	2.5

Crosslinking with Lectins. Glycocalicin is a platelet surface glycoprotein which is solubilized during platelet homogenization and which has certain similarities to glycoprotein I which remains membrane bound (Okumura et al., 1976). Glycocalicin has been proposed as the platelet receptor for thrombin and its receptor function has been shown to reside in the carbohydrate-poor "tail" peptide (M.W. 45,000) rather than in the carbohydrate-rich macroglycopeptide (M.W. 120,000) portion (Okumura and Jamieson, 1976; Okumura et al., 1978). We reasoned that lectins might be used to crosslink the macroglycopeptide portions of the putative receptor while still permitting the access of thrombin.

Binding experiments were carried out using blocked thrombin to avoid complications from the platelet release reaction. Under these conditions, the amount of thrombin bound to platelets was increased 3-4 fold in the presence of WGA, Con A and the lectin from Ricinus communis but was unaffected by the lectins of Bandieria simplicifolia and Lens culinaris (Table III).

TABLE III. High Affinity Binding of DIP-Thrombin to Washed Platelets

Lectin Added	Specificity	Sites/Platelet	Kd (nM)
None		3300	4.4
WGA	GlcNAc	14100	3.9
Con A	Glc,Man	14200	5.0
Ricinus communis	Gal	11200	2.3
Bandieria simplicifolia	Gal,GalNAc	5200	3.6
Len culinaris	Glc,Man	5800	4.3

Aggregation Studies. Studies with washed platelets and unblocked thrombin were carried out to determine whether the increased binding also manifested itself as increased reactivity in the aggregometer.

The lectins of Bandieria simplicifolia and Lens culinaris, which did not affect the amount of thrombin bound, also showed no effect on thrombin-induced aggregation. Ricinus communis lectin was also without effect with respect to thrombin-induced aggregation although it had stimulated the binding of thrombin: the reason for this is unknown. Con A inhibited aggregation induced by thrombin or by ADP but the release reaction was unaffected in agreement with previous results (Schmukler and Zieve, 1974; Jones and Evans, 1976). Aggregation by arachidonate or the calcium ionophore A23187 was unaffected by Con A.

Thrombin (50 mU/ml) showed suboptimal aggregation of platelets by itself but optimal aggregation rates were obtained in the presence of WGA (5 ug/ml). Similar synergistic interaction was seen with ADP, collagen, epinephrine and trypsin and was reversible by N-acetylglucosamine (10 mM) at any stage during the aggregation response.

DISCUSSION

Taken together, these results suggest that platelet responsiveness is somehow related inversely to the randomness of receptors in the plane of the membrane. The previous studies had shown increased responsiveness of platelets to ADP and epinephrine under conditions where the membrane microviscosity was increased (Shattil et al., 1975) but this was also accompanied by changes in adenyl cyclase levels in the membrane (Sinha et al., 1977). The present work shows, at least in the case of thrombin, that the increased membrane microviscosity was accompanied by an increased availability of membrane receptors although the affinity at these receptors was unchanged from controls. Aggregation studies with thrombin are in progress.

The results with chemical crosslinking agents, although preliminary, suggest that complete crosslinking of membrane proteins may "freeze" surface receptors in a high affinity relationship and that, in fact, all low affinity binding is converted to high affinity under these conditions. A more careful examination of this system, using more selective crosslinking agents may provide information on the nature of the conversion process and the types of macromolecules involved.

The results with lectins, particularly WGA, suggest that this may be a more generalized phenomenon since its synergistic effect on the binding of, and aggregation with, thrombin were also found in the response of platelets to all the other aggregating agents which have their initial site of reaction at the platelet surface, but not with arachidonate or ionophore which, presumably, do not. The fact that this synergism is immediately reversible with N-acetylglucosamine at any point in the aggregation response, suggests that this may be a general effect on receptor association or membrane microviscosity while the inhibition with Con A appears to be a secondary blocking of sites required for aggregation rather than at the level of the initial interaction of the agonist with the membrane.

In this context, it should be noted that fluorescence polarization studies indicate an increase in membrane microviscosity during thrombin- induced platelet aggregation (Nathan et al., 1979) and that modification in membrane microviscosity can affect the clustering of receptors through translational movements (Levitzki, 1974; de Meyts, 1976) or by passive modulation leading to vertical displacement and exposure of the membrane proteins (Borochov and Shinitzky, 1976). These results suggest that membrane microviscosity may affect the initial response of the platelet to external stimuli and that changes in it may determine the course of the activation.

ACKNOWLEDGEMENTS

This work was supported, in part, by USPHS Grants HL 20971, HL 14697 and Biomedical Research Support Grant RR 05737.

REFERENCES

Borochov, H. and Shinitzky, M., 1976. Vertical displacement of membrane proteins mediated by changes in microviscosity. Proc. Natl. Acad Sci. USA, 73, 4526-4530.

Chuang, H. Y., Mohammed, S. F., Crowther, P. E., and Mason, R. G., 1977. A concise method for study of the binding of thrombin to human platelets. Res. Commun. Chem. Pathol. Pharmacol., 18, 291-301.

de Meyts, P., 1976. Cooperative properties of hormone receptors in cell membranes. J. Supramol. Struct., 4, 241-258.

Jones, B. M. and Evans, P. M., 1976. On the susceptibility of human platelets to aggregation by concanavalin A and the effect of this lectin on their response to ADP. Biochim. Biophys. Acta, 448, 368-378.

Levitzki, A., 1974. Negative co-operativity in clustered receptors as a possible basis for membrane action. J. Theor. Biol., 44, 367-372.

Martin, B. M., Feinman, R. D. and Detwiler, T. C., 1975. Platelet stimulation by thrombin and other proteases. Biochemistry, 14, 1308-1314.

Nathan, I., Fleischer, G., Livine, A., Dvilansky, A., and Parola, A. H., 1979. Membrane microenvironmental changes during activation of human blood platelets by thrombin: A study with a fluorescent probe. J. Biol. Chem., 254, 9822-9828.

Okumura, T., Hasitz, M. and Jamieson, G. A., 1978. Platelet glycocalicin. Interaction with thrombin and role as thrombin receptor of the platelet surface. J. Biol. Chem., 253, 3435-3443.

Okumura, T. and Jamieson, G. A., 1976. Platelet glycocalicin: A single receptor for platelet aggregation induced by thrombin or ristocetin. Thromb. Res., 8, 701-706.

Okumura, T., Lombart, C. and Jamieson, G. A., 1976. Platelet glycocalicin. II. Purification and characterization. J. Biol. Chem., 251, 5950-5955.

Shattil, S. J., Anaya-Galindo, R., Bennett, J., Colman, R. W., and Cooper, R. A., 1975. Platelet hypersensitivity induced by cholesterol incorporation. J. Clin. Invest., 55, 636-643.

Shmukler, M. and Zieve, P. D., 1974. The effect of concanavalin A on human platelets and their response to thrombin. J. Lab. Clin. Med., 83, 887-895.

Sinha, A. K., Shattil, S. J. and Colman, R. W., 1977. Cyclic AMP metabolism in cholesterol-rich platelets. J. Biol. Chem., 252, 3310-3314.

Tollefsen, D. M., Feagler, J. R., and Majerus, P. W., 1974. The binding of thrombin to the surface of human platelets. J. Biol. Chem., 249, 2646-2651.

SPECIFIC BINDING OF FIBRINOGEN TO PLATELETS: RELATIONSHIP
TO SHAPE CHANGE AND AGGREGATION

Marjorie B. Zucker and Ellinor I. Peerschke

Department of Pathology, New York University Medical
Center, New York, New York, USA

ABSTRACT

Platelet shape change, fibrinogen binding, and aggregation were studied in the presence of prostaglandin E_1 (PGE_1) and cytochalasin B (CB), and after incubation with metabolic inhibitors (MI). When platelets were stimulated with ADP, shape change and fibrinogen binding were inhibited by PGE_1 or MI. CB prevented only shape change, demonstrating that fibrinogen binding can occur without shape change and suggesting that ADP-induced shape change requires actin polymerization. Chilling also induced shape change and fibrinogen binding. None of the inhibitors prevented cold-induced shape change, suggesting that depolymerization of microtubules was responsible. Since PGE_1 but not MI inhibited cold-induced fibrinogen binding, metabolic ATP is more important for ADP-induced exposure of fibrinogen receptors than cold. Induction of the fibrinogen receptor by ADP or chilling, and ADP-induced shape change probably depend upon elevation of cytoplasmic Ca^{2+}. This can be prevented by the increase in cyclic AMP caused by PGE_1. EDTA and low pH prevented fibrinogen from binding to unfixed or fixed ADP-treated platelets, indicating that external calcium is necessary. Calcium is not necessary for exposure of the receptors, however, since fibrinogen could bind to ADP-treated platelets fixed in the presence of EDTA or at low pH. Platelets aggregated when they were shaken with adequate fibrinogen under all conditions in which fibrinogen was bound, except when the temperature was very low, or the platelets were fixed. Thus, aggregation requires fibrinogen binding and membrane fluidity.

INTRODUCTION

Aggregation is the <u>sine qua non</u> for the formation of a hemostatic platelet plug and its mechanism has therefore attracted considerable interest. Primary aggregation (i.e., aggregation not associated with the release reaction) can be induced by two substances which are involved in the formation of hemostatic plugs: thrombin and ADP. We will confine ourselves here to a discussion of the mechanism of aggregation induced by ADP as well as by the rather unphysiologic stimulus of chilling.

The numerous effects of ADP on platelets have been reviewed elsewhere (Weiss, 1975; Peerschke and Zucker, 1980a). It causes the platelets to change from their usual discoid shape to spiny spheres, i.e., essentially rounded bodies with numerous projections or pseudopods. This change is not only evident from observation of the platelets with a phase or electron microscope, but also from damping of the oscillations and the decrease in light transmission in aggregometer tracings made with stirred samples, and by eye from the disappearance of the "swirls" noted when a suspension of discoid platelets is agitated while being held up to a light.

ADP causes shape change in the presence of EDTA and the absence of fibrinogen. If the ADP-treated platelets are agitated in the presence of fibrinogen and enough ionized calcium, they aggregate. Finally, if enough ADP (2-4 μM) is used to cause at least a moderate degree of aggregation, the platelets secrete the contents of their alpha granules and dense granules. With ADP, this secretory process is entirely dependent on the production of thromboxane A_2 from arachidonic acid. Hence, secretion, although not the initial steps leading to release of arachidonic acid, can be blocked by aspirin or other nonsteroidal anti-inflammatory agents.

Chilling is also a stimulus to aggregation (Zucker and Borrelli, 1960; Kattlove and Alexander, 1971). Platelets which have been chilled in an ice bath change from discs to spiny spheres and aggregate transiently if they are agitated and rewarmed in the presence of fibrinogen. Since this aggregation does not occur with thrombasthenic or EDTA-treated platelets (Zucker and Grant, 1978) or in the presence of EDTA, it is very similar to ADP-induced aggregation. However, released ADP cannot be detected, and the aggregates dissociate more rapidly than released ADP could be degraded.

Mustard et al. (1978) showed that ADP-induced aggregation is associated with binding of fibrinogen to platelets. We will review here recent data obtained in our laboratory on the binding of fibrinogen to chilled platelets, the conditions under which aggregation occurs when platelets with bound fibrinogen are agitated, and the relationship of shape change to fibrinogen binding.

METHODS

Our studies (Peerschke and Zucker, 1980b,c; Peerschke et al., 1980a) were carried out with human platelets collected into sodium citrate and aspirin (final concentrations in blood 11 mM and 50 μM, respectively) and centrifuged to prepare platelet-rich plasma (PRP). Prostaglandin E_1 (PGE_1) was added (0.1 μM), and after 20 min at 37°C the PRP was brought to pH 6.5 with citric acid and centrifuged. The platelets were resuspended in HEPES-buffered modified Tyrode's solution prepared with 0.2% bovine serum albumin and no added calcium (HBMT) containing 0.3 μM PGE_1. The platelets were gel-filtered through a column of Sepharose 2B equilibrated with HBMT and diluted promptly in this buffer. They were discoid, changed shape with ADP, and then aggregated provided they were shaken with at least 0.1 mg/ml fibrinogen. They did not release the contents of their granules since they had been treated with aspirin, which has an irreversible effect on the production of thromboxane A_2.

The platelets were treated in various ways and then exposed to highly purified fibrinogen labeled with ^{125}iodine. After various intervals, the platelet suspension was layered onto silicone oil and centrifuged rapidly to separate the platelets with bound fibrinogen from the medium with unbound fibrinogen. The radioactivity was measured in the platelet pellet and the supernatant, and the amount of bound fibrinogen per 10^8 platelets was calculated. Binding was the same in unshaken samples as in samples agitated to produce aggregation; the samples were usually not shaken because it was easier to remove representative aliquots if there were no clumps.

RESULTS

The amount of ^{125}I-fibrinogen associated with the platelets reached its maximum within 1 minute. In the absence of ADP, or in the presence of ADP with EDTA or a large excess of unlabeled fibrinogen, the amount of radiolabel associated with the platelets was proportional to the concentration of fibrinogen up to 5 mg/ml, with no evidence of saturation. With all fibrinogen concentrations, more fibrinogen was associated with the platelets in the presence of 10 μM ADP than in its absence. This ADP-induced increment became larger in a more-or-less hyperbolic fashion as fibrinogen concentrations were raised and reached a maximum (saturation) at about 0.8 mg/ml (Fig. 1). The binding curve was the same with fibrinogens of different specific activities, indicating that the labeled and unlabeled material behaved in the same way. The ADP-induced increment (i.e., specific binding) was abolished in the presence of EDTA or a large excess of unlabeled fibrinogen. The amount of radioactivity associated with unstimulated platelets or with stimulated platelets in the presence of EDTA was the same as the amount associated with stimulated platelets in the presence of excess unlabeled material. Therefore, in most of the studies to be described, the amount of fibrinogen bound nonspecifically was determined from the value in samples without ADP. In experiments on binding in the cold, it was determined in the presence of 2 mM EDTA.

Platelets from a patient with the congenital disorder known as the Bernard-Soulier syndrome bound fibrinogen in a normal manner. Platelets from 3 patients with thrombasthenia, and platelets from normal subjects which had been incubated at 37°C with EDTA for 10 min at pH 7.8 to abolish their ability to aggregate (EDTA-treated; Zucker and Grant, 1978) failed to exhibit an ADP-induced increment in fibrinogen binding. Similarly, platelets exposed to ADP at pH 6.5 did not bind fibrinogen specifically.

Various studies were carried out to investigate the mechanism which causes ADP to expose fibrinogen receptor(s). To prevent shape change without preventing aggregation, we added 0.02 to 0.2 μM cytochalasin B (White, 1971). This did not affect fibrinogen binding

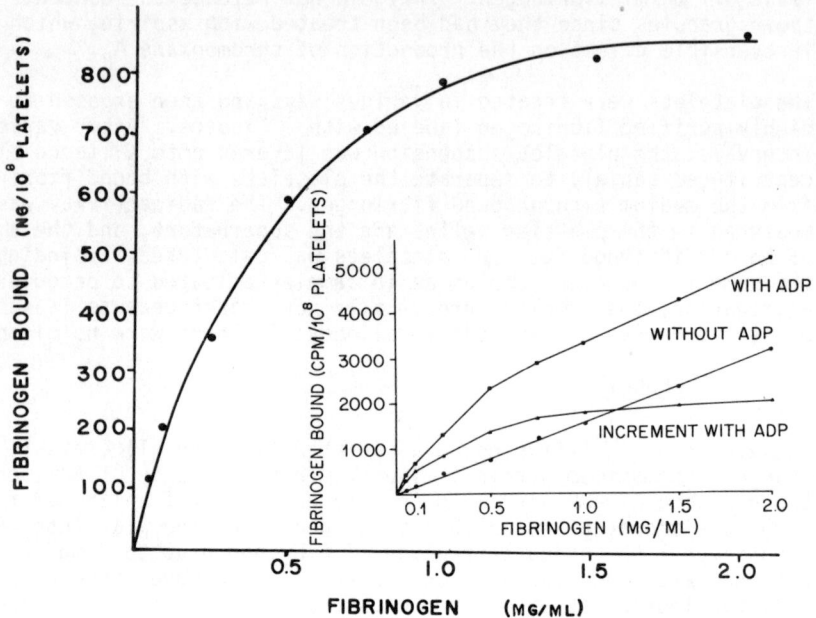

Fig. 1. Fibrinogen bound specifically per 10^8 platelets at increasing fibrinogen concentrations (2300 cpm/μg). Insert: Total fibrinogen bound per 10^8 platelets with and without ADP. Typical experiment. Taken from Peerschke et al., 1980a, by permission.

(Peerschke and Zucker, 1980b). Colchicine causes platelets to become spiny spheres because it dissociates microtubules (White, 1969); its effect was tested on the dissociation of fibrinogen from ADP-treated platelets in the presence of apyrase. With apyrase, about 75% of the platelet-associated fibrinogen dissociates from the platelets, and the platelets resume their discoid shape (Peerschke et al., 1980a). With apyrase in the presence of 208 μM colchicine, the same percentage of fibrinogen dissociated, but the platelets remained as spiny spheres (Peerschke and Zucker, 1980b). Thus, the data also indicate that platelet shape is not related to exposure of the fibrinogen receptor.

Other experiments were carried out to determine whether calcium is necessary for exposure of the fibrinogen receptor or for the actual binding of radiolabeled fibrinogen to the exposed receptor. We took advantage of the fact that platelets fixed with 2% formaldehyde and then washed could still bind fibrinogen if they were exposed to ADP before fixation. The presence of EDTA or use of a low pH (6.5) during the addition of ADP and before fixation did not affect the binding of fibrinogen to the fixed platelets, whereas EDTA or a low pH prevented binding of labeled fibrinogen to the ADP-treated, fixed, washed platelets. Thus, calcium (possibly magnesium) is not necessary for exposure of the fibrinogen receptor but for the actual binding of fibrinogen. Probably low pH prevents binding because the hydrogen ions displace the divalent cations or prevent their association with the platelets (Anderson and Foulks, 1976).

Chilled platelets do not aggregate when agitated unless they are warmed slightly. We found that they bind fibrinogen in the cold and that it dissociates rapidly as the platelets are rewarmed; about half of the bound fibrinogen had dissociated within about 15 seconds, when the platelets had warmed sufficiently to aggregate. PGE_1 (0.3 uM) and 1 mM dibutyryl cyclic AMP prevented the binding of fibrinogen and aggregation induced by chilling, but not the change in platelet shape. In contrast, these agents prevented all three responses to stimulation with ADP.

Finally, studies were carried out with metabolic inhibitors. Platelets were preincubated with 7.3 µM antimycin A (ANT) and 4.9 mM 2-deoxy-D-glucose (DG) for 20 min and then exposed either to 10 µM ADP or cold before they were used to measure the binding of labeled fibrinogen. The aggregation and fibrinogen binding induced by ADP but not by chilling were markedly decreased by the inhibitors.

DISCUSSION

It is commonly stated that ADP-induced aggregation requires two cofactors, fibrinogen and calcium. (A discussion of the extent to which magnesium can substitute for calcium is beyond the scope of this paper.) Our recent results using formalin-fixed platelets show that removal of calcium ions prevents fibrinogen from binding to ADP-stimulated platelets, but does not prevent exposure of the fibrinogen receptor. Since calcium can promote binding of fibrinogen to fixed platelets (provided they have been stimulated with ADP prior to fixation) it seems most unlikely that calcium alters the conformation of the fibrinogen receptor. Like Le Breton and Feinberg (1974), we (Peerschke et al., 1980b) failed to show an increase in the amount of calcium that became associated with calcium-deprived platelets under these conditions. Thus, it seems likely that the calcium necessary for fibrinogen binding is normally a part of the fibrinogen receptor.

Mustard et al. (1978) showed that fibrinogen not only is a necessary cofactor for aggregation but also binds to platelets previously exposed to ADP. A number of groups carried out further studies. Marguerie et al. (1979, 1980) and Bennett and Vilaire (1979) demonstrated a single class of binding sites by Scatchard analysis of their results, with apparent dissociation constants of 0.13 and 0.07 µM, and 5000 and 44,000 binding sites per platelet respectively. We (Peerschke et al., 1980a) and Niewiarowski et al. (1980) obtained evidence for two binding sites. The apparent dissociation constants were between 0.03 and 0.5 µM. The number of receptors per platelet was between 15,400 and 82,500 under optimal conditions; large differences were noted in samples from the same donor on different occasions (Marguerie et al., 1980). With different concentrations of ADP, binding was nearly maximal at 10 μM. The apparent dissociation constant calculated from aggregation curves at different fibrinogen concentrations agreed well with that obtained from data on binding of ^{125}I-fibrinogen (Marguerie et al., 1979).

Fibrinogen also bound to platelets in the cold. The amount bound at different fibrinogen concentrations was about the same as that noted for platelets stimulated with ADP. Aggregation but not fibrinogen binding apparently requires membrane fluidity since platelets fixed after ADP treatment or chilling bind fibrinogen but do not aggregate when agitated. Chilled platelets do aggregate, however, if they are warmed in the presence (O'Brien, 1962) or absence of ADP. So far, the correlation between fibrinogen binding and aggregability is perfect if the platelet membranes are sufficiently fluid, though aggregation requires agitation of the platelet suspension and the presence of more than 0.1 mg/ml fibrinogen whereas binding can be detected with concentrations of nanograms/ml. The observations are illustrated in Table I. Since fibrinogen is a dimeric molecule, it is tempting to speculate that it actually forms the "glue" between platelets. There is, however, no direct evidence that this is so.

Peerschke, Zucker and Rotman (paper in preparation) subjected platelets exposed to ADP and photoaffinity-labeled ^{125}I-fibrinogen to sodium dodecyl sulfate polyacrylamide gel electrophoresis. Reduced samples showed that the Bβ- or γ-chain of fibrinogen had bound to a membrane polypeptide of 25-35,000 daltons which was probably normally attached to a larger membrane protein by a disulfide bond.

Thrombasthenic and EDTA-treated platelets fail to bind fibrinogen (Peerschke et al., 1980a; Niewiarowski et al., 1980) although they undergo a normal shape change with ADP and a normal release reaction with thrombin (Zucker et al., 1966; Zucker and Grant, 1978). When thrombasthenic or EDTA-treated platelets were exposed to ADP plus photoaffinity-labeled ^{125}I-fibrinogen, less radioactivity was associated with the platelets. The samples were reduced and as much radioactivity was applied to a gel as was used for samples of normal platelets. Only the Bβ- and γ-chains of fibrinogen were detected after electrophoresis, with no evidence of the 80,000 dalton band seen with normal platelets. Thrombasthenic platelets exhibit deficiencies in surface glycoproteins IIb and IIIa (Nurden and Caen, 1979), and Phillips and Agin (1977) have noted that IIb normally contains a polypeptide of about 23,000 daltons (IIbβ) which is removed by reduction. These findings suggest that glycoprotein IIb is the fibrinogen receptor and that fibrinogen is attached through its β fragment.

Since platelets stimulated with both ADP and cold change their shape from discs to spiny spheres before they aggregate, we carried out experiments to determine whether shape change is necessary for exposure of fibrinogen receptors. Cytochalasin B inhibits ADP-induced shape change but not aggregation (White, 1971) or binding of fibrinogen. Studies with colchicine indicated that spiny sphered

TABLE I. Factors affecting fibrinogen binding induced by 10 uM ADP or chilling.

Platelet source or inhibitor	Response to 10 uM ADP			Response to chilling		
	Shape Change[1]	Aggreg. with fibr.[2]	Binding of fibr	Shape change[1]	Aggreg. with fibr.[3]	Binding of fibr. in cold
Normal, none	+	+	+	+	+	+
Bernard-Soulier	+	+	+	+	+	+
Thrombasthenic	+	-	-	+	-	-
EDTA-treated	+	-	-	+	-	-
EDTA present	+	-	-	+	-	-
pH 6.5	+[4]	-[4]	-[4]			
Fixed after ADP	-[5]	+	+			
Cytochalasin B	+[5]	+	+[6]	+	+	+
Colchicine	-	-	-	+	-	+
PGE₁	-	-	±			
Metabolic inhibitors	-	-	±	+	+	+

[1] Discoid platelets become spiny spheres with ADP or cold.
[2] Aggregation measured in separate samples shaken with 0.2 mg/ml fibrinogen.
[3] Aggregation measured in separate samples rewarmed and shaken with 0.2 mg/ml fibrinogen.
[4] Shape change occurred before fixation; fibrinogen binding was measured after fixation without ADP.
[5] Colchicine does not prevent ADP-induced shape change. It slowly induces shape change without ADP and, if added with apyrase after ADP-induced shape change has taken place, prevents apyrase from restoring discoid shape.
[6] Colchicine does not prevent fibrinogen from binding in the presence of ADP or from dissociating in the presence of apyrase.

platelets need not bind fibrinogen. These results may seem surprising since spiny spheres appear to have a greater surface area than discoid platelets. However, the apparent increment probably comes from the membranes of the surface-connected canalicular system, an invaginated extension of the plasma membrane that is probably always exposed to the suspension medium. For example, we showed that the same amount of sialic acid can be removed by neuraminidase from discoid platelets and from spiny spheres (Peerschke and Zucker, 1978).

Holmsen et al. (1977) summarized the evidence that shape change, aggregation and secretion are responses to increasing intensities of a single change, probably an increase in the concentration of calcium ions in the cytoplasm (see also Luscher's contribution to this volume). PGE_1 prevents the change in platelet shape and exposure of fibrinogen receptors caused by ADP. It acts by increasing the level of cyclic AMP, which in turn stimulates sequestration of calcium ions (Kaser-Glanzmann et al., 1978). In contrast, neither PGE_1 nor cytochalasin B inhibited shape change induced by chilling, reinforcing the view that it is due to depolymerization of microtubules (White and Krivit, 1967). PGE_1 also inhibited fibrinogen binding in the cold and the aggregation which occurred when chilled platelets were warmed. These responses are summarized in Figure 2.

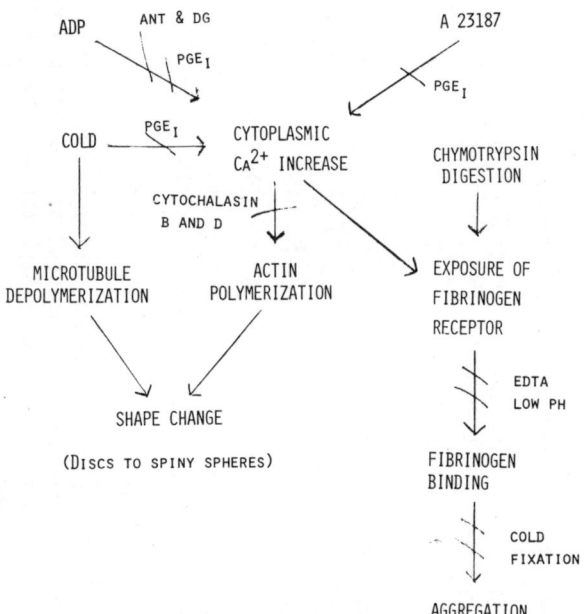

Fig. 2. Sequence of responses to platelet stimulation with ADP, cold and A23187, and response of chymotrypsin-treated platelets.

It seems likely that fibrinogen is required for aggregation induced by other stimuli of primary aggregation such as thrombin, and for aggregation associated with the release reaction such as that caused by collagen. With these stimuli, it is not necessary to add fibrinogen since the platelets can release it from the alpha granules (Kaplan et al, 1979). The release reaction is not induced by ADP unless the platelets aggregate (Zucker and Peterson, 1970; Charo et al., 1977), hence fibrinogen must be added. Thrombasthenic and EDTA-treated platelets fail to aggregate with thrombin, collagen or numerous other stimuli as well as ADP, supporting the view that aggregation always depends on fibrinogen binding.

Fibrinogen-induced binding and aggregation can be induced in an entirely different way -- by digesting the platelet surface with chymotrypsin or other proteases (Greenberg et al., 1979; Niewiarowski et al., 1980). The advantage of chymotrypsin is that it causes little if any release from platelet granules. While released ADP can enhance the reaction, it is not necessary (Grant et al., in preparation). Chymotrypsin-treated thrombasthenic platelets fail to aggregate with fibrinogen (Mustard et al., 1979), or bind this protein (Niewiarowski et al., 1980), providing evidence that the receptor is the same as that induced by ADP. EDTA prevented the aggregation of normal chymotrypsin-treated platelets but PGE_1 did not.

Platelet aggregation must be distinguished from agglutination caused by von Willebrand factor (vWF) plus ristocetin. Agglutination is readily abolished by chymotrypsin treatment. It does not require membrane fluidity since formalin-fixed platelets are active; it does not require fibrinogen; and it is normal with thrombasthenic platelets. (However, agglutination induced in citrated platelet-rich plasma from normal individuals by adding ristocetin can be followed by a release reaction with thromboxane A2 formation, release of ADP and secondary aggregation.) Platelets from patients with the Bernard-Soulier syndrome fail to agglutinate with vWF plus ristocetin and have a defect in their glycoprotein I complex (Nurden and Caen, 1979). They aggregate and bind fibrinogen normally.

Despite the distinction between aggregation and agglutination, there may be interactions between their mechanisms. Exposure of platelets to ADP inhibits vWF from binding to platelets in the presence of ristocetin (Zucker et al., 1977) and agglutinating them (Grant et al., 1976). The inhibition is also noted with thrombasthenic platelets (Cohen et al., 1975). Presumably it is a direct result of ADP, and does not require fibrinogen binding. PGE_1 can also inhibit the response to vWF plus ristocetin. Both ADP and PGE_1 are effective when added to platelets which are then fixed (Grant et al., 1976; Coller, 1979). We conclude that both ADP and PGE_1 can induce rearrangements and alterations in platelet surface glycoproteins leading to changes in the ability of platelets to bind fibrinogen or von Willebrand factor (possibly ristocetin). Binding of both vWF and fibrinogen to platelets is presumably essential for normal hemostasis. Further studies of the biochemistry, arrangement and interaction of their receptors will be necessary before we understand their mechanisms of action in vitro and in vivo.

ACKNOWLEDGEMENT

These studies were supported in part by USPHS Program Project Grant HL-15596 from the National Heart, Lung and Blood Institute.

REFERENCES

Anderson, E.R., and Foulks, J.G., 1976. The competitive inhibition by lithium and hydrogen ions of the effect of calcium on the aggregation of rabbit platelets. Thromb. Haemost., 36, 343-356.

Bennett, J.S., and Vilaire, G., 1979. Exposure of platelet fibrinogen receptors by ADP and epinephrine. J. Clin. Invest., 64, 1393-1401.

Charo, I.F., Feinman, R.D., and Detwiler, T.C., 1977. Interrelations of platelet aggregation and secretion. J. Clin. Invest., 60, 866-873.

Cohen, I., Glaser, T., and Seligsohn, U., 1975. Effects of ADP and ATP on bovine fibrinogen- and ristocetin-induced aggregation in Glanzmann's thrombasthenia. Br. J. Haematol., 31, 343-347.

Coller, B.S., 1979. Inhibition of von Willebrand factor (vWF)-dependent platelet (P) agglutination by PG E_1. Blood, 54, suppl. 1, 237.

Grant, R.A., Zucker, M.B., and McPherson, J., 1976. ADP-induced inhibition of von Willebrand factor-mediated platelet agglutination. Am. J. Physiol., 230, 1406-1410.

Greenberg, J.P., Packham, M.A., Guccione, M.A., Harfenist, E.J., Orr, J.L., Kinlough-Rathbone, R.L., Perry, D.W., and Mustard, J.F., 1979. The effect of pretreatment of human or rabbit platelets with chymotrypsin on their responses to human fibrinogen and aggregating agents. Blood, 54, 753-765.

Holmsen, H., Salganicoff, L., and Fukami, M.H., 1977. Platelet behavior and biochemistry in haemostasis, in Haemostasis: Biochemistry, Physiology, and Pathology (Eds. Ogston and Bennett), pp 241-319. Wiley, London.

Kaplan, K.L., Broekman, M.J., Chernoff, A., Lesznik, G.R., and Drillings, M., 1979. Platelet α-granule proteins: studies on release and subcellular localization. Blood, 53, 604-618.

Kaser-Glanzmann, R., Jakabova, M., George, G.N., and Luscher, E.F., 1978. Further characterization of calcium-accumulating vesicles from human blood platelets. Biochim. Biophys. Acta, 512, 1-12.

Kattlove, H., and Alexander, B., 1971. The effect of cold on platelets. I. Cold-induced platelet aggregation. Blood, 38, 39-48.

Le Breton, G.C., and Feinberg, H., 1974. ADP-induced changes in intraplatelet calcium ion concentration. Pharmacologist, 16, 313.

Marguerie, G.A., Plow, E.F., and Edgington, T.S., 1979. Human platelets possess an inducible and saturable receptor specific for fibrinogen. J. Biol. Chem., 254, 5357-5363.

Marguerie, G.A., Edgington, T.S., and Plow, E.F., 1980. Interaction of fibrinogen with its platelet receptor as part of a multistep reaction in ADP-induced platelet aggregation. J. Biol. Chem., 255, 154-161.

Mustard, J.F., Packham, M.A., Kinlough-Rathbone, R.L., Perry, D.W., and Regoeczi, E., 1978. Fibrinogen and ADP-induced platelet aggregation. Blood, 52, 453-466.

Mustard, J.F., Kinlough-Rathbone, R.L., Packham, M.A., Perry, D.W., Harfenist, E.J., and Pai, K.R.M., 1979. Comparison of fibrinogen association with normal and thrombasthenic platelets on exposure to ADP or chymotrypsin. Blood, 54, 987-993.

Niewiarowski, S., Morinelli, T., and Budzynski, A.Z., 1980. Fibrinogen receptor(s) on human platelets exposed by ADP and by chymotrypsin. Fed. Proc. 39, 543.

Nurden, A.T., and Caen, J.P., 1979. The different glycoprotein abnormalities in thrombasthenic and Bernard-Soulier platelets. Sem. Hematol., 16, 234-250.

O'Brien, J.R., 1962. Platelet aggregation. I. Some effects of the adenosine phosphates, thrombin and cocaine upon platelet adhesiveness: II. Some results from a new method of study. J. Clin. Path., 15, 446-452.

Peerschke, E.I., and Zucker, M.B., 1978. Shape change and the percentage of sialic acid removed by neuraminidase from human platelets. Proc. Soc. Exp. Biol. Med., 159, 54-56.

Peerschke, E.I., and Zucker, M.B., 1980a. Effects of ADP on blood platelets, in Contemporary Hematology (Eds. Gordon, Silber and LoBue), Vol. II, Plenum, New York. In press.

Peerschke, E.I., and Zucker, M.B., 1980b. Relationship of ADP-induced fibrinogen binding to platelet shape change and aggregation elucidated by use of colchicine and cytochalasin B. Thromb. Haemost. In press.

Peerschke, E.I., and Zucker, M.B., 1980c. Insights into the mechanism of fibrinogen receptor exposure and platelet aggregation produced by ADP and chilling. Submitted for publication.

Peerschke, E.I., Zucker, M.B., Grant, R.A., Egan, J.J., and Johnson, M.M., 1980a. Correlation between fibrinogen binding to human platelets and platelet aggregability. Blood, May, 1980.

Peerschke, E.I., Grant, R.A., and Zucker, M.B., 1980b. Decreased association of ^{45}calcium with platelets unable to aggregate due to thrombasthenia or prolonged calcium deprivation. Br. J. Haematol. In press.

Phillips, D.R., and Agin, P.P., 1977. Platelet plasma membrane glycoproteins. Evidence for the presence of nonequivalent disulfide bonds using nonreduced-reduced two-dimensional gel electrophoresis. J. Biol. Chem., 252, 2121-2126.

Weiss, H.J., 1975. Platelet physiology and abnormalities of platelet function. New Engl. J. Med., 293, 531-541.

White, J.G., 1969. Effect of colchicine and vinca alkaloids on human platelets. III. Influence on primary internal contraction and secondary aggregation. Am. J. Pathol., 54, 467-478.

White, J.G., 1971. Platelet microtubules and microfilaments. Effects of cytochalasin B on structure and function, in Platelet Aggregation. (Ed. Caen) pp 15-52. Masson, Paris.

White, J.G., and Krivit, W., 1967. An ultrastructural basis for the shape changes induced in platelets by chilling. <u>Blood</u>, 30, 625-635.

Zucker, M.B., and Borrelli, J., 1960. Viscous metamorphosis produced by chilling and by clotting; failure to find specific defect of viscous metamorphosis in PTA syndrome. <u>Thromb. Diath. Haemorrh.</u>, 4, 424-434.

Zucker, M.B., and Grant, R.A., 1978. Nonreversible loss of platelet aggregability induced by calcium deprivation. <u>Blood</u>, 52, 505-514.

Zucker, M.B., and Peterson, J., 1970. Effect of acetylsalicyclic acid, other nonsteroidal anti-inflammatory agents, and dipyridamole on human blood platelets. <u>J. Lab. Clin. Med.</u>, 76, 66-75.

Zucker, M.B., Kim, S.-J., McPherson, J., and Grant, R.A., 1977. Binding of factor VIII to platelets in the presence of ristocetin. <u>Br. J. Haematol.</u>, 35, 535-549.

Zucker, M.B., Pert, J.H., and Hilgartner, M.W., 1966. Platelet function in a patient with thrombasthenia. <u>Blood</u>, 218, 524-534.

Intracellular Platelet Response

An important aspect of intracellular platelet responses is the role of the membrane cytoskeleton interaction in the resting and activated platelet. What are the factors that control the site of polymerization and the nature of the microtubule and microfilament networks? What are the functions of such networks and their relevance to the physiology of platelets? Which are the macromolecules (if any) participating in transmembrane signalling? What is the importance of the microtubule ring to platelet shape? These are but a few of the questions raised in this part concerning the platelet cytoskeleton. In addition, other intracellular responses are considered, in particular the role of prostaglandins in platelet activation. Prostaglandins are not stored by platelet but are formed as a result of platelet stimulation. The importance of arachidonic acid and its metabolites in platelet activation and their effect on the cytoskeleton proteins is discussed. The inter-relationship between platelet aggregation and the effect of inhibitory agents, such as adenosine, PGE_1, etc., and the role of cyclic AMP, are of great importance. In particular, the function of phosphorylated proteins on the mechanism of release is discussed.

Intracellular Platelet Response

PLATELET MICROTUBULE SUBUNIT PROTEINS : ASSEMBLY AND
DISASSEMBLY FACTORS

N. Crawford,* Linda A. Amos$^{\neq}$ and A. G. Castle

*Department of Biochemistry, Royal College of Surgeons
of England, London, and $\neq$ M.R.C. Laboratory for Molecular
Biology, Cambridge, England.

INTRODUCTION

Microtubular structures have become a well recognised feature of
platelet electron micrographs provided that fixation has been
carried out rapidly and at room temperature with the platelets
suspended in a medium which maintains them in a non-activated
discoid state. The elegant electron microscopy studies of Behnke
(1965, 1970a & b), Hovig (1968), White & Krivit (1967) and White
(1971a & b) have all served to increase our knowledge of the fine
structure and intracellular disposition of platelet microtubules
which are now known to be arranged, in the equatorial plane of the
discoid cell, as a well-ordered concentric ring lying just beneath
the plasma membrane, [Figs. 1a & b]. A similar arrangement is seen
in nucleated erythrocytes of birds and cold blooded vertebrates but
although present in the primitive erythroblasts of foetal liver of
mammals they appear to be eliminated from the cells at the same
time as the nucleus, (Dustin 1978).

A marginal bundle of microtubules can be identified in the platelets
of most species so far studied but the number of tubules, seen in
section in the apices of the transversely sectioned cell, varies
from two or three to as many as thirty or more. Whether these in
section represent individual microtubules in an annular array or
are simply serial sections of the same microtubule encircling the
cell many times, has not been fully established. Some evidence
supporting the latter view has been provided by Nachmias (1976) who
showed, by detergent dissection of platelets a microtubule structure
isolated as an intact single coil of three turns with clear overlap
positions [Fig. 2a].

Platelet microtubules, unlike those in cilia and flagella, are
extremely labile structures, sensitive to calcium ions, low
temperature and pressure and to treatment with anti-mitotic drugs
such as colchicine. Following receipt of a haemostatic signal at
the surface membrane, the ring of microtubules reduces in diameter
contracting towards the centre of the cell, apparently concentrating
the granular organelles within a central cytoplasmic zone bounded by
the microtubule bundle [Fig. 2b]. Subsequent to this contractile
event the microtubules rapidly disassemble and are next seen in the
fully activated platelets in a newly polymerised and different

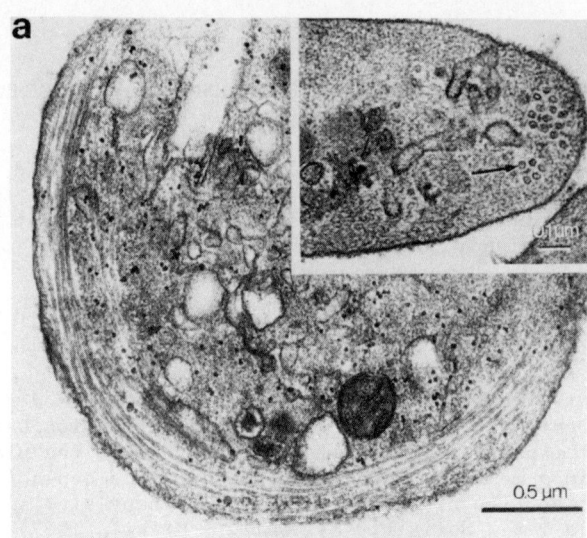

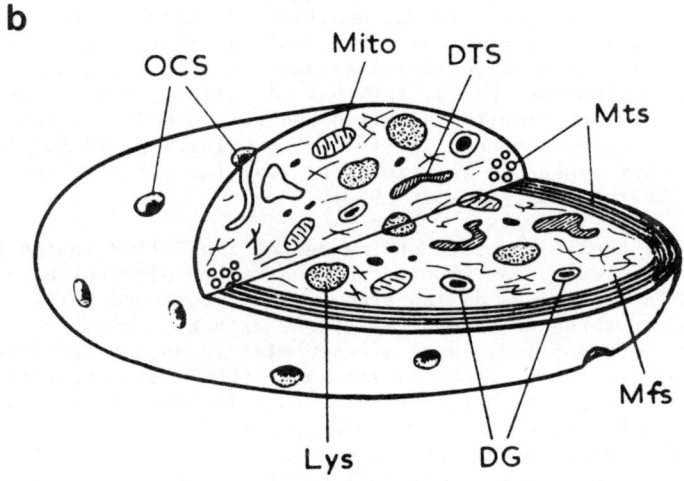

Fig. 1a. Electron microscopy of platelets sectioned in equatorial plane and in transverse section [inset] showing microtubule ring and microtubules in cross section. [taken from Behnke 1970b]

Fig. 1b. Diagrammatic representation of a discoid platelet showing location of microtubule bundle. DG = dense granules (5HT storage bodies), DTS = dense tubular system, Lys = lysosome-like organelles, Mfs = microfilaments, Mito = mitochondria, Mts = microtubules, OCS = open canalicular system.

Platelet microtubule subunit proteins 173

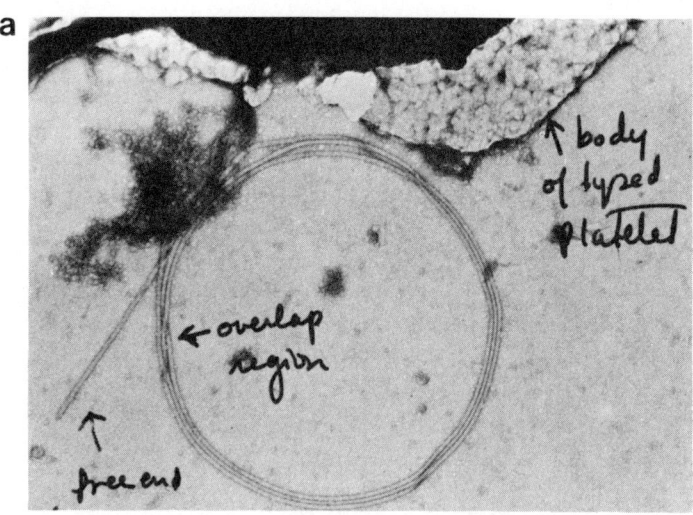

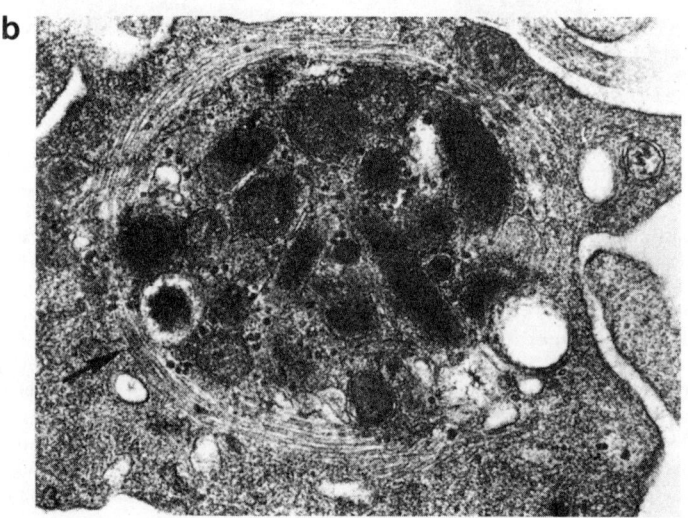

Fig. 2a. Isolated microtubule ring showing crossover points and free end. [Nachmias 1976, personal communication]

Fig. 2b. Contraction of microtubule ring towards centre of cell. [taken from White 1971b].

configuration lying in parallel array within the long pseudopodia
extending to the terminal tip [Fig. 3]. In electron microscope
studies these pseudopod-microtubules are more prominent in the wider
processes arising from the platelet surface which presumably evolve
from the initial microspike or filopodium, by a cytoplasmic flow
mechanism.

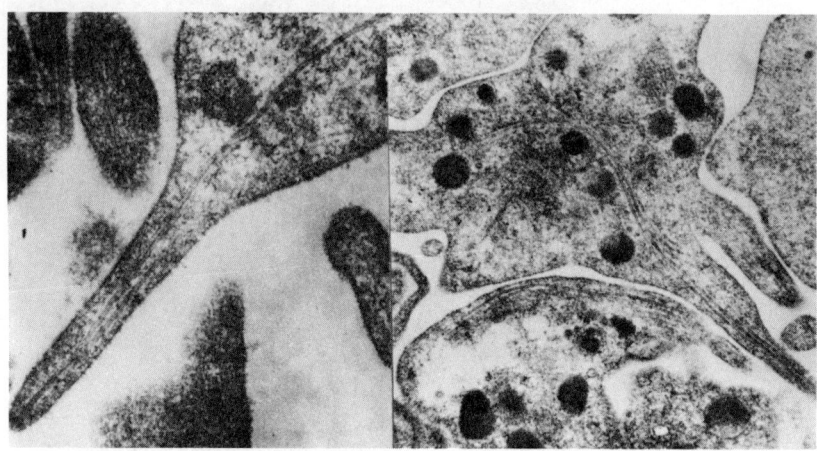

Fig. 3. Microtubules reassembled in pseudopodia of activated
platelets.

ISOLATION OF PLATELET MICROTUBULES AND SUBUNIT PROTEIN COMPOSITION

Unlike brain and other tissue, from which microtubule proteins are
readily extracted, free from other proteins, blood platelets contain
a considerable amount of actin which tends to copurify with the
microtubule proteins. Accordingly, in 1975 we developed an
isolation procedure for platelet microtubule proteins (Castle and
Crawford 1975) which, though based upon the temperature dependent
assembly method of Shelanski (1973) for brain, was modified to avoid
this actin contamination. A summarised flow diagram for this
isolation procedure is shown in Fig. 4a together with a typical SDS
polyacrylamide gel electrophoretic separation of the major
microtubule proteins which are present in the final polymer pellet
[Fig. 4b].

The gel electrophoresis patterns of platelet microtubules always
show a prominent protein of molecular weight around 55,000 together
with a number of higher molecular weight species [> 200,000
daltons]. The former subunit is analogous to tubulin, the major
subunit of microtubules of brain, cilia and flagella and the high

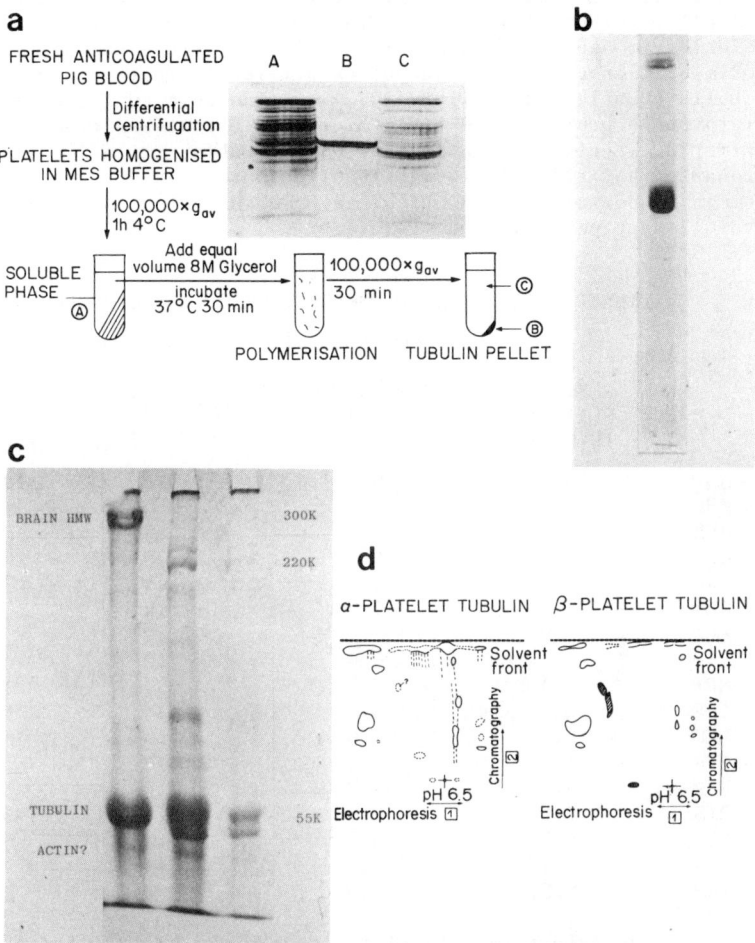

Fig. 4a. Flow diagram of platelet microtubule protein isolation with SDS polyacrylamide gel electrophoresis of platelet cytosol, microtubule pellet and supernatant.

Fig. 4b. SDS polyacrylamide gel separation of microtubule proteins after 2 cycles of assembly/disassembly showing tubulin and the two high molecular weight proteins [MAPs].

Fig. 4c. Brain and platelet microtubule proteins separated by gel electrophoresis showing mobility difference between platelet and brain MAPs and the two non-identical platelet tubulin subunits (α and β).

Fig. 4d. Two dimensional finger print of ^{125}I labelled tryptic peptides of platelet tubulin α and β monomers.

molecular weight components resemble the MAPs [microtubule associated proteins;] of brain preparations referred to later. In non-denaturing conditions platelet tubulin exists as a dimer of molecular weight of 110,000-120,000 which is the form which binds colchicine, and in the analytical ultracentrifuge the dimer has a sedimentation constant of about 6S similar to that of bovine brain tubulin (Castle and Crawford 1977). Amino acid analyses of platelet microtubule proteins and brain microtubule proteins from three different species [Table 1] show considerable similarity and it is probable that all cytoplasmic tubulins have been derived from a common ancestral protein which has been subjected to considerable evolutionary conservation.

TABLE 1. AMINO ACID COMPOSITION OF MICROTUBULE PROTEINS FROM PLATELETS AND BRAIN [moles %]

	PIG PLATELET TUBULIN	GUINEA-PIG BRAIN TUBULIN	RAT BRAIN TUBULIN	BOVINE BRAIN TUBULIN
ASP	10.4	10.0	10.4	10.6
THR	5.7	6.6	6.5	7.3
SER	6.6	7.7	7.2	7.5
GLU	12.2	12.9	12.8	12.8
PRO	6.1	5.2	5.4	7.1
GLY	15.8	7.6	8.2	7.4
ALA	8.0	7.6	7.7	7.7
VAL	7.4	6.9	7.2	6.6
MET	2.1	2.6	2.1	1.6
ILE	4.8	4.7	4.5	4.0
LEU	8.1	7.9	7.6	6.9
TYR	3.2	3.2	2.8	3.0
PHE	4.1	4.2	3.8	3.9
HIS	2.9	2.6	3.5	3.1
LYS	5.7	5.9	5.8	5.8
ARG	5.1	4.9	5.1	4.8
TRP	N.D.	N.D.	N.D.	N.D.

The values for platelets, guinea pig brain and rat brain are mean values from multiple analyses. ND = not determined

The formation of such a complex highly ordered structure as a microtubule would require regions in the protein structure of precise geometry and any slight mutation could be inhibitory towards assembly or result in bizarre microtubule forms. In discontinuous alkaline polyacrylamide gel electrophoresis platelet tubulin shows two components [53,000 and 55,000 daltons] present in approximately equal proportions [Fig. 4c]. In brain microtubules these subunits are referred to as α and β tubulins. They differ slightly in charge and it has been established by cross linking studies that dissociated tubulins exist as $\alpha\beta$ heterodimers (Luduena et al. 1975).

Comparative chemical studies of the α and β tubulins have revealed differences in amino acid analysis, peptide maps and partial sequence data. These α and β monomers of platelet tubulin also have significantly different polypeptide fingerprints when tryptic digests are made of the separated bands eluted from polyacrylamide gels [Fig. 4d].

Although the two or three high molecular weight proteins [MAPs] present in platelet microtubule preparations are similar to the dynein proteins of cilia and flagella and also to the high molecular weight proteins in brain microtubule preparations they migrate in SDS polyacrylamide gel electrophoresis much faster with apparent molecular weights of 220,000 and 240,000 [brain MAPs - 320,000 and 340,000 daltons]. More detailed studies are necessary to determine the degree of structural and functional homology between these ancillary proteins. The dynein proteins have been shown to have a divalent cation activated ATPase activity which is believed to be involved in the energetics of microtubule action during cilia and flagella beating. In our investigations no platelet microtubule preparation has had a significant ATPase activity [generally less than 10 nM Pi/mg/hour]. Unless there is some as yet unknown regulatory feature it seems improbable that this low level of ATPase could be energetically important in platelet microtubule assembly or function. Fig. 5a shows the negative stained EM. appearance of the final pellet of this "in vitro" platelet microtubule polymerisation procedure and it is clear that these structures from platelet are essentially similar in appearance to those prepared from brain showing longitudinal beaded protofilaments made up of subunits of about 5-6 nm in diameter. Negatively stained platelet microtubules show fairly smooth outer surfaces but if they are stained after light fixation with gluteraldehyde [Fig. 5b] short projections are seen at intervals along the microtubule. These surface knobs have a repeating periodicity of 960 Å and one of us [LAA] has investigated their disposition in more detail. By correlating the position of the projections with the spiral substructure of tubulin dimers previously reconstructed from optical diffraction data of flagellar and brain microtubules (Amos et al. 1976, Amos 1977) an arrangement resembling a helical super lattice decorating the microtubule outer surface seems to fit well with distribution of the projections. The projections are spaced at intervals of 12 tubulin dimers apart along each protofilament, (Figs. 5c and d).
Densitometer measurements of the proteins in SDS polyacrylamide gels of reconstituted microtubules gives a stoichometry of between 10 and 13 tubulin dimers per high molecular weight molecules and therefore these surface projections are believed to account for the high molecular weight proteins [MAPs] present in microtubule preparations. A recent paper (Sheterline 1978) in which an antibody raised to one of the high molecular weight proteins [MAP_2] from brain had been used with EM immunoperoxidase visualisation to determine the localisation of the antigen in brain microtubules [Fig. 6] confirms that at least some of the brain MAP_2 protein is surface exposed in a helical pattern. Such an arrangement could account for the surface projections on platelet microtubules too.

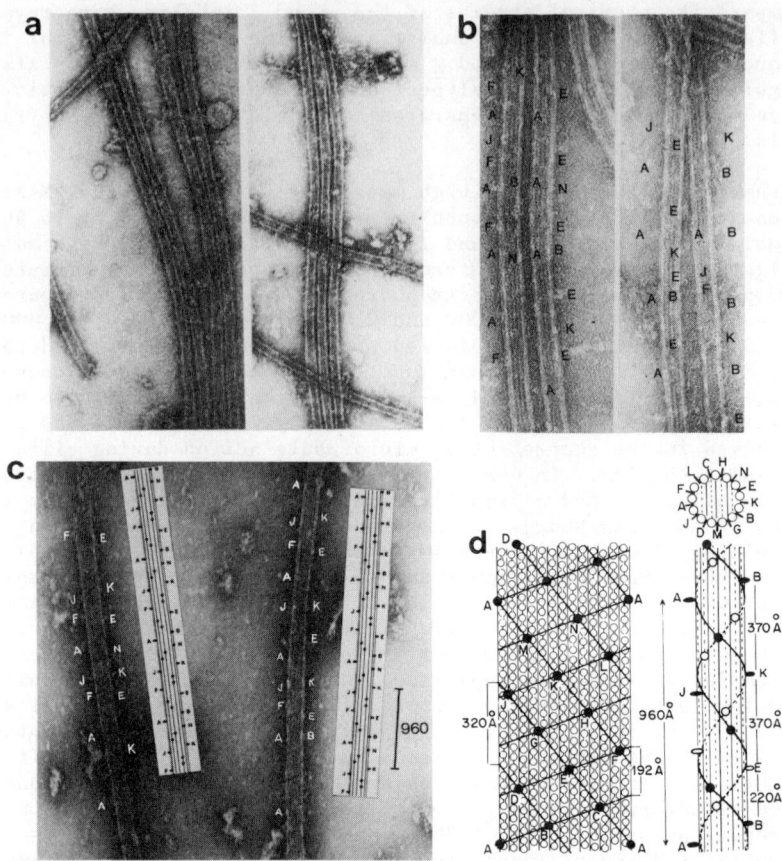

Fig. 5a. EMs, negative stained of brain microtubules (left) and platelet microtubules (right) isolated and reassembled "in vitro".

Fig. 5b. Negative-stained platelet microtubules [tubules fixed in 1% gluteraldehyde and stained with uranyl acetate] The projections show up as white spots on the tubule surface. Compare distribution with 5c.

Fig. 5c. Brain microtubules treated as in b. showing 960 Å helical superlattice arrangement of surface projections [MAPs]. The letters A to N represent projection sites associated with different tubulin protofilaments.

Fig. 5d. Representation of 960 Å superlattice superimposed on the basic tubulin lattice. The dumb bells represent tubulin dimers. Left:- Lattice opened out and viewed from outside. Right:- Rolled up to form a tube with dotted lines and projections. End on view of microtubule shown above cylinder.

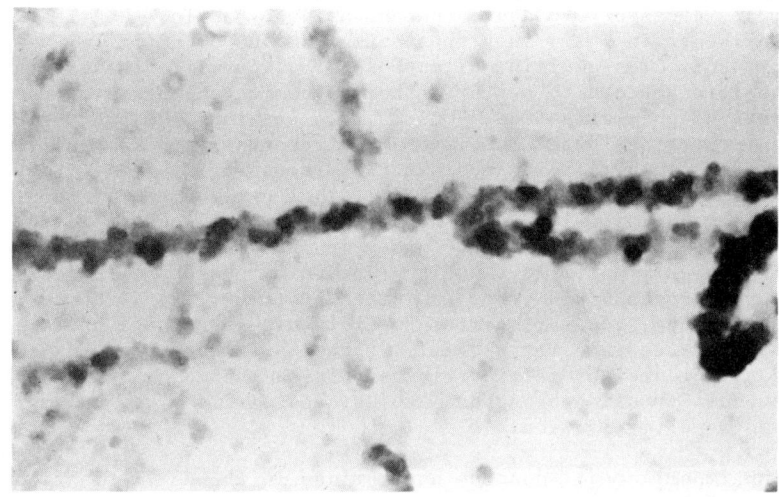

Fig. 6. Brain microtubule treated with immunoperoxidase-labelled MAP_2 antibody showing helical disposition of binding sites [Sheterline 1978].

In EMs of whole platelets sectioned equatorially, fine and often regularly spaced filaments appear to connect microtubules with each other and with the cytoplasmic face of the plasma membrane. These side arms, or bridges, may be important features in relation to general cytoskeletal properties and to the possible role of microtubules in exercising constraints upon membrane protein constituents and their freedom for movement laterally within the membrane lipid bilayer. A labile connection between platelet microtubules and the cytoplasmic face of the surface membranes could account for some of the effects seen when platelets are treated with colchicine or with the calcium ionophore A23187 both of which encourage disassembly of the microtubule polymers.

MICROTUBULE ASSEMBLY AND DISASSEMBLY FACTORS

The disappearance of the microtubules as a primary event after platelet stimulus seems to be as rapid and complete as that of the mitotic spindle microtubules at telophase in dividing cells. The dynamics of these shifts in equilibrium between a fully organised microtubular complex and a subunit protein pool have not been investigated as extensively with platelet microtubules as with those isolated from brain. The conditions which support the "in vitro" assembly of microtubules from both brain and platelets are essentially similar however, viz:- a slightly acid environment [ca pH 6.8], temperatures greater than $23°C$, normal ionic strength, a protein concentration higher than 1 mg/ml, the presence of GTP and very low concentrations of Ca^{2+}. Although low levels of Mg^{2+} appear to promote assembly of brain microtubules the addition of EDTA as well as EGTA during platelet microtubule protein isolation was found to be necessary to avoid contamination by actin, (Castle 1976). Unlike brain there is a substantial amount of actin in the platelet cytosol. The addition of sucrose or glycerol to the assembly buffers appears to act as a thermodynamic booster to increase the rate of polymerisation. One must be cautious, however, in interpreting these "in vitro" requirements since some polymerisation studies in artificial media may not necessarily relate to the dynamic situation within the colloidal environment of the intact cell. For example, under certain conditions such as in the presence of DMSO, it is possible to assemble microtubules in the test tube from highly purified tubulin prepared by phosphocellulose chromatography and free from other proteins. In more physiological conditions, however, certain microtubule-associated proteins seem to be indispensible for assembly. These assessory proteins show a constant stoichiometric relationship to the major microtubule subunit tubulin throughout many cycles of "in vivo" polymerisation and depolymerisation.

The importance of guanine nucleotides in the polymerisation process is still not entirely understood. Brain tubulin is generally agreed to have two binding sites for guanine nucleotides, one of which is more readily exchangeable than the other. This non-exchangeable site is generally occupied by GTP but whilst the presence of GTP at the exchangeable site seems to be an initiating factor for assembly, once the polymerisation process has started it can proceed with either GDP or GTP at this site (Carlier & Pantaloni 1978). The recent identification and characterisation of a nucleoside diphosphokinase (Jacobs & Huitorel 1979) associated with brain microtubule preparations may if eventually purified be useful as a tool to study these transphosphorylation reactions since the activity of the endogenous enzyme increases 7-fold during assembly. Other than an absolute requirement for GTP to initiate platelet microtubule assembly and some advantages in having the nucleotide present for the preservation of stored microtubule proteins, these transphosphorylation reactions have not been studied in platelet microtubule preparations.

A calcium chelator such as EGTA is a necessary constituent of microtubule polymerisation buffers with all mammalian tissues so far investigated and platelet microtubules are no exception in this respect. As mentioned earlier the chelation of Mg^{2+} has some advantages too. What is uncertain, however, is whether the levels of Ca^{2+} which either inhibit assembly or promote dissociation "in vitro" correlate at all with the concentration of the ion prevailing within the platelet cytoplasm. In addition to the actomyosin contractile process, the platelet contains many calcium-dependent mechanisms [ATPases, kinases, transamidases, proteases and a number of enzymes involved in cyclic nucleotide metabolism and in energy production] all competing for this second messenger cation and we know very little about its compartmentalisation and transmembrane fluxes in the platelet. Another factor which may also have a part to play in microtubule assembly dynamics is calmodulin (or CDR) the calcium dependent regulator protein. This protein is ubiquitously distributed throughout nature and present in relatively large amounts in the blood platelets (Young & Crawford 1979). It is a small molecular weight (ca 16,000) heat stable calcium binding protein which was first identified in brain as a cyclic nucleotide phosphodiesterase activating factor (Cheung 1971). It is now known to have an action in a variety of calcium dependent processes, (Cheung 1980). In most of the calmodulin sensitive systems the addition of the purified protein seems to lower the requirement for Ca^{2+} to a concentration (between 10^{-5}–10^{-7} Molar) which is more commensurate with those known to exist in cell cytosolic compartments. Our own studies with isolated platelet calmodulin added to either brain phosphodiesterase or platelet phosphorylase kinase (Young & Crawford 1979 and Gergely et al. 1979) have confirmed this low Ca^{2+} effect. Recently Marcum and his colleagues (Marcum et al. 1978) showed that brain calmodulin reduced the Ca^{2+} concentration required for brain microtubule depolymerisation, but the concentration of the regulatory protein was rather high (3.0 mg calmodulin for 2.5 mg microtubule protein) and probably outside the physiological range for such interaction. We have confirmed that such relatively large amounts of calmodulin do have a microtubule depolymerising effect but it has not been possible to reproduce this effect consistently. However, using a highly purified calmodulin we have demonstrated [Fig. 7] that microtubule assembly "in vitro" can be significantly inhibited in the presence of this protein in the microgram range.

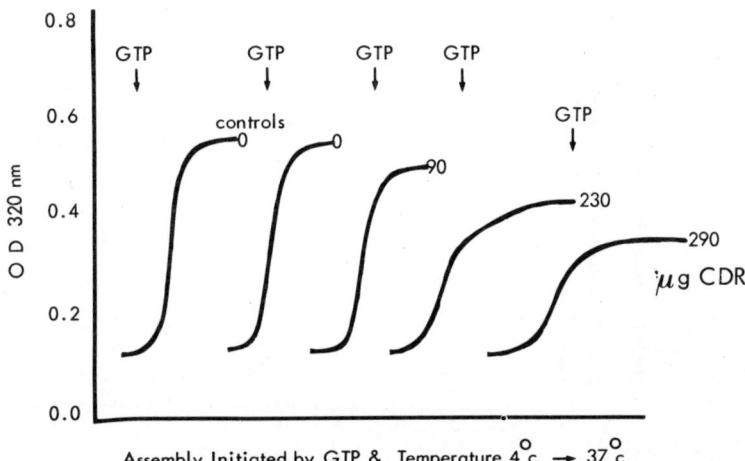

Fig. 7. Effect of purified calmodulin on assembly of brain microtubules. Conditions:- Microtubule protein concentration 1 mg/ml, optical density change recorded after GTP addition and temp. increased from $4°C$ to $37°C$.

Since in our studies with fractionated platelets we have shown that the calmodulin is substantially located in the same subcellular compartment (the cytosol) as the microtubule subunit protein pool, further studies of this calmodulin microtubule effect are perhaps warranted.

With regard to the non-tubulin assessory proteins and enzyme activities present in microtubule preparations Table 2 shows a list of those which have so far been identified in platelets and other mammalian systems. The possible location of the MAPs in the formed platelet microtubules has already been referred to and these proteins maintain a constant ratio to tubulin during cycles of polymerisation/depolymerisation. What is not known, however, is how essential they are in the assembly process itself. Like the "tau" proteins which are also identifiable in SDS polyacrylamide gels of brain microtubules they may simply associate with the tubulin dimers in a structural way but other actions as assembly initiating factors or polarity determinents are also possible. Platelet microtubules like those of brain have an endogenous protein kinase activity (Castle & Crawford 1976) which phosphorylates tubulin [Fig. 8]. In our studies using an electrophoretic gel procedure which resolves the α and β components of platelet tubulin we found that the endogenous kinase preferentially phosphorylated the β subunit.

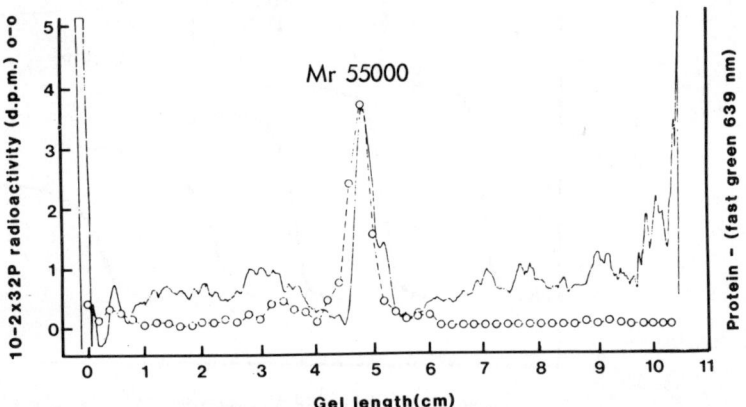

Fig. 8. Location of tubulin and protein-bound ^{32}P in SDS-polyacrylamide gel electrophoresis after phosphorylation by endogenous protein kinase. Mixture contained ^{32}P-ATP and cAMP incubated 15 min at $35°C$.

TABLE 2. MAMMALIAN (NON TUBULIN) MICROTUBULE ASSOCIATED PROTEINS AND ENZYME ACTIVITIES
(* INDICATES THOSE WHICH HAVE BEEN ESTABLISHED AS PRESENT IN PLATELET MICROTUBULE PREPARATIONS)

PROTEIN	M_r	FUNCTION	REFERENCE NO.
* MAP-1 [HMW-1] * MAP-2 [HMW-2]	350,000 300,000	PROJECTIONS ON OUTER SURFACE OF MICROTUBULES MAY LINK MICROTUBULES TO OTHER CELL STRUCTURES	23
TAU PROTEINS	55-70,000	PROMOTE MICROTUBULE ASSEMBLY	14
TUBULIN ASSEMBLY PROTEINS	66,000	ALSO PROMOTE MICROTUBULE POLYMERISATION	14
* PROTEIN KINASE	NOT KNOWN	PHOSPHORYLATE β TUBULIN AND/OR 300K MAP. ATP AS PHOSPHATE DONOR	10, 31
* ATPase	NOT KNOWN	HYDROLYSIS OF ATP – MAY BE ANALOGOUS TO DYNEIN OF CILIA AND FLAGELLA	8, 32
NUCLEOSIDE DIPHOSPHO KINASE [TRANSPHOSPHORYLASE]	NOT KNOWN	TRANSPHOSPHORYLATION OF MICROTUBULE-BOUND GDP ACTIVATED DURING POLYMERISATION	20
TYROSINE-LIGASE	NOT KNOWN	POST TRANSLATIONAL ADDITION OF TYROSINE TO THE CARBOXYL TERMINAL OF α TUBULIN	27
PHOSPHATIDYL INOSITOL PHOSPHODIESTERASE	38,000	AN ACTIVITY ASSOCIATED WITH MICROTUBULE PROTEINS PREPARED BY DEAE SEPHADEX	26

With brain microtubules, however, opinions differ on the identity of the substrate for this kinase. On the one hand, Eipper (1974) has provided evidence for β tubulin phosphorylation but others (Sloboda et al. 1975) suggest that one of the MAPs is the principle phosphate acceptor. Unlike brain we have not been able to demonstrate cAMP dependence with the platelet endogenous kinase but in other tissues this also seems to be a fugitive property and probably associated with the presence or absence of a regulatory subunit for the enzyme. A role for this kinase activity has not been satisfactorily established in assembly/disassembly studies with either platelet or brain preparations. The ATPase which is a prominent enzyme in cilia and believed to be involved in the energetics of ciliary movement is present in both brain and platelet microtubule preparations (Burns & Pollard 1974 and Crawford & Castle 1976) but its activity is so low that further work is necessary before it can be regarded as of any significance in assembly and function of mammalian microtubule systems. Other enzyme activities in the table [Table 2] are also as yet without a clearly defined functional role.

MICROTUBULES AND PLATELET SHAPE CHANGES

It is still not certain how important the microtubules are to shape maintenance in blood platelets. The marginal microtubule bundles of other disc shaped cells, bird and frog erythrocytes for example do appear to control shape but they vary in their sensitivity to experimental treatment with different temperatures and chemical agents [for review see Behnke 1970b]. In general erythrocyte microtubules of cold blooded vertebrates are much less sensitive to low temperatures than those of birds. In most mammalian platelets, low temperatures (below $10^{o}C$) result in a complete disassembly of the microtubule ring but rewarming may encourage their reappearance. If profound shape changes in the platelets have not occurred at least some of the marginal bundle may reassemble but generally the subunits appear to have been released into the cytosol pool. It is difficult to quantify such experiments since in addition to heterogeneity of the circulating platelet pool with respect to senescence and general metabolic and haemostatic competence there may well be some heterogeneity of tubulin subunits in the cytosol and what proportion of these have polymerising potential is not known. Whether dimerisation or dimer dissociation are features of the assembly and disassembly processes has also not been established. There may well be monomer-dimer equilibrium states involved in the early nucleating processes before polymer assembly. Colchicine and the vinca alkaloids promote rapid depolymerisation of platelet microtubules but it is not clear if these drugs directly attack the formed polymer or simply bind to dimer tubulin molecules in the subunit pool, thus taking them out of the equilibrium state. This would promote destabilisation and a re-equilibration by adding further subunits to the pre-existing dimer pool. A major problem is that most of the drugs and other agents which affect the integrity of platelet microtubules also interfere with certain membrane properties which are less directly related to microtubule action making interpretation difficult.

In the blood platelet most haemostatic signals to the platelet surface membrane which result in disc to sphere transformation, pseudopodia formation and release of granule stored components also produce microtubule disassembly as a primary event. Subsequently a repolymerisation process occurs with microtubules reforming in the pseudopodia and a restabilisation of the new activated platelet state is accomplished. It is significant that pseudopod microtubules are rarely seen at the early stages of microspike or filopodia formation which is to some extent reversible. Later when the pseudopodia have begun to thicken the microtubules appear throughout the length of the process to the terminal tip. It is possible that this microtubule assembly within the pseudopodia originates from some initiating site, perhaps at the tip of the pseudopod. Assembly would be encouraged by a falling Ca^{2+} gradient (tip to body of the cell) and the microtubules which form would indicate that the pseudopodia had reorganised into a non retractable state. A diagrammatic representation of the possible events which may lead to platelet pseudopodia formation and subsequent stabilization during platelet activation is presented in Fig. 9.

CONCLUDING COMMENTS

In this short review of platelet microtubular proteins some of their molecular characteristics and properties have been described in relation to our current knowledge of brain microtubules. Whilst there are many similarities there are also some significant differences not the least of which is in the way they are localised subadjacent to the surface membrane in a discoid platelet and their capacity for centripetal movement in response to haemostatic activation. Their reassembly within pseudopodia also appears to be a property not well expressed in other motile cells. Their exact function in platelets remains obscure but as part of the structural framework they have to be taken into account in relation to the control and function of other cytoskeletal equipment involved in platelet behaviour. Interactions with actomyosin subunit proteins, with constituents of surface and intracellular membranes and with important granular organelles which migrate during secretory activity are all properties deserving closer examination at the molecular level.

We gratefully acknowledge the British Heart Foundation for their generous financial support.

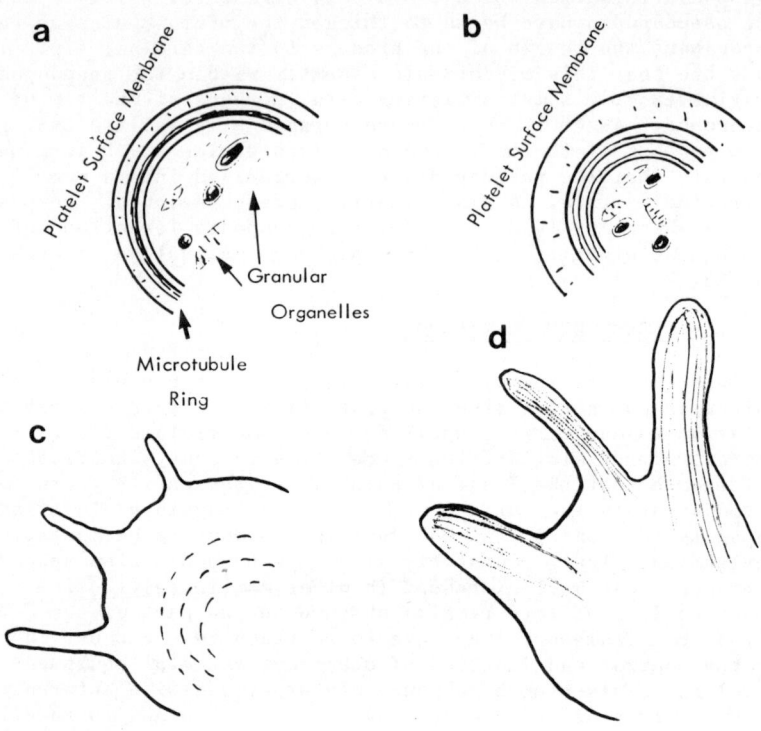

Fig. 9a. Normal arrangement of microtubules in the discoid platelet as marginal bundle lying just beneath the surface membrane.

Fig. 9b. Dislocation of bridges between microtubules and cytoplasmic face of surface membrane. Centripetal movement of microtubule bundle to centre of platelet.

Fig. 9c. Disassembly of microtubule ring and formation of surface microspikes or filopodia [possibly an actomyosin driven event, but reversible].

Fig. 9d. Thickening of pseudopods by cytoplasmic flow. Reassembly of microtubules from subunit pool [irreversible fully activated stage].

Amos, L. A., Linck, R. W., and Klug, A., 1976. Molecular structure of flagellar microtubules, in Cell Motility (Eds. R. Goldman, T. Pollard and J. Rosenbaum), pp 847-868. Cold Spring Harbor Lab.

Amos, L. A., 1977. Arrangement of high molecular weight associated proteins on purified mammalian brain microtubules. J. Cell Biol. 72, 642-654.

Behnke, O., 1970a. A comparative study of microtubules of disc-shaped blood cells. J. of Ultrastruct. Res., 31, 61-75.

Behnke, O., 1970b. Microtubules in disc-shaped blood cells. Int. Rev. Exptl. Pathol. 9, 1-92.

Behnke, O., 1965. A marginal bundle in human and rat thrombocytes. J. of Ultrastruct. Res., 13, 469.

Burns, R. G., and Pollard, T. D., 1974. A dynein-like protein from brain. Febs. Lett. 40, 274-280.

Carlier, M. F., and Pantaloni, D., 1978. Kinetic analysis of cooperativity in tubulin polymerisation in the presence of guanosine di or triphosphate nucleotides. Biochemistry, 17, 1908-1915.

Castle, A. G., 1976. Platelet tubulin : isolation and physico-chemical characterisation. Ph.D. Thesis, University of Birmingham.

Crawford, N., and Castle, A. G., 1976. Platelet microfilaments and microtubules. Chapter 6 in Platelets in Biology and Pathology (Ed. J. Gordon), Elsevier/North Holland Biomedical Press.

Castle, A. G., and Crawford, N., 1976. Phosphorylation of platelet microtubule proteins by an endogenous protein kinase. Biochem. Soc. Transactions, 4, 691-693.

Cheung, W. Y., 1971. Cyclic 3'5'Nucleotide Phosphodiesterase. Evidence for and properties of a protein activator. J. Biol. Chem., 246, 2859-2869.

Cheung, W. Y., 1980. Calmodulin plays a pivotal role in cellular regulation. Science, 207, 19-27.

Cleveland, D. W., Hwo, S-Y., and Kirschner, M. W., 1977. Preparation of "tau" a microtubule associated protein that induces assembly of microtubules from purified tubulin. J. Mol. Biol., 116, 207-225.

Dustin, P., 1978. in Microtubules, p 228, Springer Verlag, New York.

Eipper, B. A., 1974. Rat brain microtubule protein. Purification and determination of covalently bound phosphate and carbohydrate. Proc. Natl. Acad. Sci. USA, 69, 2283-2287.

Eipper, B. A., 1974. Rat brain tubulin and protein kinase activity. J. Biol. Chem., 249, 1398-1406.

Gergely, P., Castle, A. G., and Crawford, N., 1980. Platelet phosphorylase kinase activity and its regulation by the calcium-dependent regulatory protein, calmodulin. Biochim. Biophys. Acta., 612, 50-55.

Hovig, T., 1968. The ultrastructure of blood platelets in normal and abnormal states. Ser. Haematol. 1, 3-64.

Jacobs, M., Smith, H., and Taylor, E. W., 1974. Tubulin: nucleotide binding and enzymic activity. J. Mol. Biol., 89, 455-468.

Jacobs, M., and Huitorel, P., 1979. Tubulin-associated nucleoside diphosphokinase. Eur. J. Biochem. 99, 613-622.

Lagnado, J. R., Tan, L. P., and Reddington, M., 1975. The in situ phosphorylation of microtubular protein in brain cortex slices and related studies of the phosphorylation of isolated brain tubulin preparations. Ann. N.Y. Acad. Sci., 253, 577-597.

Marcum, J. M., Dedman, J. R., Brinkley, B. R., and Means, A. R., 1978. Control of microtubule assembly-disassembly by calcium-dependent regulator protein. Proc. Natl. Acad. Sci. USA, 75, 3771-3775.

Murphy, D. B., Vallee, R. B., and Borisy, G. G., 1977. Identity and polymerisation-stimulatory activity of the non tubulin proteins associated with microtubules. Biochemistry, 16, 2598-2605.

Nachmias, V., 1976. Personal communication.

Piras, M. M. and Piras, R., 1974. Phosphorylation of vinblastine-isolated microtubules from chick-embryonic muscles. Eur. J. Biochem., 47, 443-452.

Quinn, P. J., 1973. The association of phosphatidylinositol phosphodiesterase activity and a specific subunit of microtubular protein in rat brain. Biochem. J., 133, 273-281.

Rabin, D., and Flavin, M., 1977. Enzyme which specifically adds tyrosine to the α-chain of tubulin. Biochemistry, 16, 2189-2194.

Shelanski, M., Gaskin, F., and Cantor, C. R., 1973. Microtubule assembly in the absence of added nucleotides. Proc. Natl. Acad. Sci. USA, 70, 765-768.

Sheterline, P., 1978. Localisation of the major high molecular weight proteins on microtubules "in vitro" and in cultured cells. Exp. Cell Res., 115, 460-464.

Shigekawa, B. L., and Olsen, R. W., 1975. Resolution of cyclic AMP stimulated protein kinase from polymerisation-purified brain microtubules. Biochim. Biophys. Res. Comm., 63, 455-462.

Sloboda, R. D., Rudolph, S. A., Rosenbaum, J. L., Greengard, P., 1975. Cyclic AMP-dependent endogenous phosphorylation of a microtubule-associated protein. Proc. Natl. Acad. Sci. USA, 72, 177-181.

Webb, B. C., 1979. An ATPase activity associated with brain microtubules. Arch. Biochem. Biophys. 198, 296-303.

Weingarten, M. D., Lockwood, A. R., Hwo, S-Y., and Kirschner, M., 1975. A protein factor essential for microtubule assembly. Proc. Natl. Acad. Sci. USA, 72, 1858-1862.

White, J. G., and Krivit, W., 1967. An ultrastructural basis for the shape changes induced in platelets by chilling. Blood, 30, 625-635.

White, J. G., 1971a. Platelet Morphology in the Circulating Platelet. (Ed. S. A. Johnson) NY Acad. Press, p 45.

White, J. G., 1971b. Platelet Microtubules and Microfilaments: Effects of Cytochalasin B on Structure and Function, in Platelet Aggregation. (Ed. J. Caen), p 19, Masson & Cie, Paris.

Young, N. J., and Crawford, N., 1979. Isolation from blood platelets and polymorphs of a Ca^{2+}-dependent regulator protein (CDR) which activates cyclic nucleotide phosphodiesterase. Thromb. Haemostas. 42, 81.

Young, N. J., and Crawford, N., 1979. A calcium-dependent regulatory protein of leucocytes and platelets. Hoppe S.Z. 360, 1369.

PLATELET ACTIVATION AND THE CYTOSKELETON NETWORKS

C. Gitler, V. Pribluda, F. Laub and A. Rotman

Department of Membrane Research,
The Weizmann Institute of Science,
Rehovot, Israel

INTRODUCTION

There is suggestive evidence to indicate that the morphology and function of a cell depend on the nature and location of intracellular polymeric networks. In non-muscle cells, the main polymeric cytoskeletal structures are, in general terms, those of the microtubules, microfilaments and intermediate filaments. Such polymeric networks are not static structures as suggested by the term 'cytoskeleton'. Rather, it appears that cells are capable, at different stages of their development, of forming such networks at sites where they are required for specific functions. It is the purpose of this chapter to discuss briefly some of the factors that may participate in the control of the sites of polymerization and nature of the microtubule and microfilament networks that are present in normal platelets and those activated by different stimuli. In addition, an attempt will be made to define the function of such networks and their relevance to the physiology of this cell.

THE MICROTUBULAR NETWORK OF THE PLATELET

If we assume that a cell contains a fixed amount of tubulin, then the question of where microtubules are formed leads one to search for factors controlling chain initiation, direction of chain growth and control of chain termination. The studies of Behnke (1976), of White (1971), and of Nachmias et al. (1977), indicate that nucleated erythrocytes and platelets contain a ring or coil of microtubules which appears to be responsible for the discoid shape of these cells. Such a microtubular coil appears in the resting platelet to be present in close apposition with the plasma membrane (these microtubules will be referred to as *cortical microtubules*). Upon activation of the platelet, the microtubular ring appears to move from the endofacial surface of the cell towards the center entrapping within it the cellular organelles and other vesicles. It is not clear whether such a motion is due to displacement induced by the polymerization of actin normal to the plasma membrane or to an actual coil-tightening mechanism due to the sliding of apposed microtubules (see below).

In any case, it is important at this stage, even if only to speculate, to pose the factors which might control the position of the microtubule coil adjacent to the plasma membrane.

NATURE OF THE MICROTUBULE-ORGANIZING CENTERS (MTOC)

Evidence has accumulated recently to indicate that microtubules are sensitive to the concentration of Ca^{++} in their immediate vicinity (for review, see Fuller et al., 1975). Thus, an increase in the Ca^{++} concentration induces depolymerization of microtubules, while a decrease in Ca^{++} leads to their polymerization. Calcium appears not to diffuse readily within the cell (Rose and Loewenstein, 1975). This is due, perhaps, to the presence of significant concentrations of calmodulin within the cell's cytoplasm. This protein has a high affinity for calcium and might thus restrict its mobility within the cell. Furthermore, the calmodulin-Ca^{++}-complex appears to be able to control the activity of several cytoplasmic and membrane-bound systems, which in turn regulate the concentration and physiological function of the intracellular Ca^{++}.

One hypothesis has been suggested to the effect that tubulin polymerizes at sites where Ca^{++} is depleted in the cytosol. Thus, Ca^{++}-sequestering vesicles have been found to be associated with the poles of the mitotic spindle (Silver, Cole and Cande, 1980). Furthermore, Ca^{++}-ATPase activity has been found to be associated with the plasma membrane and to be part of a Ca^{++}-pump which actively excretes Ca^{++} from the cell. It is plausible to envisage that such plasma membrane-associated Ca^{++}-pumps could deplete the Ca^{++} in the vicinity of the plasma membrane, and that this could initiate the formation of cortical microtubules in platelets and nucleated erythrocytes. However, microtubules are usually rod-like in nature, so that one is faced with the problem of how a coil-like structure is formed. It is likely that microtubule-associated proteins might play an important role in the bending process and in the interaction with the plasma membrane. It is also likely that dyenin might play a role in a sliding mechanism of apposed microtubules, and that its ATPase-activity could lead to the coil having a more or less tight structure, depending on factors controlling the dyenin ATPase activity (see Nachmias et al., 1977; Phillips, 1974).

An alternative possibility is that vesicles of the 'surface-connected system' might be involved in the formation of the MTOC for the cortical microtubular ring or coil.

Irrespective of the manner in which the cortical microtubular ring forms in platelets, the next relevant question is whether it is only present to function in a structural role or whether it also plays a role in a regulatory function.

RECIPROCITY BETWEEN MICROTUBULE AND MICROFILAMENT FUNCTION

There is evidence that appears to indicate that the presence of cortical microtubules might inhibit actin-containing microfilament formation and/or function. Thus, in lymphocytes, addition of concanavalin A, which appears to induce or stabilize microtubules, inhibits the capping of surface receptors, such as surface immunoglobulins. Addition of colchicine restores the capping of such immobilized receptors. Capping is believed in some way to be mediated by microfilaments. This system, extensively studied by Yahara and Edelman (1975), suggests that microtubules prevent microfilament function. A second example is that of the amoeba-flagellate *Nagleria*, extensively studied by Fulton (1977a). This protozoan functions as an amoeba (actin-mediated functions) as long as food is available. Upon deprivation of nutrients, it undergoes a transformation to a flagellate. It forms, in addition to a flagellum, a cortical microtubular system which gives it an elongated shape. As long as the microtubular system is present, amoeboid motion is inhibited. Upon collapse of the microtubular cytoskeleton, amoeboid motion is resumed within a few seconds. This implies that the actin-mediated system was potentially present all the time in the flagellate, but was inhibited as long as the microtubules were intact (see Fulton, 1977b, for a more extensive discussion of this microtubule-microfilament reciprocity).

THE ACTIN-MICROFILAMENT SYSTEM OF THE PLATELET

It has been suggested (Edelman, 1976; Nicholson, 1976) that the mobility of surface determinants depends on their interaction with microfilaments in the endofacial surface of the plasma membrane. These authors envisaged that in the normal cell many surface receptors are attached to microfilaments. However, such a model poses many problems since the many microfilaments, that would have to exist as attached to all the various receptors, would represent a serious packing problem in the cell surface region. Singer et al. (1976) proposed that not all receptors are attached to microfilaments. Rather, some component 'X' was that associated with the microfilaments, and a receptor in order to cap would have to become associated with the 'X' component. To date no solid evidence for this hypothesis exists.

An alternative possibility appears more likely to us. It is that the interaction of effector molecules with receptors leads to a membrane state, which induces actin polymerization in the immediate vicinity of the activated receptor. This model envisages a change in actin from G-like actin to F-actin to be mediated by receptor aggregation, and the microfilaments thus formed would then couple with the receptor microaggregate leading eventually to capping. Such a model envisages the membrane as a site for a microfilament-organizing center (MFOC), similar to that discussed for microtubules.

This model requires that actin exist in the cytoplasm mainly or at least to a significant extent in a non-polymerized state. Striated muscle G-actin is known to polymerize in the presence of $\sim$100 mM KCl, 2 mM ATP, 2-5 mM Mg^{++} and a sulfhydryl compound, such as dithiothreitol at 1-2 mM. These are exactly the conditions found in the cytosol of cells. Thus, it would be expected that 99% or more of the actin in non-muscle cells should exist as F-actin. However, available measurements indicate that in most cells at least half of

the actin is present as 'G'-actin (Bray and Thomas, 1976; Tilney et al., 1973; Taylor, Rhodes and Hammond, 1976; Laub, unpublished observations studied in *Dictyostelium discoideum*).
It appeared, therefore, that mechanisms must exist within the cell that prevent actin from polymerizing. Association of actin with profilin is at least one of the means available to the cell to prevent such a polymerization (Harris and Weeds, 1978). Spectrin-like high molecular weight actin-binding proteins might also function in this respect (Pollard, 1976; Stossel and Hartwig, 1976; Weng, Ash and Singer, 1975).
In order to study the state of the actin within cells and to determine whether surface-mediated stimuli could alter the equilibrium G→F, we developed a sensitive DNAse I assay (Laub, 1980). This assay is similar, in principle, but apparently some 10-fold more sensitive to an equivalent assay developed by Blikstad et al. (1978). This assay is based on the fact that the degradation of double-stranded DNA by DNAse I is inhibited by G-actin which forms an inhibitory complex with DNAse I with very rapid kinetics (less than 10 sec). On the other hand, F-actin inhibits DNAse I activity but only upon distortion or depolymerization with a half-time for inhibition of some 5 to 10 min (Hitchcock et al., 1976). The actin in actomyosin, in the absence of ATP, is not inhibitory to DNAse I. That is, the rigor complex is not dissociated by the presence of

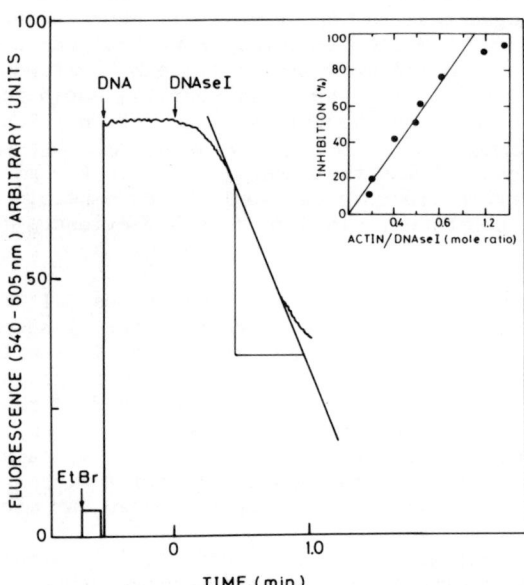

Fig. 1. DNAse I fluorescence assay. Enhanced fluorescence of ethidium bromide upon addition of DNA and decrease in fluorescence upon addition of DNAse I. Inset : Inhibition of G-actin by DNAse I.

DNAse I. However, ATP which dissociates actin from myosin leads to F-actin depolymerization by DNAse I. Our DNAse I assay is based on an ethidium bromide-double-stranded DNA complex. The enhanced fluorescence of ethidium bromide, upon intercalation into the DNA, allows the monitoring of the breakdown of the DNA (Fig. 1) by the fall in the fluorescence of the dye as its sites of intercalation are destroyed. Under the assay conditions developed, as little as 2 ng of DNAse I/ml can be assayed. This means that some 1 ng of G-actin can lead to an assay of the actin-state within the cell. In experiments using radioactive phalloidin, which binds to F-actin and not to G-actin, Laub (1980) has shown that the DNAse I inhibition assay and the phalloidin-binding assay lead to equivalent results. Studies of Pribluda, Laub and Rotman (1980) indicated that, when resting platelets were lyzed in Triton X-100 solutions (see Fig. 2 for conditions), some 80% of the total actin of the cell was found

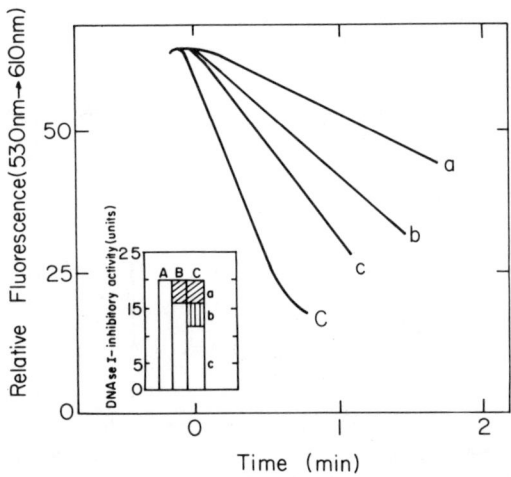

Fig. 2. Inset : A : Total platelet actin (Guanidine.HCl DNAse inhibitory actin); B : Resting platelet actin (a : non-inhibitory actin, 20% of total actin); C : Thrombin-activated platelet (b : mobilized actin; c : actin inhibiting the DNAse I).
C = Control (slope 25); a = Total actin (slope 5); b = Resting platelet (slope 9); c = Thrombin-activated platelet (slope 13).

Total actin = $\frac{C-a}{c} = \frac{25-5}{20}$ = 80% inhibition units.

Resting platelet = $\frac{C-b}{c} = \frac{25-9}{25}$ = 64% inhibition units.

Thrombin-activated platelet = $\frac{C-c}{c} = \frac{25-13}{25}$ = 48% inhibition units.

Actin mobilized = $(\frac{64-48}{64})100$ = 25% of resting platelet actin.

to immediately inhibit the DNAse I activity. Thus, under our assay conditions, some 4/5 of the resting platelet actin is found to exist in the cytoplasm in a 'G'-like state. Upon addition to gel-filtered platelets of 1 unit of thrombin, some 25% of this 'G'-actin is found within 10 seconds to be converted into a form (referred to as mobilized actin), which no longer inhibits the DNAse I even upon prolonged exposure to the enzyme. Fig. 3A shows that this change in the state of the actin precedes secretion of serotonin to the medium, as well as platelet aggregation as monitored by light scattering in an aggregometer. The presence of EDTA, which inhibits aggregation to a significant extent, increases the amount of actin which does not behave as 'G'-actin. Under these conditions, 10 min after thrombin addition, some 45% of the actin which in the resting platelet leads to inhibition of DNAse I activity was found to be mobilized into a form no longer inhibitory. In the presence of aspirin, which blocks prostaglandin formation and therefore decreases secretion due to vesicle exocytosis, the actin mobilization still occurs to an extent equivalent to that in the absence of aspirin (compare Fig. 3C with Fig. 3A).

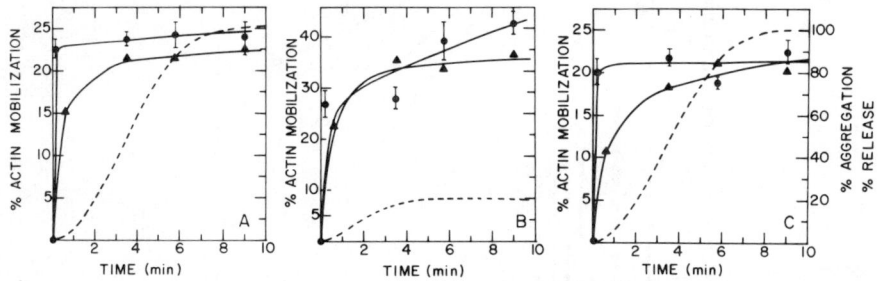

Fig. 3. Actin mobilization (●), release of serotonin (▲) and aggregation (---) when platelets were activated by thrombin (A), thrombin in the presence of EDTA (B) and thrombin in the presence of aspirin (C).

These results indicate that actin mobilization occurs very rapidly, following thrombin activation and precedes vesicle exocytosis and aggregation.

When platelet-rich plasma was exposed to ADP (Fig. 4A), actin mobilization of some 10% of that found to inhibit DNAse I in the resting platelet was observed to occur in the shortest time in which a measurement could be performed (10-15 sec). This was followed by a slower increase in the fraction no longer inhibitory to DNAse I, such that by 5 min some 30% of the actin no longer behaved as 'G'-like. Addition of EDTA to the platelets, which prevents serotonin secretion and agglutination due to ADP stimulation, did not affect the immediate actin polymerization but decreased markedly the slower rise in polymerized actin (Fig. 4B). Aspirin, which inhibits vesicle exocytosis, did not affect the change in the state of actin induced by ADP (Fig. 4C).

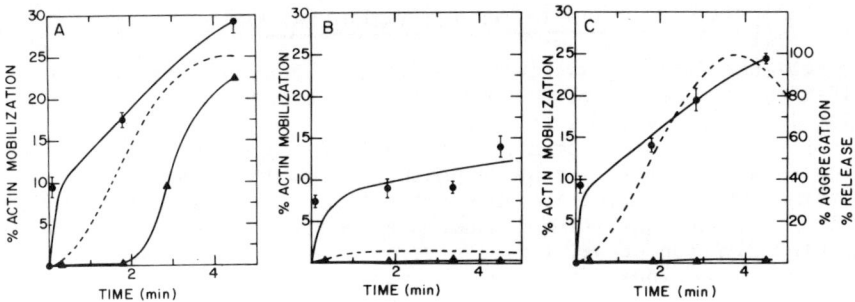

Fig. 4. Actin mobilization (●), release of serotonin (▲) and aggregation (---) when platelets were activated by ADP (A), ADP in the presence of EDTA (B), and ADP in the presence of aspirin (C).

STATE OF ACTIN IN RESTING PLATELETS

Carlsson et al. (1979) reported that lysis of resting platelets with solutions containing Triton X-100 and EGTA resulted in an extract which showed 45-75% of the total actin being capable of immediately inhibiting DNAse I. The results presented above showed consistently that some 80% of the actin of the resting platelet reacts rapidly with DNAse I. The difference in the values reported could be due to partial activation of the platelets during purification or due to the conditions of the extraction medium. Since Carlsson et al. (1979) obtained in some cases nearly equal values to those of ours, different degrees of activation during preparation appear as most likely to explain the differences recorded.

It is likely that the 'G'-like actin in the platelet exists as soluble profilactin and perhaps in a loose association with other actin-binding proteins. Electron microscopic examination of resting platelets (Behnke, 1971; Nachmias et al., 1977) shows mainly amorphous actin and some lattice-like short filaments. Similar findings have been reported by Edds (1977) for the platelet-like coelomocyte of the sea urchin, *Strongylocentrotus droebachiensis*. Whatever structure is observed in the EM pictures of the resting platelet, it probably represents the 20% of the actin not reactive with DNAse I. However, further work is required to determine whether the gels formed from the interaction of actin with actin-binding proteins allow the actin present within them to react with DNAse I. The only available evidence (Laub, 1980) shows that the majority of the actin interacting with spectrin in the erythrocyte is not readily accessible to bind to DNAse I. Indeed, it may be questioned whether or not spectrin is typical for other actin-binding proteins (Bray, 1976). Clearly, extraction of resting platelets, under differing conditions and fractionations, will have to be performed to clarify this point.

STATE OF ACTIN IN THE ACTIVATED PLATELET

As mentioned before, within the shortest period we could measure (15-25 sec), some 25% of the DNAse I inhibitory form in the resting platelet is converted into a non-inhibitory form. Thus, some 40% of the total platelet's actin is not available to inhibit DNAse a few seconds after activation by thrombin. When EDTA is present in the external medium during thrombin activation, the total actin unavailable for DNAse inhibition reaches a value as high as 60% of the total. Carlsson et al. (1979) have obtained similar results at longer time periods after thrombin activation.

Electron microscopy of activated platelets and especially the beautiful pictures of Edds (1977) with the coelomocyte clearly show that actin in the activated platelet changes from the gel-lattice filament form to actin cables or fibers. These findings are similar to those described by Tilney (1976) for Thyone sperm.
De Rosier et al. (1977) have shown that the actin cables formed are due to apposition of F-actin filaments and a 55 Kd protein. Phillips (this volume) has found that the triton X-100 pellet of thrombin-activated platelets contains actin, myosin and a 58 Kd protein. Extracts in relaxing solutions of many non-muscle cells have shown the property that upon warming they undergo a sol-to-gel transition. In the presence of ATP, such gels show fiber formation and contraction (Condeelis and Taylor, 1977). It is plausible to envisage that adjacent to the cell membrane, actin exists associated with actin-binding proteins and forming a gel-like structure and short stretches of lattice filaments (F-actin). A stimulus acting on the plasma membrane may then lead to a change in the accessibility of Ca^{++} and/or of protons which might trigger alignment of actin to form actin cables which might grow by the addition of actin coming from profilactin and/or from actin-ABP complexes. These changes would then involve loss of the gel-form adjacent to the membrane and a shape change due to the bundle formation leading to microspikes or filopodia. As mentioned above, these changes may be preceded by microtubule 'contraction' or might induce the displacement of the MT's. At the same time as actin is mobilized, it has been reported that the 20 Kd light chain of myosin is phosphorylated (Adelstein, et al., 1975; Haslam et al., in these proceedings). Thus, the actin bundles might then react with myosin to form actomyosin capable of contraction.

One interesting aspect of our findings is that the actin 'mobilized' during activation is not inhibitory to DNAse I even after prolonged incubation. Thus, it cannot be part of a reversible actomyosin complex, since it would be expected to inhibit the DNAse I with a half-life of some 5 to 10 min. An actomyosin rigor complex, however, would not be available to the DNAse I. It is known that during platelet activation, the ATP level drops markedly; thus, a rigor complex might indeed explain the above findings. Treatment with relaxing solutions after thrombin activation is required to clarify this point (these changes are depicted schematically in Fig. 5).

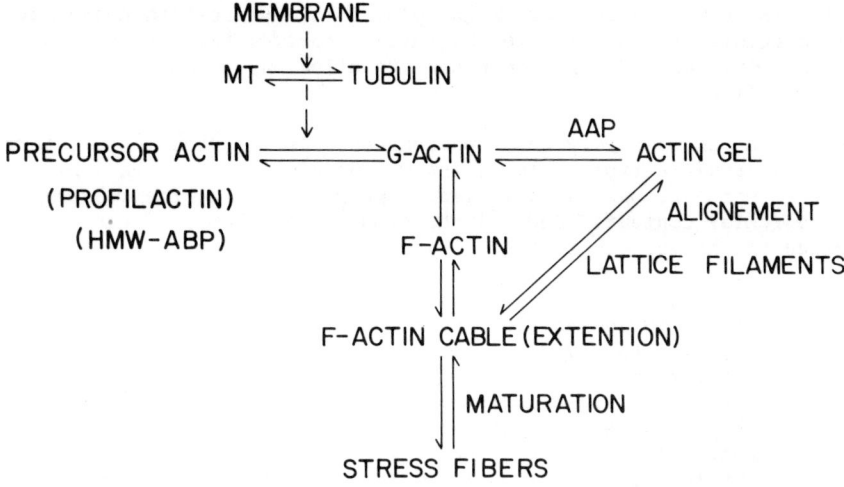

Fig. 5. Different forms of actin in platelets.

The above discussion is plausible but requires further work to pass from hypothesis to accepted findings.

It may be asked, what is the relevance of the changes in actin state observed to occur immediately upon activation. The formation of filopodia and microspikes could alter the curvature of the plasma membrane and thus expose, at the tips, proteins not normally available for cell-cell interaction. The important findings of Phillips, Jennings and Edwards (1980), that the post-Triton X-100 pellet of aggregated platelets also contains glycoproteins IIb and III, might suggest that perhaps these glycoproteins are involved in the activation of actin from precursor actin to F-actin and that the actin upon polymerizing might become attached to these proteins forming a fibrous network, at the tips of which these glycoproteins are exposed for cell-cell interaction.

Upon activation of platelets, intracellular vesicles fuse with the plasma membrane. One might ask, what is the relevance of actin in this process. Vesicle fusion appears in some cells, such as granulocytes, to be stimulated by low levels of cytochalasin B (<5 µg/ml). Hartwig and Stossel (1976) were first to observe that the gel present in lung macrophages, due to the interaction of actin with HMW-ABP, breaks down or its formation is inhibited in the presence of cytochalasin B (see also Weihing, 1976; Pollard, 1976; Condeelis and Taylor, 1977). It is plausible to envisage then, that actin mobilization, as observed here, which might involve a gel-fibrous network conversion, might lead to the removal of gel-lattice filament network from the endofacial surface of the plasma membrane and thus expose this surface for vesicle fusion to occur. Alternatively, the actin cable, 58 Kd-myosin complex, might play an active role in conveying the intracellular vesicles to the surface towards their subsequent fusion. Our knowledge is too meager to allow any definite statement to this effect.

Vesicle fusion is a very rapid phenomenon. In the granulocyte, three different vesicle types release their contents in less than 1 min. Vesicle fusion accomplishes at least two roles : (a) the release of the vesicular contents, and (b) the exposure of the endofacial surface of the vesicle to the outside or exofacial surface of the cell. In the platelet at least two types of vesicles have been described. These are the dense granules and α-granules. It is plausible that fibrinogen containing vesicles could exist and that the liberation of this molecule might then bridge between platelets leading to the formation of aggregates (Kaplan et al., 1979).It is not clear whether all vesicle fusion events are inhibited by compounds which block prostaglandin synthesis. It is clear that, in addition to conformational changes and those involving sulfhydryls, vesicle fusion might lead to the exposure of proteins in the cell surface. For this reason, they must be taken into account in any hypothesis of activation.

The gel to actomyosin rigor complex in the form of a fibrous structure could also change the viscoelastic properties of the platelet. A deformable cell is best suited to pass unhindered through capillaries. A rigid cell, on the other hand, might be capable of effectively plugging such vesicles.

ACKNOWLEDGEMENT

The generous financial support of the Gatsby Foundation (London, England) is highly appreciated.

Avner Rotman is incumbent of the Samuel and Isabelle Friedmann Career Development Chair.

REFERENCES

Adelstein, R.S., Conti, M.A., Daniel, T.L., and Anderson, W., Jr., 1975. The interaction of platelet actin, myosin and myosin light chain kinase, in Biochemistry and Pharmacology of Platelets, Ciba Foundation Symposium No.35, pp.101-119. Elsevier-Excerpta Medica, North-Holland.
Behnke, O., 1976. The blood platelet, a potential smooth muscle cell, in Contractile Systems in Non-Muscle Tissues (Eds. Perry, S.V., Margreth, A., and Adelstein, R.S.), pp.105-115. North-Holland Publishing Co.
Blikstad, I., Markey, F., Carlsson, L., Persson, T., and Lindberg, U., 1978. Selective assay of monomeric and filamentous actin in cell extracts, using inhibition of deoxyribonuclease I. Cell, 15, 935-943.
Bray, D., 1976. Spectrin-like proteins. Nature, 260, 16.

Condeelis, J.S., and Taylor, D.L., 1977. The contractile basis of ameboid movement : V. The control of gelation, solation and contraction in extracts from *Dictyostelium discoideum*. J.Cell Biol. 74, 901-927.

De Rosier, D., Mandelkow, E., Silliman, A., Tilney, L., and Kane, R., 1977. Structure of actin-containing filaments from two types of non-muscle cells. J.Mol.Biol., 113, 679-695.

Edds, K.T., 1977. Dynamic aspects of filopodial formation by reorganization of microfilaments. J.Cell Biol., 73, 479-491.

Edelman, G.M., 1976. Surface modulation in cell recognition and cell growth. Science, 192, 218-226.

Fuller, G.M., Ellison, J.J., McGill, M.S., Surdohl, L.A., and Brinkley, B.R., 1975. Studies on the inhibitory role of calcium ions in the regulation of microtubule assembly *in vitro* and *in vivo*, in Microtubules and Microtubule Inhibitors (Eds. Borgers,M., and De Brabander, M.), pp.379-392. North-Holland Publishing Co.

Fulton, C., 1977a. Intracellular regulation of cell shape and motility in *Naegleria*:First insights and a working hypothesis. J.Supramol.Struct., 6, 13-43.

Fulton, C., 1977b. Cell differentiation in *Naegleria gruberi*. Rev.Microbiol., 31, 597-629.

Harris, H.E., and Weeds, A.G., 1978. Platelet actin : Sub-cellular distribution and association with profilin. FEBS Lett., 90, 84-88.

Hartwig, J.H., and Stossel, T.P., 1976. Interactions of actin, myosin and an actin-binding protein of rabbit pulmonary macrophages : III. Effects of cytochalasin B. J.Cell Biol., 71, 295-303.

Haslam, R.J., Salama, S.E., Fox, J.E.B., Lynham, J.A., and Davidson, M.M.L. (in press) Roles of cyclic nucleotides and of protein phosphorylation in the regulation of platelet function, in Platelets - Cellular Response Mechanisms and Their Biological Significance (Eds. Rotman, A., Meyer, F.A., Gitler, C., and Silberberg, A.). J. Wiley & Sons, London.

Hitchcock, S.E., Carlsson, L., and Lindberg, U., 1976. Depolymerization of F-actin by deoxyribonuclease I. Cell, 7, 531-542.

Kaplan, K.L., Broekman, K.M., Chernoff, A., Lesznik, G.R. and Drillings, M., 1979. Platelet α-granule proteins : Studies on release and sub-cellular localization. Blood, 53, 604-618.

Laub, F., 1980. Ph.D. Thesis to be submitted to the Feinberg Graduate School, The Weizmann Institute of Science, Rehovot.

Nachmias, V., Sullender, J., and Asch, A., 1977. Shape and cytoplasmic filaments in control and lidocaine-treated human platelets. Blood, 50, 39-53.

Nicolson, G.L., 1976. Transmembrane control of the receptors in normal and tumor cells : I. Cytoplasmic influence. Biochim. Biophys.Acta, 457, 57-108.

Phillips, D.M., 1974. in Cilia and Flagella (Ed. Sleigh, M.A.), p.379. Academic Press, London.

Phillips, D.R., Jennings, L.K., and Edwards, H.H., 1980. Identification of membrane proteins mediating the interaction of human platelets. J.Cell Biol., in press.

Pollard, T.D., 1976. The role of actin in the temperature-dependent gelation and contraction of extracts of Acenthemoeba. J.Cell Biol., 68, 579-601.

Pribluda, V., Laub, F., and Rotman, A., 1980. The state of actin in activated platelets. Submitted.

Rose, B., and Loewenstein, W.R., 1975. Calcium ion distribution in cytoplasm visualized by *Aequorin* : Diffusion in cytosol restricted by energized sequestering. Science, 190, 1204-1206.

Silver, R.B., Cole, R.D., and Cande, W.Z., 1980. Isolation of mitotic apparatus containing vesicles with calcium sequestration activity. Cell, 19, 505-516.

Singer, S.J., Ash, J.F., Bourguinon, L.Y.W., Heggeness, M.H., and Louvard, D., 1976. Transmembrane interaction and the mechanisms of transport of proteins across membranes. J.Supramol.Struct., 9, 373-389.

Stossel, T.P., and Hartwig, J.H., 1976. Interaction of actin and a new actin-binding protein of rabbit pulmonary macrophages : II. Role in cytoplasmic movement and phagocytosis. J.Cell Biol., 68, 602-619.

Taylor, D.L., Rhodes, J.A., and Hammond, S.A., 1976. The contractile basis of ameboid movement : II. Structure and contractility of motile extracts and plasmalemma-ectoplasm ghosts. J.Cell Biol., 70, 123-143.

Tilney, L.G., 1976. The polymerization of actin : III. Aggregates of nonfilamentous actin and its associated proteins : A storage form of actin. J.Cell Biol., 69, 73-89.

Weihing, R.R., 1976. Cytochalasin B inhibits actin-related gelation of the He La cells extracts. J.Cell Biol., 71, 303-307.

Weng, K., Ash, J.F., and Singer, S.J., 1975. Filamin, a new high molecular weight protein found in smooth muscle and non-muscle cells. Proc.Natl.Acad.Sci.USA, 72, 4483-4486.

White, J.G., 1971. Platelet morphology, in The circulating Platelet (Ed. Johnson, S.A.), pp.45-121. Academic Press, New-York.

Yahara, I., and Edelman, G.M., 1975. Modulation of lymphocytes receptor mobility by concanavalin A and colchicine. Ann.N.Y. Acad.Sci., 253, 455-469.

PROSTAGLANDINS IN PLATELET ACTIVATION

J.G. White, G.H.R. Rao and J.M. Gerrard

University of Minnesota Health Sciences Center,
Minneapolis, Minnesota USA

INTRODUCTION

Platelet stimulus-activation-contraction-secretion coupling involves a complex sequence of biochemical and physical events resulting in formation of stable hemostatic plugs at sites of vascular injury (White, Rao and Gerrard, 1980). Initial steps in these reactions primarily involve the platelet surface membrane and its many chemical constituents. Lipids are important components of the cell wall and their involvement in the earliest phases of the platelet response has been recognized for many years (Moncada and Vane, 1978). Recently, attention has been focused on membrane phospholipids rich in arachidonic acid, liberation of this fatty acid following stimulation of the cell and subsequent conversion of free arachidonate into a variety of active products important in the regulation of platelet hemostatic function (Moncada and Vane, 1978; Marcus, 1978; Moncada and Vane, 1979). The present discussion will be concerned with certain aspects of the role of these products in platelet activation.

ARACHIDONIC ACID (AA) METABOLISM

Before embarking on the subject of this paper, it is well to briefly review current concepts of platelet AA metabolism (Moncada and Vane, 1978; Marcus, 1978; Moncada and Vane, 1979; Gerrard and White, 1978). Two different enzyme systems are involved in conversion of AA. The lipoxygenase pathway transforms AA to 12L-hydroperoxy-5,8,10,14-eicosatetraenoic acid (HPETE) which is reduced to 12L-hydroxy-5,8,10,14-eicosatetraenoic acid (HETE) by glutathione peroxidase. The role of these products in platelet physiology is uncertain, although HPETE can inhibit the second pathway of prostaglandin synthesis in platelets by blocking cyclo-oxygenase (Siegel, McConnell, Abrahams et al, 1979) and also prevent formation of PGI_2 by inhibiting prostacyclin synthetase in blood vessels (Marcus 1978). The final product, HETE, does not appear to influence platelet function, but has been shown to stimulate neutrophil chemotaxis (Turner, Tainer and Lynn, 1975).

Prostaglandin endoperoxide synthetase, the primary enzyme of the second pathway, converts AA into unstable endoperoxides (Moncada and Vane, 1978; Marcus, 1978; Moncada and Vane, 1979; Gerrard and White,

1978). The first product is PGG_2, a cyclic endoperoxide with a hydroperoxy group on carbon 15. Reduction of the 15-hydroperoxy to a hydroxy group transforms PGG_2 into PGH_2. Both endoperoxides are rapidly converted to thromboxane A_2 (TxA_2) through the action of thromboxane synthetase. In addition to the major endoperoxides, small amounts of AA are also transformed into PGE_2, PGD_2 and $PGF_{2\alpha}$. PGD_2, like PGE_1, stimulates platelet adenylate cyclase, elevates endogenous levels of cyclic 3',5'-adenosine monophosphate (cAMP), and inhibits platelet aggregation. $PGF_{2\alpha}$ has no apparent effect on platelet physiology, while PGE_2 can promote the second wave of ADP induced aggregation. The major alternative pathway for metabolism of PGG_2 and PGH_2 is degradation to the hydroxy fatty acid, HHT, and maldonialdehyde (MDA). Under same conditions the cyclic endoperoxides formed in platelets can be utilized by blood vessels as an alternate substrate for synthesis of PGI_2 (Moncada and Vane, 1978; Moncada and Vane, 1979). However, endoperoxides are converted so rapidly to TxA_2 in normal platelets that it is doubtful whether they provide a significant source for vessel wall prostacyclin synthesis. Like the endoperoxides, TxA_2 is highly unstable and is hydrolyzed rapidly into thromboxane B_2 (TxB_2). The stable end products of the cyclo-oxygenase-thromboxane synthetase pathway, including HHT, MDA and TxB_2, have little or no influence on platelet function (Moncada and Vane, 1978; Marcus 1978; Moncada and Vane, 1979; Gerrard and White, 1978). It is the unstable intermediates, PGG_2, PGH_2 and TxA_2, which are powerful mediators of the platelet activation process (Nugteren, 1978).

AA, the essential substrate for all of the stable and unstable hydroperoxy and hydroxy fatty acids, endoperoxides, thromboxanes and prostaglandins, is not available for enzymatic transformation in unaltered discoid platelets. Stimulation of platelets by any of a variety of potent agents capable of triggering the release reaction results in cleavage of free AA from membrane phospholipids. The precise mechanism involved in liberation of AA, the specific enzymes, kinetics of the reaction, modulating influences and exact type and localization of phospholipids providing the AA are still being clarified. Early work suggested that phospholipase A_2 was the principal enzyme involved and, following activation by calcium ions, cleaved AA primarily from phosphatidyl choline and partly from phosphatidyl inositol (Bills, Smith and Silver, 1976). Despite objections regarding its primary involvement, this pathway may prove to be a major or an important auxillary source of AA for prostaglandin synthesis (Lapetina, Billah and Cuatrecasas, 1980).

Recent investigations have suggested that phosphatidyl inositol is the major phospholipid source for AA in activated platelets (Rittenhouse-Simmons, 1979). Within a few seconds after exposure to thrombin or the divalent cation ionophore, A23187, phosphatidyl inositol is hydrolyzed to 1,2 diacylglycerol by the action of a calcium dependent phosphotidyl inositol specific phospholipase C (Lapetina, Billah and Cuatrecasas, 1980; Rittenhouse-Simmons, 1979). The diglyceride does not accumulate in activated platelets. A diglyceride lipase associated with the particulate fraction can degrade 1,2 diacylglycerol to a monoglyceride and AA, providing sufficient amounts of the fatty acid substrate for all pathways of AA transformation in platelets (Bell, Kennerly, Stanford et al, 1979). There are, however, reasonable objections to the concept that this route is the only source of AA in activated platelets, and further studies are required before the role of phospholipase A_2 can or should be eliminated (Lapetina, Billah and Cuatrecasas, 1980).

In addition to conversion by diglyceride lipase into monoglyceride and AA, 1,2 diacylglycerol can also be phosphorylated to phosphatidic acid by a diacylglycerol kinase. Phosphatidic acid accumulates in activated platelets before AA is released, and can induce the dissociation of AA from various phospholipids (Lapetina and Cuatrecasas, 1979). Thus, there are at least two different calcium dependent enzymes and three different routes whereby AA can be made available for prostaglandin synthesis in activated platelets.

PROSTAGLANDINS AND PLATELET FUNCTION

Platelets do not store endoperoxides, thromboxanes or prostaglandins. These products are formed as a result of platelet stimulation. Therefore, it may seem of dubious value to discuss their role in platelet activation, since formation follows the precipitating event (Marcus, 1978). Yet, activation is not a single, clearly defined step or an all or none phenomenon. It involves multiple stages of stimulus response coupling, increasing degrees of physical and biochemical alteration by more and more platelets, heightening of individual responses and interplatelet interactions until a level of total activation by enough cells is reached to sustain irreversible aggregation (Gerrard and White, 1978). In discussing the phenomena involved we have used the collective term: stimulus-activation-contraction-secretion coupling, to describe it (White, Rao and Gerrard, 1980). Within the context of this broader definition, a discussion of prostaglandins and their role in platelet activation seems to be appropriate. To facilitate the presentation, we will discuss the involvement of prostaglandins in each phase of the platelet response as a series of questions.

CAN AA AND ITS UNSTABLE METABOLITES STIMULATE PLATELETS?

The possibility that prostaglandins might be involved in platelet hemostatic physiology stemmed from the work of Smith and Willis which showed that thrombin stimulated the formation of PGE_2 and $PGF_{2\alpha}$ in platelets, and aspirin pretreatment blocked the synthesis of prostaglandins caused by exposure of the cells to thrombin (Smith and Willis, 1970; Smith and Willis, 1971). In subsequent years it was demonstrated that the unstable intermediates, PGG_2, PGH_2 and TxA_2, as well as the fatty acid precursor, AA, could all cause direct stimulation when added to samples of stirred platelets (Moncada and Vane, 1978; Marcus, 1978; Moncada and Vane, 1979; Gerrard and White, 1978). Aspirin blocked the response of platelets to AA, but did not inhibit stimulation by the endoperoxides or TxA_2. Inhibition of the response to AA was found to be due to acetylation of cyclo-oxygenase by aspirin, (Roth and Majerus, 1975) but inactivation of this enzyme did not influence conversion of endoperoxides to thromboxanes or the action of TxA_2 on aspirin treated cells. The endoperoxides and thromboxanes were found to interact with specific receptors which mediated their stimulation of platelets (Mills and Macfarlane, 1979). Stable analogs of the endoperoxides which are unable to trigger platelet activation could compete with active intermediates for the receptor sites and block platelet stimulation. Stimulation of platelets by AA, PGG_2, PGH_2 and TxA_2 could also be blocked by agents which stimulated adenylate cyclase and caused elevations in endogenous levels of cyclic 3'5' adenosine monophosphate (cAMP) (Gerrard and White, 1978). Recently, we have found that the sensitivity of platelets to stimulation by AA, endoperoxides or TxA_2 is more susceptible to inhibition by slight elevations in cAMP than the response of the cells to other aggregating agents.

Species differences in response to stimulation by prostaglandins are intriguing. Platelets from about 70% of dogs do not aggregate when stirred with AA, even though they synthesize the same quantities of endoperoxides and thromboxanes as human platelets (Chignard and Vargaftig, 1977). However, the arachidonate resistant (AR) dog platelets do change shape when stirred with the fatty acid. About 30% of dogs possess platelets which do aggregate when exposed to AA on the aggregometer (Johnson, Leis, Rao et al, 1979). No differences have been observed in the types or amounts of endoperoxides and thromboxanes generated by arachidonate sensitive (AS) dog platelets compared to AR canine cells. Unstable prostaglandin products detectable in the supernatant above samples of AR dog cells stirred with AA will cause aggregation when transferred to samples of AS canine platelets. AR and AS dog platelets do not differ in their sensitivity to other aggregating agents, and both types are unresponsive to epinephrine. However, pretreatment of AR platelets with epinephrine will make them as sensitive to aggregation by AA as are AS dog platelets (Chignard and Vargaftig, 1977; Johnson, Leis, Rao et al, 1979). Exposure of AS dog platelets to amounts of adenylate cyclase stimulators or phosphodiesterase inhibitors too small to raise endogenous levels of cAMP or affect the response to most aggregating agents, converted the AA sensitive platelets into AR platelets (Johnson, Rao, Leis, et al, 1980). Thus, the response of canine platelets to stimulation by AA, PGG_2, PGH_2 and TxA_2 is closely regulated by the adenylate cyclase-cAMP-phosphodiesterase complex, (Gerrard, Peller, Krick et al, 1977) even though significant differences in levels of cAMP in AR and AS dog platelets have not been identified.

CAN AA AND ITS UNSTABLE METABOLITES ACTIVATE PLATELETS?

The experiments discussed above indicate that AA, PGG_2, PGH_2 and TxA_2 can bind to unaltered discoid platelets and stimulate the cells. Depending on the state of the adenylate cyclase-cAMP-phosphodiesterase complex and other factors the stimulus is usually coupled to activation (Gerrard and White, 1978). Examination of platelets in the electron microscope after stirring with AA, PGG_2, PGH_2 or TxA_2 reveals physical alterations essentially identical to those which develop in platelets following exposure to potent aggregating agents such as thrombin, collagen and the calcium ionophore, A23187

(Gerrard and White, 1978; Gerrard and White, 1975; Gerrard, Townsend, Stoddard et al, 1977). Treated cells lose their discoid shape, extrude bulky and spiky pseudopods and develop concentration dependent waves of internal contraction. The process of internal contraction is visualized as a movement of organelles toward platelet centers where they are enclosed by tight fitting webs of microtubules and contractile microfilaments. With progression of the contractile wave granule contents transferred to channels of the surface connected open canalicular system are squeezed out of the cells, leaving behind a contracted mass of microfilaments and broken microtubules. Changes of this extent are associated with irreversible platelet transformation.

The similarity of the physical changes caused by endoperoxides and TxA_2 to those induced by A23187 led us to compare the effects of a variety of inhibitors on the responses of platelets activated by either A23187 or PGG_2 (Gerrard and White, 1978). Agents that acted by elevating intracellular cAMP levels or mimicking cAMP inhibited platelet activation by both PGG_2 and the ionophore. A combination of inhibitors which blocked glycolytic metabolism as well as oxidative phosphorylation and depleted the cell of ATP required for contraction resulted in inhibition of platelet activation by both agents. N-ethyl-malemide, a sulfhydryl inhibitor reputed to inhibit superprecipitation of contractile protein prevented activation of platelets by PGG_2 and A23187. The strong parallelism in the ultrastructural response of platelets to endoperoxide and A23187, and the similar effects of inhibitors on the activation of platelets by the two agents suggested that they might couple stimulation to activation through similar mechanisms (Bereziat, 1979).

CAN AA OR ITS UNSTABLE METABOLITES CAUSE CONTRACTION?

The electron microscopic studies referred to above suggested that AA, PGG_2, PGH_2 and TxA_2 activated platelets by triggering the contractile mechanism (Gerrard and White, 1978; Gerrard and White, 1975; Gerrard, Townsend, Stoddard et al, 1977). Comparison of the morphological changes caused by PGG_2 and A23187, which is known to trigger platelet contraction by elevating the level of cytoplasmic calcium, (White, Rao, Gerrard, 1974) and the effects of inhibitors on the response of platelets to either agent suggested that endoperoxides and TxA_2 might stimulate platelet activation and trigger contraction through similar mechanisms. Two types of experiments supported this hypothesis. Phorbol myristate acetate (PMA), the active principle of croton oil, is a powerful platelet aggregating agent, but causes substantially less release of granule associated substances than collagen, thrombin or A23187 (Gerrard and White, 1978; Rao, White and Estensen, 1974). Effects of PMA on platelet ultrastructure differed markedly from the changes caused by more potent release inducing agents (Estensen and White, 1974). Instead of triggering internal contraction, PMA caused selective labilization and swelling of platelet storage organelles. Microtubules and microfilaments remained dispersed in most PMA aggregated cells, despite their loss of discoid shape. Since PMA appeared to cause granule labilization but not contraction, we compared the effects of

PMA and PGG$_2$ on platelet secretion separately and together. The study demonstrated that half the threshold concentration of PGG$_2$ causing secretion and half the amount of PMA necessary to initiate release, when added together, resulted in marked augmentation of the release reaction (Gerrard, Townsend and Stoddard, 1977). These findings supported the concept that the endoperoxide acted as a stimulus for platelet contraction resulting in a squeezing out of the contents of granules labilized by PMA. The possibility that PGG$_2$, other endoperoxides and TxA$_2$ triggered platelet contraction by elevating the level of cytoplasmic calcium has been studied intensively in our laboratory (Gerrard and White, 1978). Results of these investigations indicate that the endoperoxides, PGG$_2$ and PGH$_2$, may exert their effects by mobilizing calcium, since they selectively cause release of calcium from platelet membrane vesicles (Gerrard, Butler, Graff et al, 1978). Thus, our findings suggest that AA and its unstable metabolites can cause contraction and do so by elevating the level of calcium in platelets (Gerrard, Peterson, Rao et al, 1980).

CAN AA AND ITS UNSTABLE METABOLITES CAUSE SECRETION?

Early studies with aspirin (Weiss, Aledort and Kochwa, 1968; Evans, Packham Nishizawa et al, 1968) or AA (Silver, Smith and Ingerman, 1973) and evaluation of the time course of endoperoxide production and the release reaction (Silver, Smith and Ingerman, 1973) had suggested that products generated during prostaglandin synthesis were involved in platelet secretion. However, it was difficult in such studies to separate events sufficiently well to be certain that endoperoxide or TxA$_2$ generation was coupled to the secretory process. In 1972, we described an experiment which demonstrated that endoperoxides and TxA2 synthesized in a population of platelets that had no storage pool could trigger secretion of stored products from a second population of platelets whose release mechanism had been paralyzed by aspirin (White and Witkop, 1972).

The storage pool deficient platelets were from patients with the Hermansky-Pudlak syndrome (HPS), which includes the triad of tyrosimore positive oculo-cutaneous albinism, storage of lipofuchsin or ceroid-like material in macrophages of the bone marrow and other tissues and a mild bleeding disorder due to platelet dysfunction (Hermansky and Pudlak, 1959). Thin sections of HPS platelets revealed a virtual absence of electron-dense organelles which are the storage sites for the secretable pool of adenine nucleotides and serotonin. Measurements of 5-HT and adenine nucleotides by biochemical procedures demonstrated profound deficiencies of these substances in HPS cells. Characteristically, HPS platelets develop only single waves of aggregation when stimulated with concentrations of ADP, epinephrine and thrombin that cause biphasic, irreversible aggregation in samples of normal platelets. The monophasic responses of HPS platelets are essentially identical to the single waves which develop in samples of aspirin-treated normal platelets after stirring with the same group of agents causing biphasic reactions in untreated samples of normal platelets. However, aspirin merely acetylates cyclo-oxygenase thereby blocking synthesis of endoperoxides and thromboxanes (Roth and Majerus, 1975). The drug has no effect on levels of adenine nucleotides or serotonin, or on the number of dense bodies present in normal platelets. Thus, even though the two different populations, storage pool deficient HPS cells and aspirin-treated normal platelets, react in a similar manner to aggregating agents, the basis for their failure to develop biphasic, irreversible waves of aggregation when stimulated by agents which produce this effect in normal platelet samples is quite different.

It was fascinating, therefore, when mixtures of HPS platelets and aspirin-treated normal cells responded in a perfectly normal, biphasic manner to concentrations of epinephrine, thrombin and ADP which caused only single waves on stirring with either population alone (White and Witkop, 1972). Improvement was noted when the mixture contained 20% HPS and 80% aspirin-treated normal cells, and the response to epinephrine, ADP and thrombin was entirely normal when the sample consisted of 50% HPS and 50% aspirin platelets. Since the numbers of platelets were constant the correction could not have been due to more frequent cell-cell contacts. Interaction between the two populations during the first wave of the aggregation response might have stimulated a second wave. However, this seemed unlikely since single waves of similar magnitude achieved with either population alone, were not followed by second waves. The possible role of a plasmatic factor was quickly eliminated by washing and resuspension experiments. That the corrective influence in the mixed system was a product of prostaglandin synthesis was first suggested by the observation that treatment of the HPS cells with aspirin blocked secretion by the normal aspirin treated cells and development of the second wave (Gerrard, White, Rao et al, 1975). Subsequent studies revealed that HPS platelets were capable of synthesizing endoperoxides and thromboxanes, though intact HPS platelets are less efficient than normal platelets. Evidence that the aspirin labile factor causing secretion of the storage pool from aspirin-treated normal platelets was provided by labelling the aspirin cells with ^{14}C-serotonin and following the release reaction (Gerrard and White, 1978; Gerrard, White, Rao et al, 1975). More recently we have followed the secretion of ADP directly on the lumiaggregometer. The studies demonstrate that ADP and 5-HT are secreted by the aspirin platelet population and that the release is associated with development of an irreversible second wave of aggregation. Thus, the initial phase of correction in the mixed system is accomplished by synthesis of endoperoxides and thromboxanes by HPS platelets following stimulation. The ability of prostaglandin products produced by HPS cells to act on a second population of unrelated platelets is a clear cut example of intercellular communication, and demonstrates that endoperoxides and thromboxanes can act as intercellular messengers. Secretion of ^{14}C-5-HT and ADP from aspirin-treated platelets in the mixed system demonstrates that endoperoxides and thromboxanes can cause the release reaction. Since the levels of prostaglandin products produced by HPS platelets when stirred alone with these amounts of aggregating agents are insufficient to support an irreversible second wave of aggregation, it is doubtful that the concentrations of endoperoxides and thromboxanes generated in the mixtures are alone sufficient to cause the correction. It is more likely that the ADP secreted by the aspirin platelets alone, or in combination with the prostaglandin products, is responsible for causing a second wave of aggregation in the mixed system. Another possibility, suggested by others, (Detwiler and Huang, 1980) is that interaction between aspirin normal and HPS platelets during the first wave caused the secretion, prostaglandin synthesis and second wave of aggregation as simultaneous but unrelated phenomena. However, since the ability of the HPS platelets to synthesize prostaglandins and of aspirin-treated platelets to secrete products from their storage pool appear critical to correction in the system, it seems reasonable to conclude that, under the conditions of this experiment, prostaglandin synthesis and secretion are causually linked to the second wave of aggreggation.

SUMMARY AND CONCLUSIONS

This presentation has dealt with the subject of prostaglandins in platelet activation. Based on work reported by others and experiments carried out in our laboratory, it is reasonable to suggest that AA endoperoxides and TxA_2 can stimulate platelets, cause activation, trigger contraction, produce secretion and result in irreversible platelet aggregation. However, we have not considered another very important question in this discussion. Are products of prostaglandin synthesis required for irreversible platelet aggregation? The answer to that question is no. Packham and her associate (Packham, Kinlough-Rathbone, Reimers et al, 1977) demonstrated some time ago that thrombin induced aggregation is not dependent on generation of endoperoxides and thromboxanes. On the basis of current studies in our laboratory it is possible to state that, under certain conditions nearly every agent, including AA, can cause irreversible aggregation of platelets, even though the cells cannot synthesize prostaglandins or secrete serotonin or ADP (Rao, Johnson and White, 1980). Secreted products, endoperoxides and thromboxanes facilitate activation and recruitment of platelets and markedly amplify the stickiness and contraction that lead to irreversible aggregation. However, they are not absolutely required for biphasic irreversible platelet aggregation.

REFERENCES

Bell, R.L., Kennerly, D.A., Stanford, N. and Majerus, P., 1979. Diglyceride lipase: A pathway for arachidonate release from human platelets. Proceedings of the National Academy of Sciences, 76, 3238-3241.

Bereziat, G., 1979. Are phospholipase involved in platelet activation? Agents and Actions 9, 390-399.

Bills, T.K., Smith, J.B., and Silver, M.J., 1976. Metabolism of (^{14}C) arachidonic acid by human platelets. Biochimica et Biophysica Acta 424, 303-314.

Chignard, M., and Vargaftig, B.B., 1977. Synthesis of thromboxane A_2 by non-aggregating dog platelets challenged with arachidonic acid or with prostaglandin H_2. Prostaglandins 14, 222-227.

Detwiler, T.C., and Huang, E.M., 1980. The interrelationship of platelet aggregation, secretion and prostaglandin synthesis, in The Regulation of Coagulation (Eds. Mann and Taylor), pp 377-383. Elsevier/North-Holland, New York.

Estensen, R.D., and White, J.G., 1974. Ultrastructural features of the platelet response to phorbol myristate acetate. American Journal of Pathology, 74, 441-452.

Evans, G., Packham, M., Nishizawa, E.A., and Mustard, J.F., 1968. The effect of acetylsalicylic acid on platelet function. Journal of Experimental Medicine, 128, 877-894.

Gerrard, J.M., Butler, A.M., Graff, G., Stoddard, S.F., and White, J.G., 1978. Prostaglandin endoperoxides promote calcium release from a platelet membrane fraction in vitro. Prostaglandins and Medicine, 1, 373-385.

Gerrard, J.M., Peller, J.D., Krick, T.P., and White, J.G., 1977. Cyclic AMP and platelet prostaglandin synthesis. Prostaglandins, 14, 39-50.

Gerrard, J.M., Peterson, D.A., Rao, G.H.R., and White, J.G., 1980. Some recent advances in understanding the tangle of biochemical events involved in thromboxane dependent and independent aggregation, in The Regulation of Coagulation (Eds. Mann and Taylor), pp 399-404. Elsevier/North-Holland, New York.

Gerrard, J.M., Townsend, D., Stoddard, S.F., Witkop, C.J., and White, J.G., 1977. The influence of prostaglandin G_2 on platelet ultrastructure and platelet secretion. American Journal of Pathology, 86, 99-116.

Gerrard, J.M., and White, J.G., 1975. The influence of prostaglandin endoperoxides on platelet ultrastructure. American Journal of Pathology, 80, 189-202.

Gerrard, J.M., and White, J.G., 1978. Prostaglandins and thromboxanes: "middlemen" modulating platelet function in hemostasis and thrombosis. Progress in Hemostasis and Thrombosis, 4, 87-125.

Gerrard, J.M., White, J.G., Rao, G.H.R., Krivit, W., and Witkop, C.J., 1975. Labile aggregation stimulating substance (LASS): The factor from storage pool deficient platelets correcting defective aggregation and release of aspirin treated normal platelets. British Journal of Haematology 29, 657-664.

Hermansky, F., and Pudlak, P., 1959. Albinism associated with hemorrhagic diathesis and unusual pigmented reticular cells in the bone marrow: report of two cases with histochemical studies. Blood, 14, 162-171.

Johnson, G.J., Leis, L.A., Rao, G.H.R., and White, J.G., 1979. Arachidonate-induced platelet aggregation in the dog. Thrombosis Research, 14, 147-154.

Johnson, G.J., Rao, G.H.R., Leis, L.A., and White, J.G., 1980. Effect of agents which alter cyclic AMP on arachidonate-induced platelet aggregation in the dog. Blood, in press.

Lapetina, E.G., Billah, M.M., and Cuatrecasas, P., 1980. Stimulation of the phosphatidylinositol-specific phospholipase C and the release of arachidonic acid in activated platelets, in The Regulation of Coagulation (Eds. Mann and Taylor), pp 491-497. Elsevier/North-Holland, New York.

Lapetina, E.G., and Cuatrecasas, P., 1979. Stimulation of phosphatidic acid production in platelets precedes the formation of arachidonate and parallels the release of serotonin. Biochimica et Biophysica Acta, 573, 394-402.
Marcus, A.J., 1978. The role of lipids in platelet function: with particular reference to the arachidonic acid pathway. Journal of Lipid Research, 19, 793-826.
Mills, D.C.B., and Macfarlane, D.E., 1979. Evidence for two separate receptors mediating the stimulation of platelet adenylate cyclase by prostaglandin I_2 (PGI_2), PGD_2 and PGE_1. Thrombosis and Haemostasis, 42, 118-121.
Moncada, S., and Vane, J.R., 1978. Unstable metabolites of arachidonic acid and their role in hemostasis and thrombosis. British Medical Bulletin, 34, 129-135
Moncada, S., and Vane, J.R., 1979. Arachidonic acid metabolites and the interaction between platelets and blood-vessel walls. New England Journal of Medicine, 300, 1142-1147.
Nugteren, D.H., 1978. Platelets and prostaglandins. Agents and Actions, 8, 296-298.
Packham, M.A., Kinlough-Rathbone, R.L., Reimers, H.J., Scott, S., and Mustard, J.F., 1977. Mechanisms of platelet aggregation independent of adenosine diphosphate, in Prostaglandins in Hematology (Eds. Silver, Smith and Kocsis), pp 247-276. Spectrum Publications, New York.
Rao, G.H.R., Johnson, G.J., and White, J.G., 1980. Influence of epinephrine on the aggregation response of aspirin-treated platelets. Prostaglandins and Medicine, in press.
Rittenhouse-Simmons, S., 1979. Production of diglyceride from phosphatidylinositol in activated human platelets. Journal of Clinical Investigation, 63, 580-587.
Roth, G.J., and Majerus, P.W., 1975. The mechanism of the effect of aspirin on human platelets. I. Acetylation of a particulate fraction protein. Journal of Clinical Investigation, 56, 624-632.
Siegel, M.I., McConnell, R.T., Abrahams, S.L., Porter, N.A., and Cuatrecasas, P., 1979. Aspirin-like drugs interfere with arachidonate metabolism by inhibition of the 12 hydroperoxy-5,8,10,14-eicosatetraenoic acid peroxidase activity of the lipoxygenase pathway. Biochemical and Biophysical Research Communications, 89, 1273-1280.
Silver, M.J., Smith, J.B., Ingerman, C., and Kocsis, J.J., 1973. Arachidonic acid-induced human platelet aggregation and prostaglandin formation. Prostaglandins, 4, 863-875.
Smith, J.B., Ingerman, C., Kocsis, J.J., and Silver, M.J., 1974. Formation of an intermediate in prostaglandin biosynthesis and its association with the platelet release reaction. Journal of Clinical Investigation, 53, 1468-1472.
Smith, J.B., and Willis, A.L., 1970. Formation and release of prostaglandins in response to thrombin. British Journal of Pharmacology, 40, 545P.
Smith, J.B., and Willis, A.L., 1971. Aspirin selectively inhibits prostaglandin production in human platelets. Nature (New Biology), 231, 235-237.
Turner, S.R., Tainer, J.A., and Lynn, W.S., 1975. Biogenesis of chemotactic molecules by the arachidonate liposygenase system

of platelets. Nature, 257, 680-681.
Weiss, H.J., Adeldort, L.M., and Kochiwa, S., 1968. The effects of salicylates on the hemostatic properties of platelets in man. Journal of Clinical Investigation, 47, 2169-2180.
White, J.G., Rao, G.H.R., and Estensen, R.D., 1974. Investigation of the release reaction in platelets exposed to phorbol myristate acetate. American Journal of Pathology, 75, 301-314.
White, J.G., Rao, G.H.R., and Gerrard, J.M., 1974. Effects of the ionophore, A23187 on blood platelets. American Journal of Pathology, 77, 135-150.
White, J.G., Rao, G.H.R., and Gerrard, J.M., 1980. A. Platelet stimulus activation contraction secretion coupling: A frequently fractured chain of events, in The Regulation of Coagulation (Eds. Mann and Taylor), pp 363-376. Elsevier/North-Holland, New York.
White, J.G., and Witkop, C.J., 1972. Effects of norman and aspirin platelets on defective secondary aggregation in the Hermansky-Pudlak syndrome: A test for storage pool deficient platelets. American Journal of Pathology, 68:57-66.

ROLES OF CYCLIC NUCLEOTIDES AND OF PROTEIN PHOSPHORYLATION IN THE REGULATION OF PLATELET FUNCTION

R.J. Haslam, S.E. Salama, J.E.B. Fox, J.A. Lynham, and M.M.L. Davidson

Department of Pathology, McMaster University, Hamilton, Ontario, Canada L8N 3Z5

ABSTRACT

The inhibitory effects of prostaglandins (e.g. PGE_1) and of adenosine on platelet function are mediated by cyclic AMP, presumably via the activation of cyclic AMP-dependent protein kinases. Two such enzymes, containing cyclic AMP-binding subunits similar to those of type I and type II protein kinases from other tissues, were found in platelets. Addition of PGE_1 to platelets labelled by preincubation with $[^{32}P]P_i$ enhanced incorporation of ^{32}P into at least four platelet polypeptides (P50, P36, P24, P22). Two of these, P24 and P22, were enriched in membrane fractions capable of the ATP-dependent uptake of Ca^{2+} ions. As membranes from PGE_1-treated platelets took up Ca^{2+} ions more rapidly than control membranes, the results suggest that phosphorylation of P24 and/or P22 may mediate a stimulation by cyclic AMP of the active transport of Ca^{2+} ions out of the platelet cytosol. Although aggregating agents increase platelet cyclic GMP, the ability of SNP, a potent inhibitor of aggregation, to increase platelet cyclic GMP even more markedly, has suggested that cyclic GMP may mediate an inhibition of aggregation. 8-Bromo-cyclic GMP and SNP rapidly increased the phosphorylation of two polypeptides in intact platelets (P50 and P49). SNP also increased platelet cyclic AMP and the phosphorylation of P24 and P22, but insufficiently to account for its inhibitory effects. Experiments with ^{32}P-labelled platelets have shown that inducers of the release reaction increase the phosphorylation of another group of polypeptides. Most ^{32}P was incorporated into P47, a major polypeptide distinct from actin, and into P20a and P20b, which are probably variants of the 20,000 mol. wt. light chain of myosin. These phosphorylation reactions were suppressed by drugs that inhibit Ca^{2+} movements across membranes. PGE_1 inhibited the phosphorylation reactions induced by collagen but not by ionophore A23187, which may thus short-circuit the cyclic AMP-activated Ca^{2+} pump. The results suggest that Ca^{2+}-activated phosphorylation of platelet proteins may play an important role in the release of platelet granule contents.

Abbreviations: PGE_1, prostaglandin E_1, SDS, sodium dodecylsulphate; P82, P75, P50, P49, P47, P40, P36, P27, P24, P22, P21, P20a, P20b, P19 and P18 are platelet phosphopolypeptides, the numerical values indicating their apparent mol. wts. $\times 10^{-3}$; SNP, Na nitroprusside.

INTRODUCTION

Abundant evidence now indicates that the effects of inhibitory agonists, such as adenosine, PGE_1 and prostacyclin, on the responses of platelets to aggregating agents are mediated by cyclic AMP (for review see Haslam et al., 1978a). Thus, these compounds activate adenylate cyclase in platelet particulate fractions, they increase platelet cyclic AMP before inhibitory effects are observed and their actions are potentiated by inhibitors of cyclic AMP phosphodiesterase and are suppressed by inhibitors of adenylate cyclase. The role, if any, of cyclic AMP in platelets at times when they are not exposed to inhibitory agonists has been more controversial. However, it is now clear that under these conditions inhibitors of adenylate cyclase, such as 2',5'-dideoxyadenosine, do not cause or potentiate platelet aggregation (Haslam et al., 1978b). This suggests that cyclic AMP need not be present in platelets for them to remain in their normal disaggregated state and that decreases in platelet cyclic AMP play no role in the effects of aggregating agents. Thus, in the platelet, cyclic AMP can be regarded as a unidirectional mediator of inhibitory effects. We report here some studies on the mechanism of action of cyclic AMP in platelets.

In contrast with cyclic AMP, the role of cyclic GMP in the platelet remains an enigma. Several studies have indicated that aggregating agents can increase platelet cyclic GMP but this is probably an effect rather than a potential cause of the aggregation process (Haslam et al., 1978a). In principle, cyclic GMP could be a feedback inhibitor of platelet responses. A similar concept has been advanced for the role of cyclic GMP in smooth muscle, in which both stimulatory agonists and some relaxant drugs, notably SNP, increase cyclic GMP levels (Schultz et al., 1977). Thus, it is of interest that SNP inhibits platelet aggregation (Glusa et al., 1974) and increases platelet cyclic GMP to very high levels (Haslam et al., 1978a, 1979a; Böhme et al., 1978). We report here further findings relevant to the possible role of cyclic GMP in the mechanism of action of SNP on platelets.

Both platelet aggregation and the release reaction appear to be mediated by an increase in the Ca^{2+} ion concentration in the platelet cytosol (for review see Feinstein, 1978). These Ca^{2+} ions may exert their effects on a variety of enzymes that are activated by the Ca^{2+}-binding protein, calmodulin, including phosphorylase kinase, phospholipase A_2 and myosin light chain kinase (Cheung, 1980), as well as by other mechanisms. As the actin-activated ATP-ase activity of platelet myosin depends on myosin phosphorylation (Adelstein and Conti, 1975), the activation of myosin light chain kinase by Ca^{2+} ions and calmodulin (Hathaway and Adelstein, 1979) may be of particular importance. However, correlation of myosin phosphorylation with specific platelet responses is required to define the functions of myosin in platelets. With this as one objective, several workers have studied the effects of aggregating agents on the incorporation of ^{32}P into proteins in intact platelets that have been preincubated with $[^{32}P]P_i$ (Lyons et al., 1975; Haslam and Lynham, 1977, 1978;

Daniel et al., 1977; Haslam et al., 1979b; Fox et al., 1979;
Bennett et al., 1979; Lyons and Shaw, 1980). These experiments have
shown that at least one major protein besides myosin undergoes Ca^{2+}-
dependent phosphorylation in intact platelets and that both proteins
could play a role in the mechanism of release of platelet granule
contents. Recent results related to these findings are reported.

METHODS

Human platelets were used in all the experiments described. In
studies of the effects of various agents on the phosphorylation of
proteins in intact platelets, suspensions of washed platelets in
phosphate-free Tyrode's solution containing 0.35% bovine serum
albumin and apyrase were incubated with carrier-free $[^{32}P]P_i$
(0.8 mCi/ml) for 1 h at 37°C and, after a further wash, were finally
resuspended in albumin-free Tyrode's solution containing apyrase
at about 4×10^8 platelets/ml (Haslam and Lynham, 1977). After
incubation of samples of labelled suspension with appropriate
additions (total vol. 1 ml), which was carried out in an
aggregometer (Payton Associates) in experiments in which aggregating
agents were studied, protein was precipitated with 0.1 ml of 3 M
$HClO_4$, redissolved in a buffered solution containing 3% SDS and 5%
mercaptoethanol and heated at 100°C for 2 min (Haslam et al., 1979b).
Platelet polypeptides were then separated by discontinuous SDS-
polyacrylamide gel electrophoresis with 13% acrylamide in the
separating gel as described by Haslam et al. (1979b), except that
20 cm slab gels rather than 10 cm cylindrical gels were used. Gels
were stained with Coomassie Brilliant Blue R, destained and dried
under vacuum on Whatman 3MM chromatography paper. ^{32}P-Labelled
polypeptides were detected by autoradiography. Details of other
methods used are given in the Table and Figure legends.

RESULTS AND DISCUSSION

<u>Cyclic AMP-Dependent Protein Kinases in Platelets</u>. Chromatography
of the soluble proteins from many tissues on DEAE-cellulose has led
to the recognition of two principal types of cyclic AMP-dependent
protein kinase that are eluted at different salt concentrations and
are present in varying proportions in different tissues (Corbin et
al., 1975). Both isoenzymes were found in platelets; the type I
enzyme was eluted with around 0.08 M NaCl and the type II enzyme
with around 0.17 M NaCl. When the platelet soluble fraction was
prepared from freshly isolated platelets that had been frozen and
thawed in a medium containing EDTA, much less type I than type II
activity was found in the fractions eluted from DEAE-cellulose, at
least when both enzymes were assayed using histone IIA as the
substrate (Fig. 1). However, in experiments in which clinically
outdated platelets that had been stored for 3 days at room
temperature were used, the type I activity eluted was usually much
greater and approached that of the type II enzyme. Binding of
cyclic $[^3H]AMP$ by the fractions containing the type I and type II
enzymes roughly paralleled their cyclic AMP-dependent protein kinase
activities (Fig. 1). However, in many experiments with fresh
platelet material an additional cyclic $[^3H]AMP$ binding peak that was

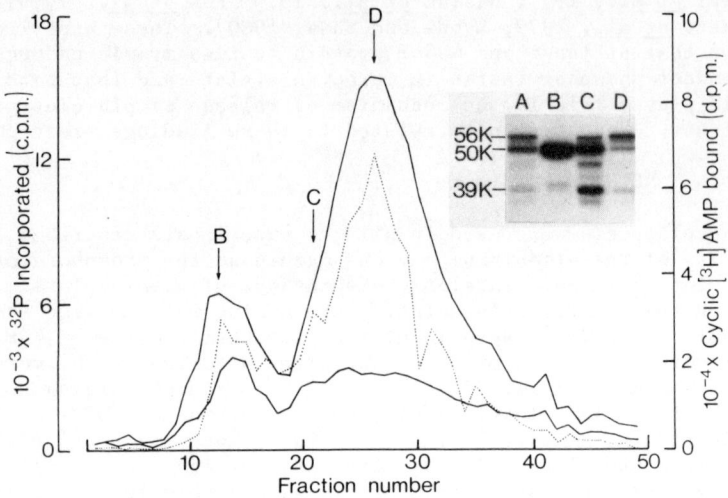

Fig. 1. DEAE-cellulose chromatography of soluble cyclic AMP-dependent protein kinases from platelets. Washed platelets in a medium (pH 6.5) containing 135 mM NaCl, 5 mM glucose, 13 mM citrate and 1 mM EDTA were lysed by rapid freezing and thawing. The 49,000 g x 20 min supernatant was dialysed against 10 mM K phosphate buffer, pH 7.0, containing 1 mM EDTA and 2 mM mercaptoethanol and applied to a DEAE-cellulose column equilibrated with the same buffer. Protein kinases were eluted with a linear gradient of 0-0.4 M NaCl. The cyclic AMP-dependent and independent protein kinase activities (upper and lower solid lines, respectively) and the cyclic [^{3}H]AMP binding capacity (broken line) of the fractions were measured at 30°C, as described elsewhere (Salama and Haslam, 1980). Samples of dialysed platelet supernatant (A) and of the column fractions indicated (B, C and D) were mixed with 0.088 μM 8-azido-cyclic [^{32}P]AMP and irradiated for 10 min at 0°C with a Mineralight UVS-11 held at a distance of 4 cm. Photoaffinity-labeled polypeptides were separated by SDS-polyacrylamide gel electrophoresis and detected by autoradiography (see inset).

not associated with catalytic activity was eluted between the type I and type II enzymes.

To characterize the regulatory cyclic AMP-binding subunits present in the platelet cyclic AMP-dependent protein kinases, we have labelled them covalently with the photoaffinity reagent, 8-azido-cyclic [^{32}P]AMP (Haley, 1977). With fresh whole platelet lysate at least two cyclic AMP-binding polypeptides were detected, a heavily labelled one with an apparent mol. wt. of 50,000 that was resolved into a doublet under optimal electrophoretic conditions, and a

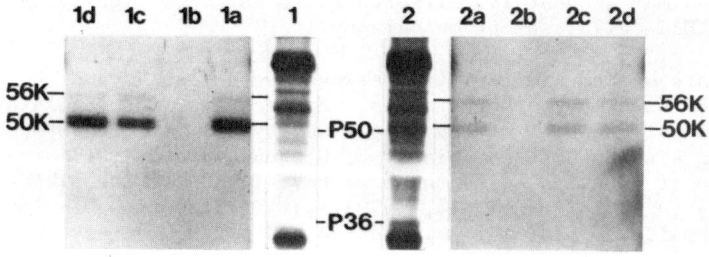

Fig. 2. Photoaffinity labelling of cyclic AMP-binding proteins in platelet lysates. Washed platelets suspended in Tyrode's solution containing 5 mM HEPES, pH 7.4, and apyrase were incubated for 10 min at 37°C with and without 2 μM PGE$_1$. EDTA (10 mM) and diisopropylfluorophosphate (1 mM) were added to the incubation mixtures which were then rapidly cooled to 0°C and sonicated. Samples of the sonicate from (1) the control and (2) the PGE$_1$-treated platelets were incubated for 20 min at 0°C with (a) no addition, (b) 10 μM cyclic AMP, (c) 10 μM cyclic GMP and (d) 10 μM AMP. 8-Azido-cyclic [^{32}P]AMP (0.78 μM) was then added and the samples were irradiated (see legend to Fig.1). Labelled polypeptides were separated by SDS-polyacrylamide gel electrophoresis and detected by autoradiography. Intact platelets were also labelled with [^{32}P]P$_i$ and then incubated (1) without PGE$_1$ and (2) with PGE$_1$; protein from these incubations was electrophoresed (central tracks) in parallel with the photo-affinity-labelled samples.

weakly labelled one with an apparent mol. wt. of 56,000 (Fig. 2). Labelling of both was abolished by preincubation of the lysate with 10 μM cyclic AMP but was unaffected by 10 μM AMP, indicating that specific cyclic AMP-binding sites were present. Cyclic GMP (10 μM) only partly prevented labelling of the 50,000 mol. wt. polypeptide. When lysate was prepared from platelets that had been incubated with PGE$_1$, photoaffinity labelling of the 50,000 mol. wt. polypeptide was markedly inhibited (Fig. 2), indicating occupation of these cyclic AMP-binding sites by endogenously generated cyclic AMP. Photoaffinity labelling of fractions from DEAE-cellulose chromatography of platelet soluble proteins showed that the type I and type II cyclic AMP-dependent protein kinases contained the 50,000 and 56,000 mol. wt. cyclic AMP-binding polypeptides, respectively (Fig. 1). Substantial amounts of the 50,000 mol. wt. polypeptide and of a 39,000 mol. wt. cyclic AMP-binding polypeptide that was sometimes detected in whole platelet lysates, were found in fractions between the type I and type II enzymes. Photoaffinity labelling of the platelet particulate fraction that remained after removal of the soluble proteins for chromatography showed that it contained a high concentration of the 50,000 mol. wt. (type I) cyclic AMP-binding polypeptide. This suggests that variations in the release of type I enzyme from the particulate into the soluble fraction may account for differences in the type I activity found after DEAE-cellulose chromatography.

There are marked similarities between these results and those obtained with many other tissues. For example, the regulatory subunit polypeptides of the type I and type II cyclic AMP-dependent protein kinases have invariably been found to have mol. wts. that are almost identical with those we have found for the platelet enzymes (e.g. Zoller et al., 1979). It is also probable that the 39,000 mol. wt. platelet polypeptide and other minor cyclic AMP-binding polypeptides (see Fig. 1) are related to the proteolytic fragments of the regulatory subunits that have often been observed in other tissues (e.g. Potter and Taylor, 1979). However, the platelet cyclic AMP-binding proteins seem atypical in other respects. Thus, the 56,000 mol. wt. polypeptide incorporated much less ^{32}P from 8-azido-cyclic [^{32}P]AMP relative to the 50,000 mol. wt. polypeptide than expected, considering the amounts of cyclic [^{3}H]AMP bound by the fractions containing the type I and type II enzymes. Secondly, it was surprising to find that the 50,000 mol. wt. rather than the 56,000 mol. wt. cyclic AMP-binding polypeptide existed as a doublet, as it is the latter that is usually present in two forms consisting of the phosphorylated and non-phosphorylated polypeptide (Zoller et al., 1979). Finally, the platelet particulate fraction contained the 50,000 mol. wt. (type I) cyclic AMP-binding polypeptide, rather than the 56,000 mol. wt. (type II) polypeptide that is more commonly found in membrane fractions (e.g. Corbin et al., 1977). However, erythrocyte plasma membranes have recently been shown also to contain the type I enzyme (Rubin, 1979).

<u>Physiological Substrates of Platelet Cyclic AMP-Dependent Protein Kinases</u>. These were identified after addition of PGE_1 to platelets that had been preincubated with [^{32}P]P_i. Previous studies using this method, but followed by a less complete electrophoretic separation of ^{32}P-labelled phosphopolypeptides, showed that PGE_1 increased ^{32}P incorporation into two phosphopolypeptides, P24 and P22, within 1.5 min (Haslam et al., 1978a, 1979b). In the present experiments, additional phosphopolypeptides of interest were resolved. Increased labelling of two (P50 and P24) was readily detected within 0.5 min and reached a maximum within 3 min, whereas increased labelling of two others that incorporated less ^{32}P (P36 and P22) occurred more slowly and peaked later (Fig. 3). Less easily detectable and more variable increases in ^{32}P incorporation into some other phosphopolypeptides (e.g. P82 and P49) were also noted. Whereas P50 and P36 contained no detectable ^{32}P in control platelets, the other phosphopolypeptides affected by PGE_1 were always labelled to some extent (Fig. 3). On 13% polyacrylamide gels, P50 had virtually the same electrophoretic mobility as the 50,000 mol. wt. cyclic AMP-binding polypeptide (Fig. 2), but a significant difference in mobility was detected using 7.5% polyacrylamide. As inhibition of platelet aggregation by PGE_1 develops within 0.5 min, phosphorylation of P50 or P24 is more likely to play a major role in the inhibition of platelet function than are the slower phosphorylation reactions. All other compounds

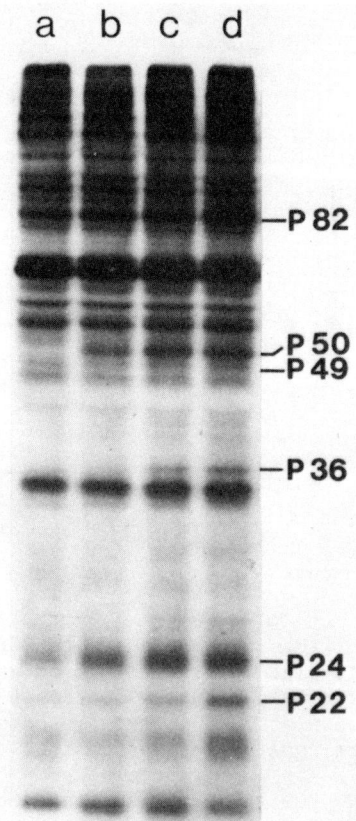

Fig. 3. Effects of PGE_1 on the phosphorylation of polypeptides in intact ^{32}P-labelled platelets. Samples of a suspension of labelled platelets in Tyrode's solution containing apyrase were incubated at 37°C with 2 μM PGE_1 for (a) 0 min, (b) 0.5 min, (c) 3 min and (d) 10 min. Platelet protein was then precipitated with acid and redissolved for SDS-polyacrylamide gel electrophoresis. An autoradiograph of the dried gel is shown.

investigated that increase platelet cyclic AMP, including prostacyclin, adenosine, papaverine, 3-isobutyl-1-methyl xanthine and $N^6,2'$-O-dibutyryl cyclic AMP, also increased ^{32}P incorporation into the same phosphopolypeptides as did PGE_1.

A rapid fractionation of ^{32}P-labelled platelets that had been incubated with PGE_1 was carried out to determine the subcellular distribution of these phosphopolypeptides (Fox et al., 1979). The platelets were sonicated in the presence of EDTA and PP_i to inhibit protein kinases, Ca^{2+}-activated neutral protease and phosphoprotein phosphatases, and were separated by differential centrifugation into 1,300-19,000 g_{av} and 19,000 g_{av}-90,000 g_{av} particulate fractions and a 90,000 g_{av} supernatant. Whereas ^{32}P-labelled P50 and P36 were found in the supernatant fraction, ^{32}P-labelled P24 and P22 were most highly enriched in the 19,000 g_{av}-90,000 g_{av} fraction, which consisted of both plasma and intracellular membranes. Because of published evidence that addition of cyclic AMP and cyclic AMP-dependent protein kinase to a similar membrane fraction from platelets increases the ATP-dependent uptake of Ca^{2+} ions

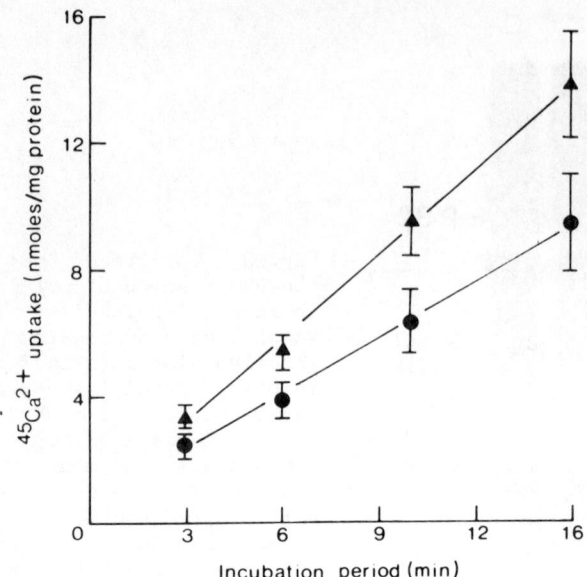

Fig. 4. Effect of incubation of intact platelets with PGE_1 on the uptake of $^{45}Ca^{2+}$ by a platelet membrane fraction. Washed platelets suspended in Tyrode's solution containing 5 mM EDTA were incubated for 2 min at 37°C in the presence and absence of 2 μM PGE_1. After cooling the suspensions to 0°C, they were sonicated for 4 x 15s in presence of proteinase inhibitors and 19,000-90,000 g_{av} membrane fractions were then prepared by differential centrifugation. Uptake of $^{45}Ca^{2+}$ by these membranes was measured at 25°C in a medium containing 5 mM ATP, 5 mM oxalate and a free $^{45}Ca^{2+}$ concentration of 0.75 μM. The values shown are means ± S.E.M. from 6 experiments in each of which membranes were prepared from both control (●) and PGE_1-treated (▲) platelets. Analysis of variance showed that PGE_1 significantly enhanced Ca^{2+} uptake ($P < 0.05$). Full experimental details are given elsewhere (Fox et al., 1979).

(Käser-Glanzmann et al., 1977), we have investigated the relationship between phosphorylation of P24 and P22 and Ca^{2+} transport. Membranes prepared from PGE_1-treated platelets showed a significantly faster rate of ATP-dependent, oxalate-stimulated, $^{45}Ca^{2+}$ uptake than control membranes (Fig. 4). Moreover, when ^{32}P-labelled membrane vesicles that had taken up $^{45}Ca^{2+}$ ions in the presence of oxalate were centrifuged through a discontinuous sucrose density gradient, the $^{45}Ca^{2+}$ bound/mg of protein correlated with the enrichment of ^{32}P-labelled P24 and P22 in the three membrane fractions obtained and were both greatest in the most dense membrane fraction. However, when unlabelled platelet membranes were incubated with $[\gamma\text{-}^{32}P]$ATP in the presence and absence of cyclic AMP, a cyclic AMP-dependent phosphorylation of P22 was observed but little or no radioactivity was incorporated into P24 and no increase in $^{45}Ca^{2+}$ uptake was detected. Käser-Glanzmann et al. (1979) have also noted the phosphorylation of a 22,000 mol. wt. polypeptide in platelet membrane preparations on addition of partially purified type I platelet cyclic AMP-dependent protein kinase in the presence of cyclic AMP and $[\gamma\text{-}^{32}P]$ATP, but in their experiments an increase in $^{45}Ca^{2+}$ uptake was observed. The requirement for exogenous enzyme for phosphorylation of P22 in the latter study could reflect loss of type I enzyme from the membrane preparation due to the use of less fresh platelet preparations or to differences in the method of membrane isolation. It is also possible that the added enzyme fraction contained factors that promote Ca^{2+} transport in addition to cyclic AMP-dependent protein kinase. It is not yet known why P24 is not easily phosphorylated in isolated membrane preparations but this phosphopolypeptide could be present in a different membrane fraction from P22, perhaps at sites within sealed membrane vesicles that are inaccessible to added ATP. The results of Käser-Glanzmann et al. (1977, 1979) indicate that the cyclic AMP-dependent phosphorylation of P22 may stimulate the active transport of Ca^{2+} ions out of the platelet cytosol. However, the available evidence, though circumstantial, also suggests a similar function for P24, phosphorylation of which in intact platelets correlates better with the inhibition of aggregation than does phosphorylation of P22.

Roles of Cyclic Nucleotides and of Protein Phosphorylation in the Inhibitory Actions of SNP. We have compared the biochemical changes and inhibition of platelet responses caused by SNP with those caused by PGE_1 to determine whether there may be common features in their mechanisms of action (Table 1). Both compounds were potent inhibitors of platelet aggregation and the release reaction, though with strong stimuli inhibition of release was incomplete. With washed platelets, 1 μM SNP was more effective than 2 μM PGE_1 in inhibiting the effects of collagen (Table 1). As reported previously (Haslam et al., 1978a, 1979a), SNP caused large increases (up to 50-fold) in platelet cyclic GMP and much smaller increases (up to 2-fold) in platelet cyclic AMP. Because basal levels of platelet cyclic GMP were much lower than cyclic AMP (approx. 1 and 18 pmol/10^9 platelets, respectively), the final concentrations of the two cyclic nucleotides were similar after platelets were incubated with optimal concentrations of SNP (Table 1). These results suggested that the accumulation of cyclic AMP, probably formed with cyclic GMP by the SNP-activated guanylate cyclase (Mittal and Murad, 1977), might contribute to the inhibitory action of SNP. In contrast with SNP, PGE_1 did not affect platelet cyclic GMP levels but, as expected, markedly increased platelet cyclic AMP. Quantitation of the effects of the increases in cyclic AMP observed with SNP by comparison with the effects of PGE_1 on platelet function and cyclic AMP is difficult because PGE_1 caused a rapid increase in cyclic AMP followed after 0.5 min by a decline (Haslam et al., 1978a), whereas SNP caused a slow progressive increase. Moreover, collagen (i.e. released ADP) inhibited the increase in cyclic AMP caused by PGE_1 much more than

TABLE 1. Effects of PGE1 and of SNP on platelet function, cyclic nucleotides and protein phosphorylation.

Additions		Extent of aggregation ΔT(%)	Release of ATP + ADP (%)	Cyclic nucleotides (pmol/10^9 platelets)		Relative amounts of ^{32}P in phosphopolypeptides				
Inhibitor	Aggregating agent			cAMP	cGMP	P50	P49	P47	P24	P20a,b
None	None	-	-	18	0.9	10	11	26	46	2
	Collagen	37	42	18	2.2	-	-	200	54	56
PGE1(0.1 μM)	None	-	-	34	1.1	22	13	25	59	4
	Collagen	24	38	20	0.8	-	-	170	60	56
PGE1(2.0 μM)	None	-	-	159	0.5	42	20	27	61	5
	Collagen	8	29	38	1.3	-	-	107	62	33
SNP(1 μM)	None	-	-	33	5.2	30	17	20	57	2
	Collagen	3	19	29	7.5	-	-	85	57	24
SNP(100 μM)	None	-	-	37	21.8	48	21	24	57	3
	Collagen	3	17	30	31.9	-	-	80	56	26

Samples of washed platelet suspension containing 4.3 x 10^8 platelets that had been labelled by pre-incubation with [^{32}P]Pi were stirred in an aggregometer for 2.5 min with the additions indicated (final vol. 1 ml). Inhibitors were added at 0 min and collagen (25 μg/ml) after 0.5 min. Cyclic nucleotides were extracted with 0.2 ml of 30% trichloracetic acid, separated and purified by chromatography on Dowex 50 and alumina and measured by radioimmunoassay (Harper and Brooker, 1975). The acid-precipitated protein was redissolved in buffered SDS solution and analysed by SDS-polyacrylamide slab gel electrophoresis. The relative amount of ^{32}P in the phosphopolypeptides studied were estimated from the peak heights on densitometric scans of autoradiographs of the dried gels. Values for cyclic nucleotides and ^{32}P in phosphopolypeptides are means from 3 identical incubation mixtures. Release of adenine nucleotides was determined in separate incubations terminated by addition of 0.2 ml of 9% formaldehyde. After removal of the platelets by centrifugation, the supernatants were extracted with HClO4 and their absorption at 256 nm determined. Released ATP + ADP are expressed as percentages of the storage-pool adenine nucleotides.

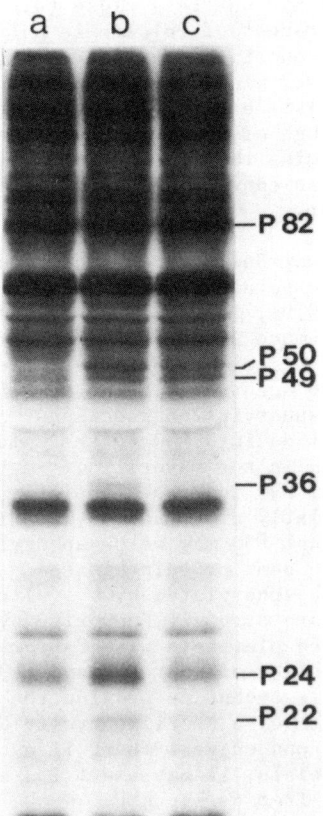

Fig. 5. Effects of SNP and of 8-bromo-cyclic GMP on the phosphorylation of polypeptides in intact ^{32}P-labelled platelets. Samples of a suspension of labelled platelets in Tyrode's solution containing apyrase were incubated for 9 min at 37°C with (a) no addition, (b) 100 μM SNP and (c) 2 mM 8-bromo-cyclic GMP. Platelet protein was then precipitated with acid and redissolved for SDS-polyacrylamide gel electrophoresis. An autoradiograph of the dried gel is shown.

that caused by SNP (Table 1). However, despite these problems, it is clear that the increases in cyclic AMP observed with SNP cannot account for more than a fraction of its inhibitory activity. For example, in the experiment shown in Table 1, the final cyclic AMP level with 1 μM SNP was significantly lower than with 2 μM PGE$_1$ even in the presence of collagen, although the SNP was the more potent inhibitor. Thus, additional effects, perhaps including the formation of cyclic GMP, must mediate the actions of SNP. It is of interest that collagen not only caused a small increase in platelet cyclic GMP by itself but also greatly potentiated the increase caused by SNP. In support of a role for cyclic GMP, we have observed a good correlation between the effects of SNP on platelet aggregation and platelet cyclic GMP under a variety of conditions. For example, a substantial accumulation of cyclic GMP always preceded inhibition of platelet aggregation by SNP, even when both of these effects were delayed for several minutes as on addition of low SNP concentrations to platelet-rich plasma. However, the correlation between increases in platelet cyclic GMP and the inhibition of the release reaction by SNP was less close (e.g. Table 1), perhaps because a substantial component of release is not susceptible to inhibition. In this connection, Weiss et al. (1978) found that several agents that increased platelet cyclic GMP, including SNP and ascorbic acid, had little or no effect on the release reaction induced by a wide range of thrombin concentrations. Further studies are required to determine the reasons for these apparent discrepancies and to establish convincingly that cyclic GMP can function as an inhibitory mediator.

Addition of SNP to intact platelets that had been preincubated with $[^{32}P]P_i$ was found to increase ^{32}P incorporation into the same polypeptides as PGE_1 (Haslam et al. 1979a; Table 1 and Fig. 5). However, labelling of P24 and P22 was much slower and less marked with 100 μM SNP than with 2 μM PGE_1, suggesting that the increases in platelet cyclic AMP caused by these agents may alone be responsible for stimulating these phosphorylation reactions. In contrast, SNP increased ^{32}P incorporation into P50 to the same extent and as rapidly as did PGE_1, and in the majority of experiments increased the labelling of P49 to a substantially greater extent than did PGE_1, particularly after short (0.5 min) incubations. These results suggest that P50 may be phosphorylated by both cyclic AMP and cyclic GMP-dependent protein kinases, whereas P49 may be more selectively phosphorylated by a cyclic GMP-dependent enzyme. These conclusions are strongly supported by the finding that incubation of ^{32}P-labelled platelets with 8-bromo-cyclic GMP led to enhanced phosphorylation of only P50 and P49 (Fig. 5). The results obtained by this technique provide the only evidence yet available for the presence of a specific cyclic GMP-dependent protein kinase in platelets and suggest that, if cyclic GMP is an inhibitory mediator in platelets, it may exert its effects by mechanisms that differ in emphasis from cyclic AMP.

Phosphorylation of Specific Platelet Proteins in Relation to the Platelet Release Reaction. Published studies have shown that when washed platelets labelled by preincubation with $[^{32}P]P_i$ were stimulated by concentrations of thrombin, collagen or the divalent cation ionophore, A23187, that induced platelet aggregation and the release of platelet 5-HT, ^{32}P was selectively incorporated into phosphoserine residues in platelet polypeptides with apparent mol. wts. of about 47,000 (P47) and 20,000 (P20) (Lyons et al., 1975; Haslam and Lynham, 1977; Haslam et al. 1979; Lyons and Shaw, 1980). As addition of ADP and fibrinogen, which caused a comparable extent of platelet aggregation without release of 5-HT, did not increase ^{32}P incorporation into these polypeptides, it appears that their phosphorylation is specifically associated with the platelet release reaction (Haslam and Lynham, 1977). Moreover, as ^{32}P incorporation into P47 and P20 commenced before any aggregation or release of 5-HT could be detected, these phosphorylation reactions could play a role in the mechanism of release. The enhancement of protein phosphorylation by A23187, which is believed to release Ca^{2+} ions from intracellular storage sites, together with the finding that drugs that interfere with the movement of Ca^{2+} ions across cell membranes (tetracaine and verapamil) prevented the collagen-induced phosphorylation of P47 and P20 (Haslam and Lynham, 1978), suggest that these phosphorylation reactions are probably mediated by Ca^{2+}-dependent protein kinases. This conclusion is supported by the finding that in rabbit platelets phosphorylation of these polypeptides is, like the release reaction, partly dependent on extracellular Ca^{2+} ions (Lyons and Shaw, 1980), though studies with rat platelets have suggested that extracellular Ca^{2+} ions are also required for the release of 5-HT from platelets in which protein phosphorylation has already occurred (Bennett et al., 1979). The identity of P47 is unknown, though it is clearly not actin (Haslam and Lynham, 1977; Lyons and Atherton, 1979), but P20 has been shown to contain the phosphorylated 20,000 mol. wt. light chain of platelet myosin (Daniel et al., 1977).

We have recently reinvestigated the effects of collagen on protein phosphorylation in intact ^{32}P-labelled platelets using techniques (see Methods) that gave a considerably better resolution of individual ^{32}P-labelled phosphopolypeptides than was obtained in our earlier studies (e.g. Haslam et al., 1979). In particular, P20 was resolved into four separate components, which we have now designated P21, P20a, P20b and P19, all of which showed an increased incorporation of ^{32}P (Fig. 6). At least two of these, P20a and P20b, appear to represent the phosphorylated forms of variants of the 20,000 mol. wt. light chain of platelet myosin, which stained as a doublet under these electrophoretic conditions. In addition to the above changes and the greatly enhanced phosphorylation of P47, collagen also increased ^{32}P incorporation into three other polypeptides (P75, P40, P27) and decreased labelling of one (P18). Incorporation of ^{32}P into P47, P20a and P20b led to very small but reproducible decreases in the electrophoretic mobilities of the associated polypeptides, indicating that net changes in protein-bound phosphate had occurred. Little or no ^{32}P was found in platelet actin, tropomyosin or profilin, either in the presence or absence of collagen.

Rapid subcellular fractionation of ^{32}P-labelled platelets that had been stimulated by ionophore A23187 and sonicated in the presence of EDTA and PP_i (Fox et al., 1979), followed by slab gel electrophoresis of the protein in the fractions, indicated that most of the phosphopolypeptides that showed ionophore-dependent changes in labelling, including P47, P27, P21 and P18, were recovered in the soluble fraction. However, one minor phosphopolypeptide of interest (P40) was membrane-bound. The subcellular distribution of ^{32}P-labelled P20a, P20b and P19 could not be determined, as they were almost completely dephosphorylated during fractionation of the platelets, suggesting that they are substrates for a specific phosphoprotein phosphatase, presumably the platelet myosin light chain phosphatase (Barylko et al., 1977). In the absence of EDTA and presence of Ca^{2+} ions, a generalized loss of protein-bound ^{32}P was observed, involving most of the phosphopolypeptides that did not participate in the phosphorylation reactions described in this paper, as well as P50 and P36. However, ^{32}P-labelled P47 was not dephosphorylated under these conditions, though its phosphorylation is reversible in the intact platelet (Haslam and Lynham, 1977). These

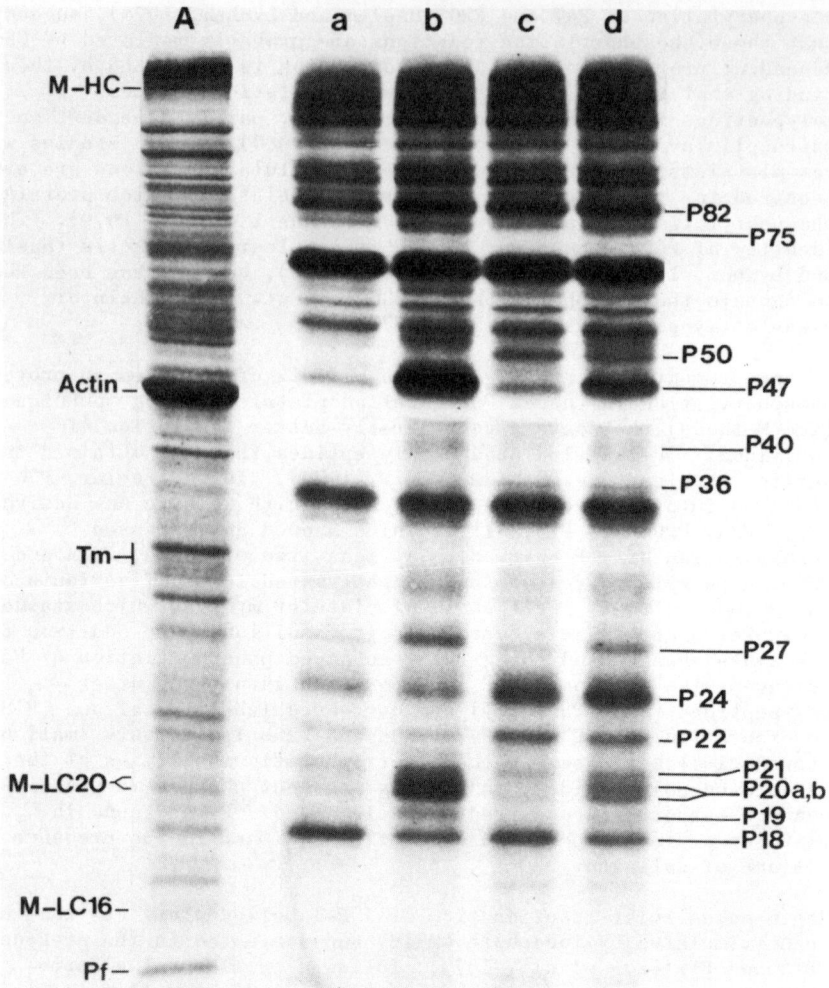

Fig. 6. Effects of collagen added either alone or after PGE_1 on the phosphorylation of polypeptides in intact ^{32}P-labelled platelets. Suspension of labelled platelets in Tyrode's solution containing apyrase was stirred at 37°C with (a) no additions, (b) collagen (50 μg/ml) added after 1 min, (c) PGE_1 (2 μM) added at 0 min and (d) both PGE_1 and collagen. After 3 min, platelet protein was precipitated with acid and then redissolved for SDS-polyacrylamide gel electrophoresis. An autoradiograph of the dried gel (a-d) and the stained polypeptide pattern (A) corresponding to (a) are shown. The positions of platelet polypeptides identified by parallel electrophoresis of purified platelet proteins are shown: M-HC, myosin heavy chain; Tm, tropomyosin; M-LC20 and M-LC16, 20,000 and 16,000 mol.wt. light chains of myosin; Pf, profilin.

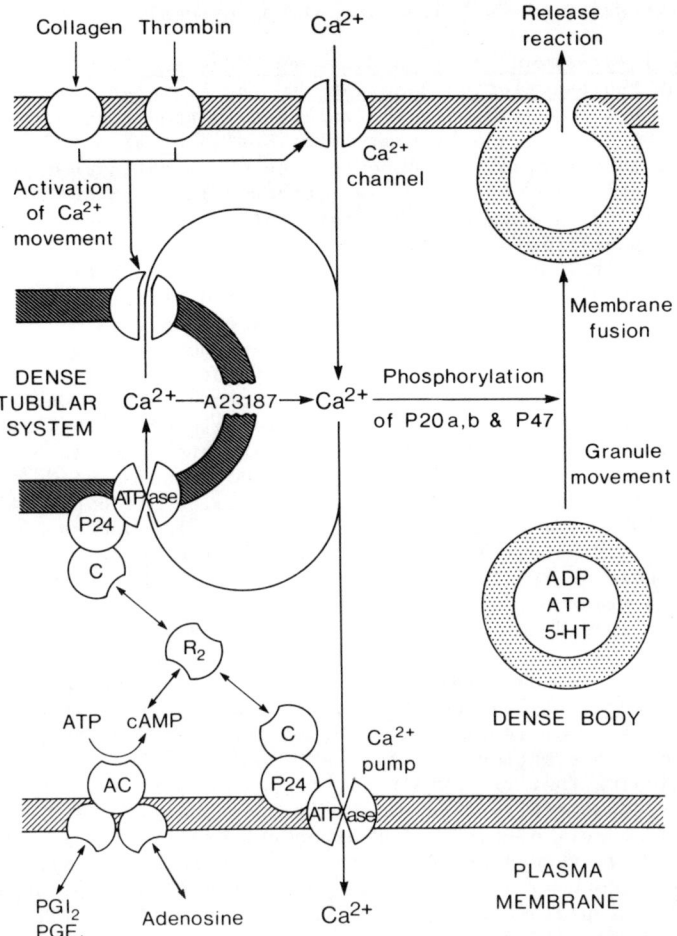

Fig. 7. Schematic representation of some of the possible roles for Ca^{2+} ions, cyclic AMP and protein phosphorylation in the regulation of platelet function. The additional abbreviations used are: AC, adenylate cyclase; R and C, regulatory and catalytic subunits of cyclic AMP-dependent protein kinase.

findings suggest that platelets may contain at least three distinct phosphoprotein phosphatase activities. Finally, we found that fractionation of ^{32}P-labelled platelets in the presence of Ca^{2+} ions led to an enhanced phosphorylation of P24 and P22, suggesting that these phosphopolypeptides may be substrates for a Ca^{2+}-activated protein kinase, as well as for the cyclic AMP-dependent enzymes. This raises the possibility of a negative feedback mechanism by which an increase in cytosol Ca^{2+} concentration might promote the active transport of Ca^{2+} ions out of the cytosol.

Possible Interactions between Ca^{2+}-Dependent and Cyclic AMP-Dependent Phosphorylation Reactions in the Platelet.

We have reported that PGE_1 inhibits the collagen-induced phosphorylation of P47 and P20 (Haslam and Lynham, 1978; Haslam et al., 1979) and have now found that PGE_1 also suppresses the other collagen-induced phosphorylation reactions we have detected in the platelet (Fig. 6). The inhibition by PGE_1 of ^{32}P incorporation into these polypeptides, and particularly into P47 and the P20a,b doublet, correlates closely with the inhibition of the release reaction (e.g. Table 1), which supports the view that these phosphorylation reactions may have specific roles in the mechanism of release. In view of the evidence that Ca^{2+}-dependent protein kinases are responsible for the collagen-induced phosphorylation of platelet proteins and that PGE_1 (i.e. cyclic AMP) may promote the active transport of Ca^{2+} ions out of the platelet cytosol, it is plausible to suggest that PGE_1 may inhibit the phosphorylation of P47, P20a,b etc. and, as a result, the release reaction, by reducing the concentration of Ca^{2+} ions available to Ca^{2+}-dependent protein kinases. This hypothetical scheme is shown diagrammatically in Fig. 7. In support of this view, PGE_1 did not inhibit the phosphorylation reactions induced by the ionophore A23187 (Haslam et al., 1979), which may short-circuit the active transport of Ca^{2+} ions out of the platelet cytosol. This hypothesis should not be regarded as exclusive, and it is indeed likely that Ca^{2+} ions exert important effects in the release reaction that are not mediated by activation of protein kinases (Bennett et al., 1979) and that cyclic AMP inhibits platelet function by mechanisms additional to the activation of a Ca^{2+} pump. One further possible action of cyclic AMP in the platelet is suggested by the finding that the myosin-light chain kinase from smooth muscle is inhibited as a direct result of its phosphorylation by the catalytic subunit of cyclic AMP-dependent protein kinase (Adelstein et al., 1978), though as yet we have not detected the cyclic AMP-dependent phosphorylation of a polypeptide with an appropriate mol. wt. in intact platelets (105,000; Hathaway and Adelstein, 1979). Moreover, we have found that PGE_1 can to some extent inhibit the ionophore-induced release reaction in the absence of any inhibition of ionophore-induced protein phosphorylation (Haslam et al., 1979). In this connection, we still do not know the identity and function of P50, phosphorylation of which correlates closely with the inhibition of aggregation by PGE_1 or SNP. Another observation not explained by the scheme in Fig. 7 is the finding that SNP was a potent inhibitor of the collagen-induced phosphorylation reactions (Table 1), although it was much less effective than PGE_1 in inducing the phosphorylation of P24 and P22. Finally, it must be emphasized that with the exception of the myosin light chain, we know nothing of the functions of the polypeptides that are phosphorylated during the release reaction. However, now that the descriptive phase of our studies on protein phosphorylation in the blood platelet is approaching completion, the purification of individual phosphoproteins and the analysis of their interactions with the membrane systems and granular organelles of the platelet and with components of the platelet cytoskeletal system has become a realistic target.

ACKNOWLEDGEMENTS

This research was supported by grants from the Medical Research Council of Canada (MT 5626) and the Ontario Heart Foundation (T.15-6). J.E.B.F. and S.E.S. were supported by Research Fellowships from the Canadian Heart Foundation. The authors thank Dr. R. S. Adelstein of the National Institutes of Health, Bethesda, MD, for a sample of platelet myosin and Dr. L. B. Smillie of the University of Alberta, Edmonton, Alberta for a sample of platelet tropomyosin.

REFERENCES

Adelstein, R. S., and Conti, M. A., 1975. Phosphorylation of platelet myosin increases actin-activated myosin ATP-ase activity. Nature, 256, 597-598.

Adelstein, R. S., Conti, M. A., Hathaway, D. R., and Klee, C. B., 1978. Phosphorylation of smooth muscle myosin light chain kinase by the catalytic subunit of adenosine 3':5'-monophosphate-dependent protein kinase. J. Biol. Chem., 253, 8347-8350.

Barylko, B., Conti, M. A., and Adelstein, R. S., 1977. Properties of platelet myosin light chain phosphatase. Biophys. J., 17, 270a.

Bennett, W. F., Belville, J. S., and Lynch, G., 1979. A study of protein phosphorylation in shape change and Ca^{2+}-dependent serotonin release by blood platelets. Cell, 18, 1015-1023.

Böhme, E., Graf, H., and Schultz, G., 1978. Effects of sodium nitroprusside and other smooth muscle relaxants on cyclic GMP formation in smooth muscle and platelets. Adv. Cyclic Nucleotide Res., 9, 131-143.

Cheung, W. Y., 1980. Calmodulin plays a pivotal role in cellular regulation. Science, 207, 19-27.

Corbin, J. D., Keely, S. L., and Park, C. R., 1975. The distribution and dissociation of cyclic adenosine 3':5'-monophosphate-dependent protein kinases in adipose, cardiac and other tissues. J. Biol. Chem., 250, 218-225.

Corbin, J. D., Sugden, P. H., Lincoln, T. M., and Keely, S. L., 1977. Compartmentalization of adenosine 3':5'-monophosphate and adenosine 3':5'-monophosphate-dependent protein kinase in heart tissue. J. Biol. Chem., 252, 3854-3861.

Daniel, J. L., Holmsen, H., and Adelstein, R. S., 1977. Thrombin-stimulated myosin phosphorylation in intact platelets and its possible involvement in secretion. Thrombos. Haemostas., 38, 984-989.

Feinstein, M. B., 1978. The role of calcium in blood platelet function, in *Calcium in Drug Action* (Ed. Weiss, G. B.), pp. 197-239, Plenum, New York.

Fox, J. E. B., Say, A. K., and Haslam, R. J., 1979. Subcellular distribution of the different platelet proteins phosphorylated on exposure of intact platelets to ionophore A23187 or to prostaglandin E_1. Possible role of a membrane phosphopolypeptide in the regulation of calcium-ion transport. *Biochem. J.*, 184, 651-661.

Glusa, E., Markwardt, F., and Stürzebecher, J., 1974. Effects of sodium nitroprusside and other pentacyanonitrosyl complexes on platelet aggregation. *Haemostasis*, 3, 249-256.

Haley, B. E., 1977. Adenosine 3',5'-cyclic monophosphate binding sites. *Methods Enzymol.*, 46, 339-346.

Harper, J. F., and Brooker, G., 1975. Femtomole sensitive radioimmunoassay for cyclic AMP and cyclic GMP after 2'O-acetylation by acetic anhydride in aqueous solution. *J. Cyclic Nucleotide Res.*, 1, 207-218.

Haslam, R. J., and Lynham, J. A., 1977. Relationship between phosphorylation of blood platelet proteins and secretion of platelet granule constituents. I. Effects of different aggregating agents. *Biochem. Biophys. Res. Commun.*, 77, 714-722.

Haslam, R. J., and Lynham, J. A., 1978. Relationship between phosphorylation of blood platelet proteins and secretion of platelet granule constituents. II. Effects of different inhibitors. *Thromb. Res.*, 12, 619-628.

Haslam, R. J., Davidson, M. M. L., Davies, T., Lynham, J. A., and McClenaghan, M. D., 1978a. Regulation of blood platelet function by cyclic nucleotides. *Adv. Cyclic Nucleotide Res.* 9, 533-552.

Haslam, R. J., Davidson, M. M. L., and Desjardins, J. V., 1978b. Inhibition of adenylate cyclase by adenosine analogues in preparations of broken and intact human platelets. Evidence for the unidirectional control of platelet function by cyclic AMP. *Biochem. J.*, 176, 83-95.

Haslam, R. J., Davidson, M. M. L., and Lynham, J. A., 1979a. Functional significance of the effects of sodium nitroprusside (SNP) and prostaglandin E_1 (PGE_1) on cyclic nucleotides and protein phosphorylation in human platelets. *Fed. Proc.*, 38, 232.

Haslam, R. J., Lynham, J. A., and Fox, J. E. B., 1979b. Effects of collagen, ionophore A23187 and prostaglandin E_1 on the phosphorylation of specific proteins in blood platelets. *Biochem. J.*, 178, 397-406.

Hathaway, D. R., and Adelstein, R. S., 1979. Human platelet myosin light chain kinase requires the calcium-binding protein calmodulin for activity. Proc. Natl. Acad. Sci. USA, 76, 1653-1657.

Käser-Glanzmann, R., Gerber, E., and Lüscher, E. F., 1979. Regulation of the intracellular calcium level in human blood platelets : cyclic adenosine 3',5'-monophosphate dependent phosphorylation of a 22,000 dalton component in isolated Ca^{2+}-accumulating vesicles. Biochim. Biophys. Acta, 558, 344-347.

Käser-Glanzmann, R., Jakábová, M., George, J. N., and Lüscher, E. F., 1977. Stimulation of Ca^{2+} uptake in platelet membrane vesicles by adenosine 3',5'-cyclic monophosphate and protein kinase. Biochim. Biophys. Acta, 466, 429-440.

Lyons, R. M., and Atherton, R. M., 1979. Characterization of a platelet protein phosphorylated during the thrombin-induced release reaction. Biochemistry, 18, 544-552.

Lyons, R. M., and Shaw, J. O., 1980. Interaction of Ca^{2+} and protein phosphorylation in the rabbit platelet release reaction. J. Clin. Invest., 65, 242-255.

Lyons, R. M., Stanford, N., and Majerus, P. W., 1975. Thrombin-induced protein phosphorylation in human platelets. J. Clin. Invest., 56, 924-936.

Mittal, C. K., and Murad, F., 1977. Formation of adenosine 3':5'-monophosphate by preparations of guanylate cyclase from rat liver and other tissues. J. Biol. Chem., 252, 3136-3140.

Potter, R. L., and Taylor, S. S., 1979. Relationships between structural domains and function in the regulatory subunit of cAMP-dependent protein kinases I and II from porcine skeletal muscle. J. Biol. Chem., 254, 2413-2418.

Rubin, C. S., 1979. Characterization and comparison of membrane-associated and cytosolic cAMP-dependent protein kinases. J. Biol. Chem., 254, 12439-12449.

Salama, S. E., and Haslam, R. J., 1980. In preparation.

Schultz, K.-D., Schultz, K., and Schultz, G., 1977. Sodium nitroprusside and other smooth muscle relaxants increase cyclic GMP levels in rat ductus deferens. Nature, 265, 750-751.

Weiss, A., Baenziger, N. L., and Atkinson, J. P., 1978. Platelet release reaction and intracellular cGMP. Blood, 52, 524-531.

Zoller, M. J., Kerlavage, A. R., and Taylor, S. S., 1979. Structural comparisons of cAMP-dependent protein kinases I and II from porcine skeletal muscle. J. Biol. Chem., 254, 2408-2412.

UNIQUE SPECIALIZATIONS FOR THE SUBCELLULAR COMPARTMENTATION OF AMINES IN PIG AND HUMAN PLATELETS

Jonathan L. Costa and Dennis L. Murphy

Clinical Neuropharmacology Branch
National Institute of Mental Health
Bethesda, Maryland 20205 U.S.A.

ABSTRACT

Platelets appear to store the bulk of their intracellular amine in membrane-bound vesicles containing high concentrations of divalent cations and phosphate groups. This paper examines the amine-storing mechanisms of pig and human platelets, which exhibit significant differences in vesicular elemental and molecular composition, the maximal amount of amine stored per vesicle (maximal packet size), and the degree to which storage of amine is coupled to the storage of other vesicular components. Nuclear-magnetic resonance examination of ring-fluorinated amines and phosphate resonances in intact platelets suggests that the contents of human-platelet vesicles are highly restricted in motion (essentially in a solid phase), while pig vesicles enclose a much more fluid internal environment. Some of the data presented explore the roles of intravesicular pH and the formation of an amine-nucleotide-metal macromolecular complex in the maintenance of high intra-vesicular amine concentrations. In human platelets, but not in pig platelets, amines may also accumulate in two types of extra-vesicular storage sites not releasable by thrombin. Amines can be induced to move from vesicles into an extra-vesicular compartment by treatment with certain drugs or during prolonged incubation with extracellular amines. Amines newly taken up across the plasma membrane can also accumulate extra-vesicularly at what appears to be a separate intracellular site. Extra-vesicular amines lost from vesicles can move relatively slowly into the extracellular medium by a non-exocytotic process, whereas extra-vesicular amine newly taken up from the extracellular medium appears to move relatively rapidly into vesicles but not into the extracellular medium. In addition, exchange of amines between the two extra-vesicular compartments does not appear to occur. At present, the location, functional significance, and storage mechanisms of the two extra-vesicular amine pools in human platelets are unclear.

Platelets are highly structured cells whose internal space contains both membrane-enclosed organelles and structures not specifically segregated from the cytoplasmic ground substance (for reviews see Fukami and Salganicoff, 1977, Holmsen and Weiss, 1979, White, 1971, White and Gerrard, 1976). Evidence has been accumulating for several years that the bulk of intra-platelet amine (predominantly serotonin in most species) is sequestered in a specific membrane-surrounded entity, usually termed the storage vesicle but also known as the "dense body" (White, 1971, White and Gerrard, 1976). Storage vesicles from all species examined to date appear to be capable of storing considerable quantities of amine (Pletscher et al., 1971). Nevertheless, recent work suggests that extra-vesicular sequestration of amine may occur, and that the vesicular storage process is not accomplished by a single mechanism. It is the purpose of this paper to explore two amine storing systems, those of pig and human platelets, in which this type of diversity occurs. Understanding the unique mechanisms in each species should serve as a framework within which to place current concepts about amine storage in platelets and possibly other tissues.

I. Vesicular Storage

In all amine-storing vesicles examined to date, the amine appears to be packaged together with divalent cations and phosphate-containing moities (usually adenine nucleotides). This rather striking coincidence, plus the existence of relatively high intra-vesicular amine concentrations (often in excess of 0.5 M), has been incorporated into the hypothesis that amines and ATP are stored with metal ions as a macromolecular complex with a lowered solubility and osmotic strength (Pletscher et al., 1971). It is instructive to examine this hypothesis in the light of what is currently known about the storage vesicles of pig and human platelets.

First, storage vesicles from each species differ appreciably in molecular and elemental composition--a phenomenon which one assumes contributes at least in some measure to other differences enumerated below. As summarized in Table 1, human platelet storage vesicles contain large amounts of calcium with essentially no magnesium; pig vesicles contain magnesium and little calcium. As anionic groups, vesicles from human platelets apparently contain ADP, ATP, and pyrophosphate in the approximate molecular ratios of 1:0.67:0.50, while pig vesicles have been reported to contain only ADP and ATP in the ratio 1:1.23. The evidence for these differences comes from a number of diverse studies. As early as 1969, Holmsen and co-workers and other groups had concluded that human platelets contained a "storage pool" of ATP and ADP (Holmsen et al., 1969, Holmsen and Day, 1971). Pyrophosphate was subsequently reported to be a thrombin-releasable component of human platelets (Silcox et al., 1973). In 1973, Kinlough-Rathbone and collaborators noted that pig platelets released magnesium following stimulation with thrombin (Kinlough-Rathbone et al., 1973), while Detwiler and Feinman pointed out that under similar circumstances human platelets released calcium (Detwiler and Feinman, 1973). Localization of these substances to specific structures has been facilitated by the observation of electron-opaque structures in whole mounts of platelets from both species, with differences in opacity which correspond to compositional differences as determined by electron microprobe X-ray analyses (Costa et al., 1977d, Skaer et al., 1976, and unpublished observations). More recent work

TABLE 1. Comparison of the molecular composition of storage vesicles in pig and human platelets[1]

	Relative concentrations	
	Pig	Human
	Moles per platelet $\times 10^{18}$ (total vesicular pool)	
Mg	218	< 12
Ca	20.6	125
ATP	21.7	25.0
ADP	17.6	37.5
pyrophosphate	< 4	18.8
	Moles per vesicle[2] $\times 10^{18}$	
Mg	10.9	< 1.5
Ca	1.03	15.6
ATP	1.09	3.13
ADP	0.88	4.69
pyrophosphate	< 0.19	2.35

[1] Data summarized from Kinlough-Rathbone et al., 1973; Lages et al., 1975; Holmsen & Weiss, 1979; Ugurbil et al., 1979; Fukami et al., personal communication.

[2] Calculated by assuming that each pig platelet contained 20 dense bodies (unpublished observations), and that each human platelet contained 8 dense bodies (Costa et al., 1979b; Sweetman et al., 1980).

has documented the phosphate-group signature of each type of platelet storage vesicle, utilizing both classical biochemical and nuclear-magnetic resonance (NMR) techniques (Costa et al., 1979a, 1980a, Johnson et al., 1978, Ugurbil et al., 1979), and has evaluated the composition of biochemically-isolated storage vesicles (Fukami et al., 1978, Salganicoff et al., 1975, and unpublished observations). It is of interest that the NMR "analysis" of intact cells gives data which agrees well with that obtained by biochemical analysis of the same specimen (Ugurbil et al., 1979), and that the calcium and phosphorus content of the vesicles appears from electron microprobe data not to be altered by the isolation procedure (unpublished observations). It is also important to note the the vesicular magnesium concentration as estimated from literature values exceeds the estimated concentration of phosphate residues by a factor of 5. Thus pig vesicles may contain other anionic species besides adenine nucleotides.

Second, as summarized in Table 2, the two types of vesicles differ in their storage capacity for biogenic amines and the basic molecule quinacrine. Under normal circumstances, neither type of vesicle appears to be filled to its maximal storage capacity (maximal packet size) with serotonin (5HT). When each is filled to its maximal 5HT capacity by incubation with exogenous 5HT, an individual pig vesicle appears to store only about one-third the amount found in a typical human vesicle. As far as is known, neither type of vesicle contains appreciable quantities of dopamine *in vivo*. When the two types of vesicles are induced to take up considerable quantities of this amine, the concentration in the pig vesicle is only about 30% of that in the human vesicle. Quinacrine, a basic substance which has been reported to accumulate by a "passive" process in platelet storage vesicles in a variety of species (Da Prada and Pletscher, 1975, Lorez *et al.*, 1977, Picotti *et al.*, 1976), can be measured fluorometrically

TABLE 2. Comparison of the vesicular storage capacity of pig and human platelets for serotonin, dopamine, and quinacrine[1]

Component Stored	Normal Concentration Stored[2] (moles/platelet x 10^{18})				Maximal Storage Capacity[2] (moles/platelet x 10^{18})			
	In total pool		Per vesicle		In total pool		Per vesicle	
	Pig	Human	Pig	Human	Pig	Human	Pig	Human
Serotonin	16	0.5-6.6	0.80	0.06-0.83	24	30	1.20	3.75
Dopamine[3]	?	<0.05	?	<0.006	10	15	0.50	1.88
Quinacrine[3]	0	0	0	0	43	53	2.5	6.63

[1]Serotonin was measured by a radioenzymatic assay (see Costa *et al.*, 1978c), dopamine with the use of C^{14}-labelled dopamine plus liquid scintillation counting, and quinacrine by measuring the emitted fluorescence at 508 nm following excitation with light at 420 nm. Values for endogenous 5HT in the pig are in the same range as those of Minter and Crawford (1974). Other data summarized from Costa *et al.*, 1976, Holmsen and Weiss, 1979, and Eisler *et al.*, 1980.

[2]Note that human platelets average 8 dense bodies/platelet, as compared with 20 dense bodies/pig platelet (see Table 1).

[3]Maximal amount stored was determined without prior removal of endogenous 5HT, and thus may vary depending on amount of endogenous 5HT initially present.

in both pig and human platelets following incubation with 5×10^{-5}M quinacrine for periods of one hour or more. As was the case with 5HT and dopamine, the apparent maximal capacity of a single human-platelet vesicle for quinacrine exceeds that of a single pig vesicle by a factor of about 3.

Third, as summarized in Table 3, pig and human platelets differ in the extent to which stored 5HT can be displaced to the extracellular medium by incubation with certain substances, and in the response of other vesicular components to this treatment (i.e., the extent to which the storage of 5HT is coupled to the storage of other vesicular components in an obligatory fashion, possibly as a macromolecular complex whose maintenance as a complex depends on the mutual association of all the stored substances) (Pletscher et al., 1971). Both can be filled to maximal capacity with 5HT, or can add considerable quantities of dopamine, without any observed change in the peak heights or widths of the phosphate resonances (as studied by ^{31}P NMR of human and pig platelets) (Costa et al., 1980a) or in human platelets in the net calcium and phosphorus content (as observed by electron microprobe analysis of dense bodies) (Costa et al., 1979b). However, as assessed by both radioactive tracers and measurement of total 5HT, 5HT in pig vesicles appears to be less readily displaced from vesicles to the extracellular medium than is 5HT in human vesicles following incubation with either metabolic poisons (4.1 μg/ml of antimycin A plus 40 mM 2-deoxyglucose, 90 minutes at 37°C) or reserpine (10^{-6}M, 90 minutes at 37°C). Treatment with 25 μM X537A for 1 minute at 37°C releases essentially all the 5HT from the vesicles of both species. Following this treatment, human-platelet vesicles lose approximately 20% of their calcium and phosphorus content (as measured by electron microprobe X-ray analysis) (Costa et al., 1979b) without a significant change in the ^{31}P NMR appearance of their remaining phosphorus resonances (Costa et al., 1979a, 1980a). Pig-platelet vesicles, on the other hand, lose both electron opacity as studied in whole mounts (unpublished observations) and their vesicular phosphorus resonances (as seen by ^{31}P NMR) (Costa et al., 1980a). Incubation with 5×10^{-5}M quinacrine for 60 minutes at 37°C produces a 40-60% loss of 5HT from pig vesicles regardless of whether or not they are filled to their maximal 5HT storage capacity. Human vesicles can lose from 10% to 60% of their 5HT content depending on whether or not they are relatively empty (10% loss) or filled to their maximal 5HT storage capacity (50-60% loss) (unpublished observations). Furthermore, vesicular phosphate resonances (as studied by ^{31}P NMR) respond differently to incubation with quinacrine (unpublished observations). The ^{31}P NMR signal from the human-vesicle resonances is unchanged, while that from the pig-vesicle resonances is changed in a fashion consistent with an apparent increase in their molecular mobility (see below).

To this point, we have presented a series of observations characterizing differences and similarities between pig and human storage vesicles. To delineate the relationship of these observations to the "macromolecular complex" hypothesis of Pletscher and co-workers (Pletscher et al., 1971), it is helpful to examine in

TABLE 3. Effect of changes in amine content on cations and phosphate-containing molecules in storage vesicles of pig and human platelets[1]

Experiment protocol	Change in amine content	Effect on other vesicular components		Method of analysis
		Pig	Human	
Incubate with extracellular 5HT (5×10^{-5}M, 90')	fill to maximal capacity with 5HT	none	none	electron microprobe, NMR
Incubate with extracellular dopamine (10^{-4}M, 90')	fill to maximal capacity with DA	none	not done	NMR
Metabolic poisons (antimycin A plus 2-deoxyglucose) (60')	remove ~7% (pig) or ~50% (human) of 5HT	none	none	electron microprobe, NMR
Reserpine (10^{-6}M, 60')	remove ~20% (pig) or ~30% (human) of 5HT	none	not done	NMR
Treat with X537A (25 μM, 1')	remove ~90% of 5HT	loss of all components	loss of ~20% of Ca and P	transmission electron microscopy, electron microprobe, NMR
Quinacrine (5×10^{-5}M, 60')	remove ~50% of 5HT, add quinacrine	increased mobility of phosphorus resonances	none	NMR, electron microprobe

[1] Data summarized from Ugurbil et al., 1979, Costa et al., 1979a, 1979b, and 1980a, and unpublished observations.

some detail the results of recent NMR studies. In ^{31}P NMR, the phosphorus resonances of each of the intra-vesicular phosphate-containing species may present as discrete peaks (lines) at characteristic points on the spectrum. Intra-vesicular amines may be studied by ^{19}F-NMR, by examining the characteristic peaks derived from ring-fluorinated amines sequestered in storage vesicles during *in vitro* incubation of the platelets with these compounds. The fluorinated bioisosteres of 5HT and dopamine have been reported to mimic the behavior of the parent compounds in many respects, and in human platelets appear to accumulate predominantly inside storage vesicles (Costa *et al.*, 1978a, 1979a, Creveling *et al.*, 1979, Goldberg *et al.*, 1980, Joy and Maher, 1979). From examination of the linewidths and chemical-shift parameters of phosphorus or fluorine resonances, as well as from studies employing more sophisticated NMR techniques, it is possible to derive information about the relative molecular mobility of the molecule(s) bearing a phosphorus or a fluorine atom (also termed the molecular tumbling or correlation time), and in some cases the relative contribution of that atom's neighbors to its magnetic relaxation properties (i.e., the bonding relationships of that atom to atoms in its immediate environment).

The ^{31}P linewidths of the intra-vesicular adenine nucleotides and pyrophosphate in human platelets are so broad as to be essentially invisible at all temperatures examined between 0°C and 50°C, and in magnetic fields varying from 2.3 tesla to 8.45 tesla (Costa *et al.*, 1979a, 1980a, Ugurbil *et al.*, 1979). One can estimate that these substances have a molecular tumbling time of less than 10^6/second, more than three orders of magnitude less than if the molecules were moving freely in an aqueous solution. The vesicular calcium-phosphate core thus appears to exist inside the platelet essentially as a solid. Other information suggests that the solid is an amorphous one: dense bodies in platelet whole mounts give no electron diffraction pattern, and generally appear to have a spherical shape (Costa *et al.*, 1977d). It is known that simple calcium phosphate precipitates, as well as precipitates with the complex composition of the dense body, tend to form amorphous aggregates which are spherical in shape (Eanes *et al.*, 1973, Nylen *et al.*, 1972, Weber *et al.*, 1967, and unpublished observations). Since no change occurs in the ^{31}P NMR spectrum of human platelets whose vesicles are depleted of endogenous 5HT, filled to maximal capacity with 5HT, or whose composition is changed by incubation with X537A or metabolic poisons (Costa *et al.*, 1979a, 1980a), the vesicular calcium-phosphate core appears to exist as a solid regardless of concomitant storage of 5HT or of a modest compositional change. It is of interest that intra-vesicular amine, as judged from the ^{19}F NMR spectrum of human platelets containing 4,6-difluoroserotonin at 4°C, appears to be closely associated with the solid phase, since the fluorine linewidths are also too broad to see, even at relatively low magnetic field strengths (Costa *et al.*, 1980a). Experiments at higher temperatures are difficult to interpret because of leakage of the amine to the extracellular medium during the NMR observation period (Costa *et al.*, 1980a and unpublished observations).

In comparative studies of pig platelets carried out under similar experimental conditions, both adenine nucleotides and fluorinated amines in the vesicles appear to tumble as if located in a gel-like medium. The apparent intra-vesicular viscosity decreases with increasing temperature, but is sufficiently high at 4°C to make direct observation of the characteristic resonances difficult. Since these vesicles appear to contain essentially no core-associated protein, the linewidth increases seen as the temperature is lowered presumably reflect decreases in the relative freedom of motion of the amines and nucleotides (i.e., the aggregation state or the "molecular weight" of any macromolecular complex). This portion of the observed behavior is thus grossly consistent with the postulate that the vesicular contents behave similarly to an *in vitro* system in which an amine-metal-nucleotide macromolecular complex is formed by cooling appropriate solutions to 4°C (Pletscher et al., 1971). Other phenomena also consistent with this model are (a) the observed loss of nucleotides following treatment with X537A (removal of Mg^{++} followed by disaggregation of the complex?), and (b) the apparent increase in the ATP and ADP tumbling rates following the addition of quinacrine (loss of approximately 50% of the endogenous 5HT, with formation of a complex of smaller molecular weight?).

The interpretation of other NMR observations, however, suggests that in several specifics the behavior of the pig-platelet vesicles fails to parallel that of *in vitro* systems. First, based on the relative amounts of nucleotides believed to exist in pig versus human vesicles (Ugurbil et al., 1979), and on the relative metal contents of the two types of isolated vesicles (Fukami, personal communication), pig vesicles contain a molar ratio Mg/total nucleotide of approximately 5. *In vitro*, amine-nucleotide complexes have been reported to dissociate in the presence of this much magnesium (Pletscher et al., 1971). Second, in contrast to the behavior of pig vesicles as observed by NMR, amines and nucleotides *in vitro* can form a viscous gel-like phase or a precipitate at room temperature, can maintain such a phase at 20-37°C when formed at 4°C, and can exhibit a pronounced and rapid phase separation (i.e., dramatic increase in the apparent molecular weight of the complex) at lowered temperatures (which vary with the Mg/nucleotide ratio) (Berneis et al., 1970). As the temperature of pig vesicles is progressively raised to 37°C, both amines and nucleotides tumble more rapidly, so that at 37°C the apparent viscosity approaches that of unstructured cytoplasm. The temperature-dependent transitions are fully reversible, and progress in a linear fashion without any obvious sharp transitions (Costa et al., 1980a, Ugurbil et al., 1979). Third, a specific, stoichiometric macromolecular complex is unlikely to be a concomitant of storage in pig vesicles because the phosphorus linewidths vary so markedly with temperature, and because they do so in the same fashion regardless whether or not vesicles are loaded to maximal capacity with 5HT or dopamine, or are subjected to a 10-30% decrease in the amount of endogenous 5HT present by incubation with metabolic poisons or reserpine (see above). In addition, the fluorine linewidths and temperature dependence parallel those of the phosphorus resonances and are similar regardless of whether 5-fluorodopamine, 6-fluoro-5HT, or 4,6-difluoro-5HT are added to the vesicles (unpublished observations). The observed behavior is thus apparently more compatible with a model in which there exists an intra-vesicular amine binding mechanism of high affinity for 5HT, dopamine, and quinacrine, but with a relatively poor ability to distinguish between the three types of amines. One can postulate that as the amines partition into the interstices of a nucleotide matrix whose motional properties vary with temperature, they assume similar properties.

The observed differences between storage vesicles in pig and human platelets indicate that each particular cell is committed to a unique type of amine storage system, neither of which appears to fit well with a model involving the formation of a specific macromolecular complex. Human-vesicle constituents appear to exist essentially in a solid phase, which is highly restricted in motion, while pig-vesicle constituents occur in a less restricted phase whose tumbling rate (i.e., molecular viscosity) is a function of temperature. Given the close coupling of the specific motional properties of intra-vesicular amine and phosphate residues, it seems likely that intra-vesicular amine binding of some type plays a more important role than a trans-membrane pH gradient in the maintenance of the amine stores. This plus the evidence for restricted motion differentiate both systems from the chromaffin granule, whose protein, epinephrine, and ATP core appears to tumble almost as rapidly as if free in solution, and to exist at a pH of approximately 5.7 (Sen et al., 1979). It is of interest that the design of the storage mechanisms in pig and human platelets appears to influence the relative efficiency with which each can store amines. One can speculate that the pig vesicle is structured so as to permit optional storage of magnesium, and as a consequence of this choice is less well adapted to store 5HT.

II. Non-Vesicular Storage

In addition to differences in their mechanisms for vesicular storage of amines, pig and human platelets also appear to differ in their ability to hold amines in extra-vesicular compartments. Although in both types of platelets the majority of amine resides in vesicles, several lines of evidence suggest that in normal human platelets as much as 10% of the total amine present may be sequestered in extra-vesicular compartments (see text below, Table 4, and Costa et al., 1977a, 1977b, 1977c, and 1978c). The intracellular disposition of amine can be documented by comparing the fraction of total amine released from cells following brief treatment with agents which specifically release storage vesicles (i.e., thrombin or the ionophore A23187) with the fraction of storage vesicles (dense bodies) so released (Costa et al., 1977a). In practice, radiolabelled amines are added to the cells and the percent release of the label (measured by conventional liquid scintillation counting) is compared to the percent release of dense bodies (counted by electron microscopy of air-dried whole mounts). When sufficiently small amounts of radiolabelled 5HT are added to platelets, the percent release of 5HT and dense bodies is the same, and one assumes from this and other criteria that essentially 100% of the 5HT is intra-vesicular, and that the behavior of the labelled 5HT can be

TABLE 4. Evaluation of the intra-platelet distribution of labelled 5HT in pig and human platelets following various experimental procedures

Experimental Protocol	Percent Release of Vesicles Versus Radiolabelled Amine			
	Human Platelets		Pig Platelets	
	Vesicles	Radio-labelled Amine	Vesicles	Radio-labelled Amine
10^{-7}M H^{3}5HT 30' at 37°C, resuspend	80.5%[1]	79.5%	34.8%[1]	33.9%
5x10^{-5}M H^{3}5HT 90' at 37°C, resuspend	79.2%[2]	61.3%	26.7%[2]	26.4%
10^{-7}M H^{3}5HT 30' at 37°C, resuspend; 10^{-6}M reserpine 90' at 37°C	81.2%[2]	56.5%	37.1%[2]	36.7%
10^{-7}M H^{3}5HT 30' at 37°C, resuspend; 180' at 37°C	80.5%[2]	64.2%	28.5%[2]	34.3%
10^{-7}M H^{3}5HT 30' at 37°C, resuspend; 5 x 10^{-5}M 5HT 90' at 37°C	79.0%[2]	70.6%	33.9%[2]	37.1%
10^{-4}M C^{14}-dopamine 90' at 37°C, resuspend	89.2%[2]	76.3%	53.8%[2]	50.2%
5x10^{-5}M H^{3}5HT 90' at 37°C, resuspend, 60' at 37°C with releasing agent				
5x10^{-5}M quinacrine	84.2%[2]	55.2%	48.3%[2]	49.4%
10^{-4}M H75/12[3]	84.2%[2]	72.8%	48.3%[2]	48.7%
10^{-4}M fenfluramine	84.2%[2]	75.0%	48.3%[2]	53.9%
10^{-5}M fluphenazine	84.2%[2]	77.2%	48.3%[2]	51.4%
10^{-4}M tyramine	84.2%[2]	72.9%	48.3%[2]	53.6%

[1] Measured by counting dense bodies in air-dried whole mounts before and after releasing stimulus. For human platelets, release was obtained by incubation with 4 units/ml of human thrombin for 1 minute at 37°C. Vesicles in pig platelets were released by incubation with 2 μM A23187 for 1 minute at 37°C. In a separate experiment, the percent release of vesicles from washed pig platelets was the same regardless of the releasing stimulus employed (2 μM A23187, 10 μM A23187, or 4 units/ml of human thrombin) or buffer composition (Tris- or phosphate-based buffering system, with or without 2 mM Mg^{++} and 2 mM Ca^{++}).

[2] Percent release of vesicles was determined by prelabelling platelets in PRP by incubation for 30 minutes at 37°C with 10^{-8}M $H^3$5HT (for human platelets) or 10^{-7}M $H^3$5HT (for pig platelets). The pre-labelled cells were then pelleted, resuspended, and either fixed with formaldehyde (Costa and Murphy, 1975) or treated with thrombin (human platelets) or A23187 (pig platelets) for 1 minute prior to fixation.

[3] 4-methyl-α-ethyl-tyramine (Campbell and Todrick, 1976).

used as an index of the responsivity of the cells to the releasing agent (Costa et al., 1977a, 1979b). Under certain conditions, as described in Table 4, human platelets will accumulate labelled amines in a non-releasable compartment which is apparently extra-vesicular. Since non-releasable amine is not found when pig platelets are subjected to similar experimental protocols, it seems likely that pig platelets hold little or no amine extra-vesicularly.

Not only do human platelets accumulate extra-vesicular, non-releasable amine, but also they appear to assign their extra-vesicular 5HT to two distinct types of compartments, termed pools I and II, which are not in equilibrium with one another (Costa et al., 1980b). When normal platelets at 37°C are exposed *de novo* to extracellular 5HT, the 5HT accumulates rapidly in both vesicles and extra-vesicular pool I. The contents of pool I do not appear to re-enter the extracellular medium, but can either rapidly become releasable (i.e., move into vesicles over a period of seconds) when 5HT is removed from the medium, or can remain non-releasable if the vesicles have previously been filled to their maximal storage capacity for 5HT (Costa et al., 1977a, 1977c, 1978c, 1980b). Releasable vesicular 5HT, in contrast, can move into non-releasable pool II following prolonged incubation at 37°C, treatment with reserpine, or during the process of the addition of extracellular 5HT to maximally filled vesicles (Table 4 and Costa et al., 1977c, 1980b). Pool II 5HT moves relatively slowly (over a period of several minutes) into the extracellular medium, but fails to re-enter vesicles regardless of whether or not the vesicles and pool I are accumulating extracellular 5HT, or whether or not pool I 5HT is in the process of entering the vesicles (Costa et al., 1980b).

If extra-vesicular and extracellular 5HT were in equilibrium, one would expect the accumulation of significant quantities of extra-vesicular 5HT in human platelets to affect the rate at which extracellular 5HT continued to enter the cells. Since this is not in fact observed, and since 5HT in pool I does not appear to be in equilibrium with that in pool II, it seems likely that both pools I and II represent some type of unique, non-releasable storage compartments for 5HT, of uncertain location and functional significance. Furthermore, the complexity of the interrelationships between 5HT in the extracellular medium, vesicles, and the extra-vesicular pools has led to the suggestion that 5HT may enter vesicles directly from the extracellular medium, possibly through channels created by close apposition of the vesicle and plasma membranes (Costa et al., 1980b).

Although pig platelets apparently fail to accumulate 5HT in extra-vesicular pools, they may, nevertheless, move extracellular 5HT directly into vesicles. If this is so, it is of interest that over a range of initial extracellular 5HT concentrations from 10^{-7}M to 10^{-5}M, the rate of accumulation into the pig vesicular pool averages only about 20% the rate at which 5HT enters human-platelet vesicles (unpublished observations). When expressed as the rate of uptake per vesicle per unit time, the difference between pig and human uptake rates is even greater, since the typical pig platelet contains more than two times as many vesicles as the human platelet. It seems possible that differences between pig and human in vesicular composition, amine storage mechanisms, or maximal amine storage capacity may influence the rate at which new amine can accumulate at this site. Further examination of amine uptake and storage in the two types of platelets might profitably explore the relationship of these three parameters to amine uptake in both isolated vesicles and intact platelets.

ACKNOWLEDGMENTS

We wish to thank Drs. Christopher Dobson and Fleming Poulsen (Dept. of Chemistry, Harvard University) for permitting us to discuss their NMR data, Dr. Kenneth L. Kirk (Laboratory of Chemistry, National Institute of Arthritis, Metabolism, and Digestive Diseases) for supplying the fluorinated amines, Mrs. Irene Bellesky for help with the manuscript, and Ms. Denise Fay for her excellent technical assistance.

REFERENCES

Berneis, K.H., Da Prada, M., and Pletscher, A., 1970. Metal-dependent aggregation of nucleotides with formation of biphasic liquid systems. Biochimica et Biophysica Acta, 215, 547-549.

Campbell, I.C., and Todrick, A., 1976. Effects of 4-methyl-α-ethyl-tyramine, 4, α-dimethyl-tyramine and tetrabenazine on the release and uptake of 5-hydroxytryptamine by human blood platelets in vitro. Life Sciences, 18, 1091-1098.

Costa, J.L., and Murphy, D.L., 1975. Platelet 5-HT uptake and release stopped rapidly by formaldehyde. Nature, 255, 407-408.

Costa, J.L., and Murphy, D.L., 1976. Changes in human-platelet storage packet size following incubation with labelled serotonin. Life Sciences, 18, 1413-1418.

Costa, J.L., Murphy, D.L., and Kafka, M.D., 1977a. Demonstration and evaluation of apparent cytoplasmic and vesicular serotonin compartments in human platelets. Biochemical Pharmacology, 26, 517-521.

Costa, J.L., Murphy, D.L., and Reveille, J., 1977b. Evaluation of the uptake of various amines into storage vesicles of intact human platelets. British Journal of Pharmacology, 61, 223-228.

Costa, J.L., Silber, S.A., and Murphy, D.L., 1977c. Effects of reserpine and imipramine on vesicular serotonin uptake and storage in intact human platelets. Life Sciences, 21, 181-188.

Costa, J.L., Tanaka, Y., Pettigrew, K.D., and Cushing, R.J., 1977d. Evaluation of the utility of air-dried whole mounts for quantitative electron microprobe studies of platelet dense bodies. Journal of Histochemistry and Cytochemistry, 25, 1079-1086.

Costa, J.L., Joy, D.C., Maher, D.M., Kirk, K.L., and Hui, S.W., 1978a. Fluorinated molecule as an ultramicroscopic tracer: Mapping of 4,6-difluoroserotonin distribution in human platelets by electron energy-loss spectroscopy. Science, 200, 537-539.

Costa, J.L., Murphy, D.L., and Smith, M.A., 1978b. Comparison of the X537A-induced ionophoric removal of serotonin and tryptamine from intact human platelets. Research Communications in Chemical Pathology and Pharmacology, 22, 27-36.

Costa, J.L., Stark, H., Shafer, B., Corash, L., Smith, M.A., and Murphy, D.L., 1978c. Maximal packet size for serotonin in storage vesicles of intact human platelets. Life Sciences, 23, 2193-2198.

Costa, J.L., Dobson, C.M., Kirk, K.L., Poulsen, F.M., Valeri, C.R., and Vecchione, J.J., 1979a. Studies of human platelets by ^{19}F and ^{31}P NMR. FEBS Letters, 99, 141-146.

Costa, J.L., Pettigrew, K.D., and Murphy, D.L., 1979b. Electron probe microanalysis of changes in dense-body phosphorus and calcium content following alterations in platelet serotonin levels. Biochemical Pharmacology, 28, 23-26.

Costa, J.L., Dobson, C.M., Kirk, K.L., Poulsen, F.M., Valeri, C.R., and Vecchione, J.J., 1980a. Nuclear magnetic resonance studies of blood platelets. Proceedings of the Royal Society of London. Series B, in press.

Costa, J.L., Kirk, K.L., Murphy, D.L., and Stark, H., 1980b. Anomalous compartmentation of serotonin in intact human platelets. (Submitted for publication).

Creveling, C., Seifried, H., Cantacuzene, D., and Kirk, K., 1979. Fluorine-substituted catecholamines as substrates for catechol-O-methyltransferase, in Transmethylation (Eds. Usdin, Borchardt and Creveling), pp 269-276. Elsevier, New York.

Da Prada, M., and Pletscher, A., 1975. Accumulation of basic drugs in 5-hydroxytryptamine storage organelles of rabbit blood platelets. European Journal of Pharmacology, 32, 179-185.

Detwiler, T.C., and Feinman, R.D., 1973. Kinetics of the thrombin-induced release of calcium (II) by platelets. Biochemistry, 12, 282-289.

Eanes, E.D., Termine, J.D., and Nylen, M.U., 1973. An electron microscopic study of the formation of amorphous calcium phosphate and its transformation to crystalline apatite. Calcified Tissue Research, 12, 143-158.

Eisler, T., Teravainen, H., Nelson, R., Krebs, H., Weise, V., Lake, C.R., Ebert, M.H., Whetzel, N., Murphy, D.L., Kopin, I.J., and Calne, D.B., 1980. Deprenyl in Parkinson disease. Neurology, in press.

Fukami, M.H., and Salganicoff, L., 1977. Human platelet storage organelles. A review. Thrombosis and Haemostasis, 38, 963-970.

Fukami, M.H., Bauer, J.S., Stewart, G.J., and Salganicoff, L., 1978. An improved method for the isolation of dense storage granules from human platelets. The Journal of Cell Biology, 77, 389-399.

Goldberg, L.I., Kohli, J.D., Cantacuzene, D., Kirk, K.L., and Creveling, C.R., 1980. Effects of ring fluorination on the cardiovascular actions of dopamine and norepinephrine in the dog. Journal of Pharmacology and Experimental Therapeutics, in press.

Holmsen, H., Day, H.J., and Storm, E., 1969. Adenine nucleotide metabolism of blood platelets. VI. Subcellular localization of nucleotide pools with different functions in the platelet release reaction. Biochimica et Biophysica Acta, 186, 254-266.

Holmsen, H., and Day, H.J., 1971. Adenine nucleotides and platelet function. Series Haematologica, 4, 28-58.

Holmsen, H., and Weiss, H.J., 1979. Secretable storage pools in platelets. Annual Review of Medicine, 30, 119-134.

Johnson, R.G., Scarpa, A., and Salganicoff, L., 1978. Measurement of the protonmotive force in amine containing subcellular organelles, in Frontiers of Biological Energetics (Eds. Dutton, Leslie, Leigh and Scarpa), pp 534-544. Academic Press, New York.

Joy, D.C., and Maher, D.M., 1979. Inner-shell electron spectroscopy for microanalysis. Science, 206, 162-168.

Kinlough-Rathbone, R.L., Chahil, A., and Mustard, J.F., 1973. Effect of external calcium and magnesium on thrombin-induced changes in calcium and magnesium of pig platelets. American Journal of Physiology, 224, 941-945.

Lages, B., Scrutton, M.C., and Holmsen, H., 1975. Studies on gel-filtered human platelets: Isolation and characterization in a medium containing no added Ca^{++}, Mg^{++}, or K^{+}. The Journal of Laboratory and Clinical Medicine, 85, 811-825.

Lorez, H.P., Da Prada, M., Rendu, F., and Pletscher, A., 1977. Mepacrine, a tool for investigating the 5-hydroxytryptamine organelles of blood platelets by fluorescence microscopy. The Journal of Laboratory and Clinical Medicine, 89, 200-206.

Minter, B.F., and Crawford, N., 1974. Subcellular distribution of reserpine and 5-hydroxytryptamine in blood platelets after treatment with reserpine in vitro and in vivo. Biochemical Pharmacology, 23, 351-367.

Nylen, M.U., Eanes, E.D., and Termine, J.D., 1972. Molecular and ultrastructural studies of non-crystalline calcium phosphates. Calcified Tissue Research, 9, 95-108.

Picotti, G.B., Da Prada, M., and Pletscher, A., 1976. Uptake and liberation of mepacrine in blood platelets. Naunyn-Schmiedeberg's Archives of Pharmacology, 292, 127-131.

Pletscher, A., Da Prada, M., and Berneis, K.H., 1971. Aggregation of biogenic monoamines and nucleotides in subcellular storage organelles. Mem. Society Endocrinology, 19, 767-783.

Salganicoff, L., Hebda, P.A., Yandrasitz, J., and Fukami, M.H., 1975. Subcellular fractionation of pig platelets. Biochimica et Biophysica Acta, 385, 394-411.

Sen, R., Sharp, R.R., Domino, L.E., and Domino, E.F., 1979. Composition of the aqueous phase of chromaffin granules. Biochimica et Biophysica Acta, 587, 75-88.

Silcox, D.C., Jacobelli, S., and McCarty, D.J., 1973. Identification of inorganic pyrophosphate in human platelets and its release on stimulation with thrombin. The Journal of Clinical Investigation 52, 1595-1600.

Skaer, R.J., Peters, and Emmines, J.P., 1976. Platelet dense bodies: a quantitative microprobe analysis. Journal of Cell Science, 20, 441-457.

Sweetman, H.E., Costa, J.L., Vecchione, J.J., Valeri, C.R., and Shepro, D., 1980. Dense bodies and total calcium in human platelets following aspirin ingestion for a two-week period. Thrombosis Research, 17, 55-61.

Ugurbil, K., Holmsen, H., and Shulman, R.G., 1979. Adenine nucleotide storage and secretion in platelets as studied by ^{31}P nuclear magnetic resonance. Proceedings of the National Academy of Sciences, 76, 2227-2231.

Weber, J.C., Eanes, E.D., and Gerdes, R.J., 1967. Electron microscope study of noncrystalline calcium phosphate. Archives of Biochemistry and Biophysics, 120, 723-724.

White, J.G., 1971. Platelet morphology, in The Circulating Platelet (Ed. Johnson), pp 46-122. Academic Press, New York.

White, J.G., and Gerrard, J.M., 1976. Ultrastructural features of abnormal blood platelets. A review. American Journal of Pathology, 83, 590-614.

MECHANISMS OF PLATELET SECRETION

H. Holmsen

Thrombosis Research Center, Temple University,
Philadelphia, PA., USA

DEFINITION

Platelet secretion means the exocytosis of the contents of storage granules of platelets to their extracellular environment. Since platelets contain three types of storage granules, the secretory process can be subdivided into dense granule secretion, α-granule secretion and acid hydrolase secretion.

CONTENTS OF STORAGE GRANULES

This subject was recently reviewed (Holmsen and Weiss, 1979) and will briefly be summarized and provided with additional information.

Dense granules are homogeneous, containing ATP, ADP, pyrophosphate, a divalent metal and serotonin. The nature of the divalent metal is species-dependent as human platelet granules contain only Ca^{2+}, those of pig only magnesium (Holmsen, unpublished) while those of bovine origin contain equal proportions of Ca and Mg (Meyers et al., 1979). Both ATP, ADP, pyrophosphate and metal are present in concentrations above 200 mM and exchange very slowly with corresponding extragranular pools. Granule-located serotonin, exchanges very rapidly with both extragranular and extracellular serotonin. About 30% of GTP + GDP in human platelets is secretable and absent in platelets from patients with Storage Pool Deficiency, strongly suggesting a localization of GTP in the dense granules (Daniel et al., 1980). Using the same criteria, 21% of the inorganic orthophosphate in platelets is present in the dense granules (Fukami et al., 1980).

α-Granules are heterogeneous and contain only proteins: coagulation factors (fibrinogen, factor V), platelet specific-proteins (platelet factor 4, low affinity platelet factor 4-a precursor for β-thromboglobulin), cationic proteins (growth factor, permeability factor, bactericidal factor, chemotactic factor) and glycoproteins. The latter have been characterized as thrombospondin (Lawler et al., 1978) and fibronectin (Zucker et al., 1979). This subdivision is premature since both fibrinogen and particularly factor V are glycoproteins, the platelet growth factor may be platelet specific (Antoniades and Scher, 1977) and thrombospondin may also be plateletspecific. However, many of the glycoproteins (fibrinogen, factor V, fibronectin) have their counterparts in plasma. Substantial amounts of albumin are also present in platelets and secreted by thrombin (Davey and Luscher, 1961). The failure of demonstrating de novo synthesis of fibrinogen in megakaryocytes (Nachman et al., 1978) and the identity of platelet fibrinogen with plasma fibrinogen (Doolittle, et al., 1974), suggest that fibrinogen, as well as the other glyco-proteins, have entered the α-granules by receptor-mediated endocytosis of certain plasma glycoproteins.

Acid hydrolase-containing vesicles are poorly defined morphologically and subcellular fractionation has yet failed to yield preparations with particle-bound acid hydrolases in which well defined granules are present; these preparations also contain predominantly mitochondria. The fact that acid hydrolases are secreted from platelets while mitochondria are retained, shows that they must originate from specific subcellular granules. The composition of these putative granules have therefore originated from secretion studies. Table I shows some of the most prominent acid glycosidases that are released from platelets by thrombin, their level in platelets and percent secretion. Other secretable acid hydrolases are β-glycerophosphatase and aryl sulfate. Table I also shows that the most abundant acid hydrolase, aryl phosphatase (p-nitrophenylphosphate or 4-methylembelliferyl phosphate as substrate) is not secreted. This enzyme activity is present in the microsomal fractions. It is of interest to note that platelets

TABLE I. Secretion of acid glycosidases from human platelets by thrombin

	Enzyme level*	% Secretion**
β-N-acetylglucosaminidase	4.30	61
β-N-acetylgalactosaminidase	0.34	65
α-Fucosidase	0.18	54
α-Mannosidase	0.46	45
β-Glucuronidase	1.10	38
β-Galactosidase	0.80	29
α-Galactosidase	0.33	22
β-Fucosidase	0.14	29
α-Arabinosidase	0.34	27
Aryl phosphate	32.8	2

*moles/min/10^{11} platelets.
** Percent of total activity (1st column).

Human platelets were gel-filtered with Tyrode's solution containing 0.2% crystalline human albumin (Lages et al., 1975) and incubated with and without 5 μ/ml of thrombin for 5 min at 37°C. Total levels were determined directly in the suspension incubated without thrombin, and the levels secreted were determined in the supernatant after centrifugation of the thrombin-treated samples 2 min at 12000 xg. The glycosidase activities were determined with 4-methylumbelli-ferone-containing substrates (Dangelmaier and Holmsen, 1980).

have more of the endocytosable (high uptake) form of β-glucuronidase than any other tissue investigated (Brot et al., 1974). It is therefore possible that the acid hydrolases (which are glycoproteins) have been incorporated within storage vesicles by receptor-mediated endocytosis, as suggested above for the α-granules glycoproteins.

INDUCTION OF PLATELET SECRETION - INTERRELATION WITH OTHER PLATELET RESPONSES.

It was pointed out previously that the secretory responses are part of a response propagation following stimulation of platelets (Holmsen, 1978). Specifically, stimulation of platelets causes a rapid shape change, development of adhesive properties of the plasma membrane leading to platelet aggregation if the cells are brought in close contact and adhesion to foreign surfaces, liberation of aracidonate from platelet phospholipids followed by oxygenation of the free fatty acid, and secretion of the contents of dense granules, α-granules and acid hydrolase-containing vesicles. A number of hypotheses have been forwarded to explain the interrelation between the various responses and, in particular, why inhibition of one response under certain circumstances influences the manifestation of others. The four most prevailing of these hypotheses are listed below.

Hypothesis No. 1. An agonist induces arachidonate liberation in a direct fashion and thromboxane A_2 which is formed causes dense granule secretion by which ADP appears extracellularly and causes aggregation (Claesson and Malmsten, 1977; Zucker, 1980). The shape change, α-granule secretion and acid hydrolase secretion responses are not included.

Hypothesis No. 2. A weak agonist induced aggregation which in itself causes "activation". Strong agonists cause "activation" directly which results in dense granule secretion, arachidonate liberation and further ("secondary") aggregation (Charo et al.,1977). The shape change, α-granule secretion and acid hydrolase secretion responses are not included.

Hypothesis No. 3. Platelets are activated by three different mechanisms which operate independently. The first is the direct mechanism: the agonist (e.g., thrombin) induces shape change, aggregation, dense granule secretion, acid hydrolase secretion and arachidonate liberation directly. The second is the arachidonate pathway: the agonist causes arachidonate liberation directly and the thromboxane A_2 formed subsequently causes shape change, aggregation and dense granule secretion. The third mechanism is the "release" dependent one: the agonist induces shape change, aggregation and dense granule secretion, and the secreted ADP further potentiates the overall response propagation (Kinlough-Rathbone et al., 1977).

Hypothesis No. 4. This is called "the basic platelet reaction" which bridges hypothesis 2 and 3, takes all six responses into account and is based on evidence discussed in detail previously (Holmsen, 1974; 1976, 1977, 1978). Briefly, an agonist interacts with its specific receptor, which leads to release of second messenger to the cytoplasm. Each receptor controls a certain amount of second messenger, so when maximal stimulus is received, the entire amounts of receptor-controlled second messenger are released; below maximal stimulation, fractional amounts are released. Released second messenger will activate the various platelet responses according to their affinity for the second messenger. The affinities relate to each other in the order: shape change > aggregation > dense granule/α-granule secretion > arachidonate liberation > acid hydrolase secretion. Each response requires ATP availability in the opposite order. The response sequence contain two distinct positive feedback loops, appearance of thromboxane A_2 and extracellular ADP which increases the total stimulus strength by interaction with their receptors and result in activation of more responses than the original stimulus. A third less distinct positive feedback loop is the activation of arachidonate liberation and secretion by close call contact (aggregation and centrifugation - see below). The ADP and thromboxane A_2 made available act synergistically with each other or with the original agonists.

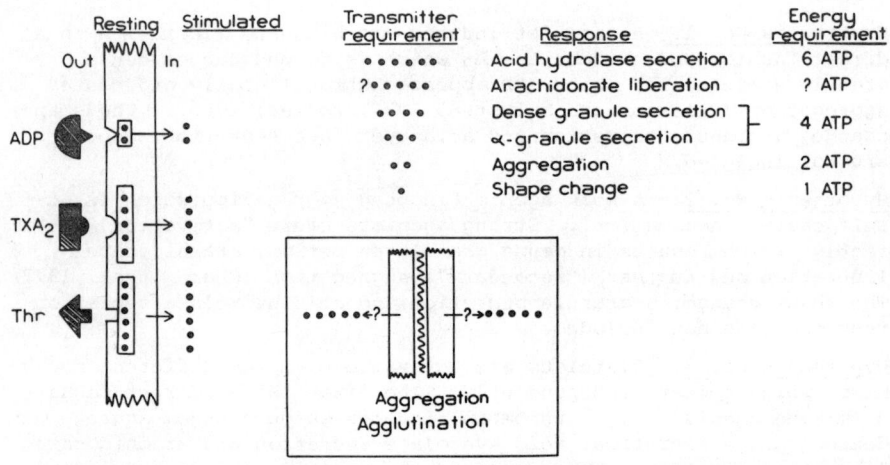

Figure 1. Receptors controlling quanta of second messenger (transmitter).

which controls sufficient amounts of second messenger to activate all responses, while a "weak" agonist has receptors which control small amounts of second messenger which, when fully released to cytoplasm, only will activate shape change and aggregation. This is illustrated in Fig. 1, where the total number of different receptors control quanta of a second messenger which relate to each other

in simple proportions. The responses, in the order given above, require increasing simple numbers of quanta.
All the thrombin receptors, for example, are shown in Fig. 1 to control a total of six quanta of second messenger, sufficient for all six responses. The putative ADP receptors, on the other hand, have a total of two quanta and only will activate shape change and aggregation, and if the latter is allowed to occur, the overall close cell contact feedback loop will cause release of three additional quanta resulting in dense granule secretion, α-granule secretion and arachidonate liberation. Platelets do, however, not secrete during ADP-induced aggregation when the synthesis of thromboxane A_2 is blocked (e.g. with aspirin), demonstrating that close cell contact induction of secretion is completely dependent on the thromboxane A_2 feedback loop. Considerable secretion can, however, occur in aspirin-treated platelets by close cell contact induced by other inducers (see below).

The three mechanisms of hypothesis No. 3 are represented by the basic platelet reaction without feedback loops (=mechanism 1), the thromboxane A_2 feedback loop (=mechanism 2) and the secreted ADP feedback loop (=mechanism 3). The activation step in hypothesis No. 2 is represented by the close cell contact feedback loop in the basic platelet reaction. Hypothesis No. 1 must be disregarded since thromboxane A_2 causes shape change and biphasic aggregation without participation of secreted ADP (Kinlough-Rathbone et al., 1976; Meyers et al., 1979).

THE NATURE OF SECOND MESSENGER - THE CLOSE CELL CONTACT FEEDBACK LOOP

The divalent cationophore A 23187 causes shape change, aggregation and, when the platelets are washed in certain media (see below), both dense granule, acid hydrolase secretion and arachidonate liberation in an apparently direct fashion; the responses to both thrombin and A 23187 are inhibited by so-called Ca-antagonists, and the inhibition is counteracted by extracellular Ca^{2+} ions. In addition, the fluorescence of chlorotetracycline decreases in platelets having absorbed this fluorophor when the cells are treated with thrombin, and the secretory responses to A 23187 take place in platelets suspended in EDTA-containing salt solutions (for references, see Holmsen, 1978). These observations indicate, but do not prove, that Ca^{2+} ions derived from stores within the platelets themselves are the second messenger.

A Ca^{2+} ionophore is thought to form a lipid-soluble complex with Ca^{2+} which can pass across biological membranes. It dissociates according to mass action at the aqueous/phospholipid interface and can thus transport Ca^{2+}-rich aqueous milieu across membranes to a Ca^{2+}-poor aqueous milieu. The experiments reported below do not support the view that induction of secretion in platelets by A 23187 occurs by a simple transport of Ca^{2+} from putative Ca stores to the cytoplasm within the platelets.

We have shown that A 23187 conditions platelets to undergo dense granule secretion when the cells are packed together during centrifugation, a procedure most often used to remove the cells so secreted substances can be determined in the supernatant. Such centrifugation-induced secretion is abolished by fixing the cells at $0°$ with 135 mM formaldehyde (Costa and Murphy, 1975). So, when a mixture of platelet-rich plasma (PRP) and A 23187 was stirred in an aggregometer, and aliquots from this mixture were withdrawn at various times, mixed with formaldehyde and centrifuged, secreted adenine nucleotides and serotonin accumulated in the supernatants of samples taken only after aggregation was well on its way (Holmsen and Setkowsky-Dangelmaier, 1977). A similar experiment, using platelets gel filtered into Ca-free Tyrode's solution (GFP) is shown in Table II. The supernatants obtained by centrifugation without formaldehyde-treatment of GFP stirred with A 23187, so aggregation occurred, contained 63.1% ATP + ADP. However, when the stir bar was omitted, the platelets did not aggregate, the supernatant contained 29.7 & ATP + ADP.

TABLE II. Dense granule secretion by A 23187. Requirement for close cell contact and active cyclo-oxygenase.

Treatment of platelet-rich plasma	+Formaldehyde		-Formaldehyde	
	+stirring	-stirring	+stirring	-stirring
No aspirin	60.6	7.1	63.1	29.7
Aspirin	12.2	0.2	25.2	24.1

Gel filtered platelets (1.0 ml portions) from platelet-rich plasma treated with and without 8 mM aspirin were incubated with 12 µM A 23187 at $37°$ C in aggregometer cuvettes with and without stirring (900 rpm). After 3 min 100 µl of the cuvette content was transferred to tubes in ice containing 50 µl 0.15 M NaCl/25 mM EDTA or 675 mM formaldehyde/25 mM EDTA. The tubes were centrifuged and the amounts of secreted ATP + ADP determined in the supernatant and expressed a % of the total ATP + ADP content.

This difference shows that aggregation markedly enhances the secretory response of A 23187-conditioned platelets above that produced by close cell contact during centrifugation. Without this effect of centrifugation, i.e., when GFP was mixed with formaldehyde before centrifugation, A 23187-aggregated GFP gave 60.6% secretion, almost the same degree of secretion as when aggregated GFP was experiencing the full effect of close cell contact by centrifugation. However, when GFP did not aggregate in response to A 23187, by omitting the stir bar, only 7.1% secretion took place when the close cell contact effects during centrifugation were prevented by formaldehyde. Blockade of thromboxane A_2 formation by aspirin reduced the centrifugation induced secretion (i.e., without formaldehyde) to about 25% irrespective of whether aggregation occurred or not. When the centrifugation-induced secretion was abolished by formaldehyde, A 23187-aggregated,

aspirin-treated GFP secreted 12.2% ATP + ADP, while no secretion
took place when their GFP was not allowed to aggregate. The same
observations were made using PRP instead of GFP. These results
show that A 23187 does not include dense granule secretion in GFP
per se, and that the secretory response depends entirely on both
the close cell contact provided by aggregation and packing during
centrifugation and on an active cyclooxygenase. Acid hydrolase
secretionary A 23187 in GFP was even more dependent than those granule secretion on close cell contact and active cyclo-oxygenase.
Furthermore, the A 23187-induced liberation of ^{14}C-arachidonate from
phospholipids in GFP prepared from ^{14}C-arachidonate-incubated PRP
depended completely on aggregation (results not shown). Therefore,
the mechanism for the interaction between A 23187 and platelets in
GFP and PRP can be written as:

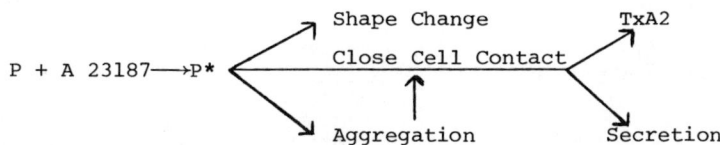

where P is a resting and P* an ionophore-stimulated platelet. It
follows from Table II that the aggregation-induced close cell contact
depends on the TxA$_2$ loop, while the centrifugation-induced process
does not.

When thrombin (0.4 u/ml) was used in these experiments, no effect of
close contact on secretion or arachidonate liberation was seen.
However, at low concentrations and reaction times less than 30 seconds, close cell contact enhanced the thrombin-induced responses.
The requirement for close cell contact in A 23187-induced dense
granule secretion was absent in platelets that had been washed at
4° with salt solution containing EDTA or had pH 6.5 (Table III),
thus confirming previous studies (Feinman & Detwilter, 1974, Murer
& Stewart, 1977). The same was found for acid hydrolase secretion
and arachidonate liberation. Considerably higher concentrations of
A 23187 were used in GFP and the two other platelet suspension in
Table II. GFP contains albumin while the others do not, and albumin
greatly counteracted the effects of A 23187, presumably by binding
the lipophilic ionophore. However, increase of the A 23187 concentration to lytic levels do not overcome the absolute requirement for
close cell in GFP. Therefore, the difference between GFP (and PRP)
and the washed platelets is qualitative. In the earlier studies
with washed platelets, secretion by A 23187 could easily be explained by A 23187-mediated translocation of Ca from intracellular
stores to cytoplasm where it directly activated the secretory process. Evidently, the GFP and PRP, this explanation does not hold,
and other factors may play a role. Our working hypothesis is that
there is a small pool of Ca^{2+} associated with the membrane while,
when released to the cytoplasm, provides sufficient second messenger to induce shape change and aggregation, but is insufficient for
the other responses. Another, large store of Ca^{2+} is thought to be

present intracellularly (dense tubular system?). A 23187 has access to the small membrane pool in unwashed cells, but not to the intracellular pool, thus explaining the induction of shape change and aggregation, and absence of induction of secretion. During close cell contact, the intracellular pool becomes partially available to the ionophore, and submaximal secretion takes place; complete secretion, however, only occurs when the thromboxane feedback loop is triggered. During washing, great morphological alterations take place under which the intracellular pool becomes fully available to the ionophore, and complete secretion is triggered directly, independent of the close cell contact and thromboxane feedback loops.

TABLE III. Dense granule secretion by A 23187 - effect of method for platelet isolation

Time with A 23187 (sec)	Stirring	% ^{14}C-Serotonin Secreted		
		Gel filtered	EDTA washed	pH 6.5 washed
90	+	8.3	76.5	72.2
	−	0.1	80.5	86.5
180	+	60.3	75.3	69.2
	−	2.1	76.3	85.6
Platelet count, 10^8 cells/ml		1.6	2.2	2.0
Concentration, A 23187, μM		8	2	2

Equal portions of platelets from one PRP labeled with ^{14}C-serotonin (Holmsen et al., 1978) were 1.) gel filtered as described in Table I, 2.) washed (4°) and suspended with 0.12 M NaCl/0.03 M Tris HCl/0.003 M EDTA/0.005 M glucose, pH 7.4 and 3.) wahsed with 0.12 M NaCl/0.03 M HEPES/0.005 M glucose, pH 6.5 and suspended in the same buffer, pH 7.4. Aliquots of the suspensions were incubated with A 23187 in the presence and absence of stirring, treated with formaldehyde before centrifugation as outlined in Table II.

ENERGY REQUIREMENTS FOR SECRETION

The secretory responses, as the other responses, are gradually inhibited and eventually abolished, when the ATP availability in platelets decreases steadily by incubating platelets with metabolic inhibitors. However, as shown in Table IV, the dense granule and α-granule secretion are inhibited to a lesser degree than is acid hydrolase secretion during incubation of GFP with 2-deoxyglucose and antimycin A. Moreover, acid hydrolase secretion is immediately inhibited upon addition of the metabolic inhibition while dense granule and α-granule secretion is unaffected of the immediate presence of the inhibitors (zero time, Table IV). This is probably related to our previous finding that acid hydrolase secretion is inhibited by antimycin A alone while dense granule secretion is not (Holmsen et al., 1980). These results suggest that acid hydrolase secretion is more dependent on available ATP than are dense granule and α-granule secretion. It also appears as if acid hydrolase secretion depends specifically on ATP produced by oxidative phosphorylation. However, other effects of blocking respiration, e.g. a change in the redox potential in the cell, could also be of importance.

Dense granule secretion occurs without simultaneous production of ATP, showing that the energy present in the cytoplasmic ATP pool is sufficient to support the process (Akkerman et al., 1979). This was shown by monitoring Ca^{2+} secretion when thrombin was added together with 2-deoxglucose and glucano-δ-lactone to antimycin A-containing GFP, which causes instantaneous abolition of platelet ATP production (Holmsen and Akkerman, 1980). This instantaneous stop of ATP production causes a rapid fall in the level of metabolic ATP, due to ongoing ATP consuming processes in the platelet. However, when

TABLE IV. Differential inhibition of the individual platelet secretory responses during ATP depletion

	Incubation time, min			
	0	5	10	15
[^{14}C-ATP], % of total ^{14}C	83	63	49	5
Adenylate energy charge	0.95	0.88	0.81	0.78
*Dense granule secretion, ATP + ADP	105	103	61	51
*α-granule secretion, fibrinogen	98	95	60	45
*Acid hydrolase secretion, β-N**	79	30	8	0

*Expressed in % of the secretion obtained at the same times in aliquots of GFP incubated concomitantly with inhibitor solvents.
**β-N-acetylglucosaminidase.

GFP (Table II), prepared from PRP which had been incubated for 1 hour at room temperature with 0.4 μM ^{14}C-adenine, was incubated at 37° with 20 mM 2-deoxyglucose (added in 0.15 M NaCl) and 5 μg/ml of antimycin A (added in 95% ethanol). At the times shown the level of radioactive ATP and the adenylate energy charge were determined (Holmsen et al., 1972) and 3 ml aliquots were stirred in an aggregometer with 0.2 u/ml of thrombin for 1 min. The sample was then centrifuged and the supernatant analyzed for ATP + ADP (Holmsen et al., 1972), fibrinogen (performed by Dr. K. Kaplan) and β-N-acetylglucosaminidase (Dangelmaier and Holmsen, 1980).

thrombin was added together with the inhibitors, a substantially more rapid ATP consumption occurred, which suggests that thrombin initiated additional ATP consumption (Akkermen et al., 1979). This is also reflected by the decrease in the steady-state level of metabolic ATP, the time course of which is superimposable on that of acid hydrolase secretion (Fukami et al., 1976) as well as by the well-established increase in ATP production of platelets in response to thrombin. Therefore, stimulation of platelets with thrombin leads to increase in ATP consumption within the period of time secretion occurs. How much extra ATP is consumed during dense granule secretion? From the above, it must be equal or less than the amounts present at any time in the platelets. Thrombin was therefore added to platelets with decreasing amounts of available ATP, i.e., at various times after arrest of ATP production, and the extent of dense granule secretion was found to be directly proportional to the level of ATP at the moment of thrombin addition, a level which represents all available ATP in the platelet. This result is in accordance with the view that ATP is consumed in processes directly related to dense granule secretion, and we found that 1.9 µmoles ATP/10^{11} platelets was sufficient for complete secretion.

MAJOR ATP CONSUMING PROCESSES INITIATED DURING THE BASIC PLATELET REACTION.

The phosphatidyl inositol (PI) response includes a rapid turnover of PI and PA (phosphatidic acid) in secretory cells in response to stimuli (Michell, 1975). It is a cyclic process (Fig. 2) and requires three ATP equivalents per cycle. The PI response has been demonstrated by Lloyd et al. (1973, 1974) in platelets during the entire basic platelet reaction induced with thrombin and to a far smaller extent, during shape change induced by ADP, and is therefore not specific for secretion in these cells. These authors also noted that PI mono- and biphosphate were formed during the thrombin-platelet interaction, a formation that also requires ATP.

The significance of the PI response is not clear, but has been thought to be connected with openings of gates in the plasma membrane specific for influx of extracellular Ca^{2+} (Michell, 1975). The counterpart of such a mechanism in platelets, in which secretion does not require extracellular Ca^{2+} would be the liberation of Ca^{2+} from intracellular stores, and in analogy, the PI response may be connected with this liberation and thus precede both the contractile (see below) and secretory processes. The PI response is conveniently monitored as the increase in the content, i.e. specific radioactivity of particularly PA and PI in cells where ATP is labelled with ^{32}P orthophosphate. This method has been successfully used in platelets by Lloyd et al. (1973, 1974), Leung et al. (1977) and Lapetina & Cuetrecassas (1979); a preliminary experiment from our laboratory is shown in Fig. 3. Here, PRP was incubated with ^{32}P-orthophosphate and gel filtered in phosphate free Tyrode's solution. The time course of ^{32}P incorporation into PA with 5 U/ml of thrombin and the ^{32}P incorporation after 2 min with increasing concentrations of thrombin are shown. Under identical conditions and use of formaldehyde to stop secretion precisely, dense granule secretion starts after 15 sec, i.e., after a period of time in which there has been a considerable uptake of ^{32}P in PA. Thus, the PI response may well precede secretion. However, dense granule secretion is terminated after 60 sec and acid hydrolase secretion after 120 sec under identical conditions, while ^{32}P uptake in PA lasts for at least 4 min. Moreover, the leveling off of ^{32}P uptake after

4 min may just mean that the phosphate in PA has attained the same specific radioactivity as the γ-phosphate of ATP, so turnover of the cycle (Fig. 2) may continue with the same rate after 4 min. The dose-response relationship for ^{32}P incorporation in PA is also slightly shifter to lower thrombin concentrations as compated with that of dense granule secretion as viewed from separate experiments in our laboratory. These preliminary studies therefore indicate that the PI response may precede secretion in platelets.

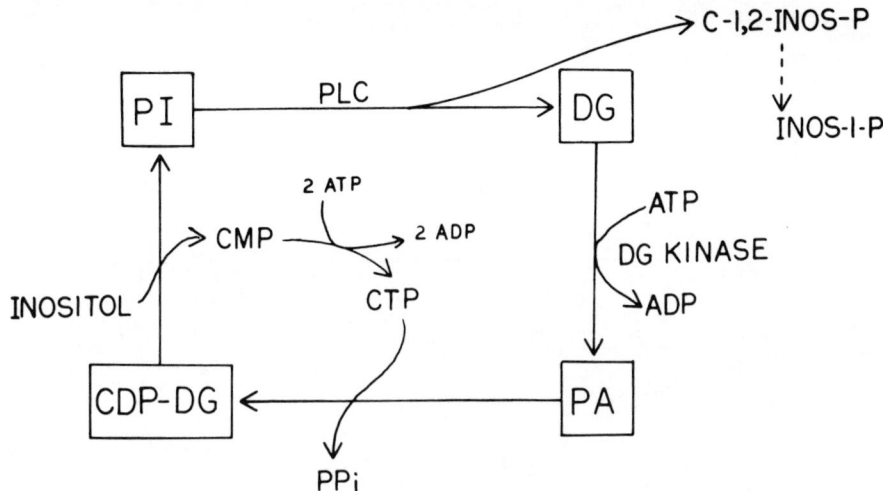

Figure 2. <u>The phosphatidyl inositol response.</u>

<u>Contractile Processes</u> A 20,000 dalton protein was shown to be phosphorylated intact platelets in response to thrombin (Lyons et al., 1975). The protein was identified as myosin light chain and the time hydrolase secretion and coincides with dense granule secretion in previous studies (Daniel et al., 1977). The phosphorylation of this 20,000 dalton protein is also inhibited in parallel with dense granule secretion (Halsam & Lynham, 1978). Phosphorylation of this myosin light chain stimulated the actin-activated ATPase of myosin (Adelstein & Conti, 1972) and enhances the development of tension in reconstituted platelet actomyosin fibers (Lebowitz & Cooke, 1978). A specific myosin light chain kinase has been isolated from platelets and shown to be regulated by Ca^{2+} through calmodulin (Hathaway & Adelstein, 1979). These observations suggest that contractile processes are connected with secretion in platelets and are triggered by phosphorylation of the 20,000 dalton myosin light chain kinase. The phosphorylation step <u>per se</u> requires minute amounts of ATP, whereas the resulting stimulation of actomyosin ATPase presumably consumes large amounts of ATP. A plausible function of contraction in platelets with regard to secretion could be to bring the storage granules in close proximity of the plasma membrane or invaginations of this. White (1971) has demonstrated that the storage granules move centripetally during secretion and seem to fuse with invaginations of the plasma membrane, the cannalicular system. Although no clear picture

of the putative fusion of the storage granules with the membrane invaginations has yet been reported, it is of great importance that a derivative, fibrin, of the secretable fibrinogen has been demonstrated in the cannicular system of platelets treated with high doses of thrombin (Holme et al., 1973).

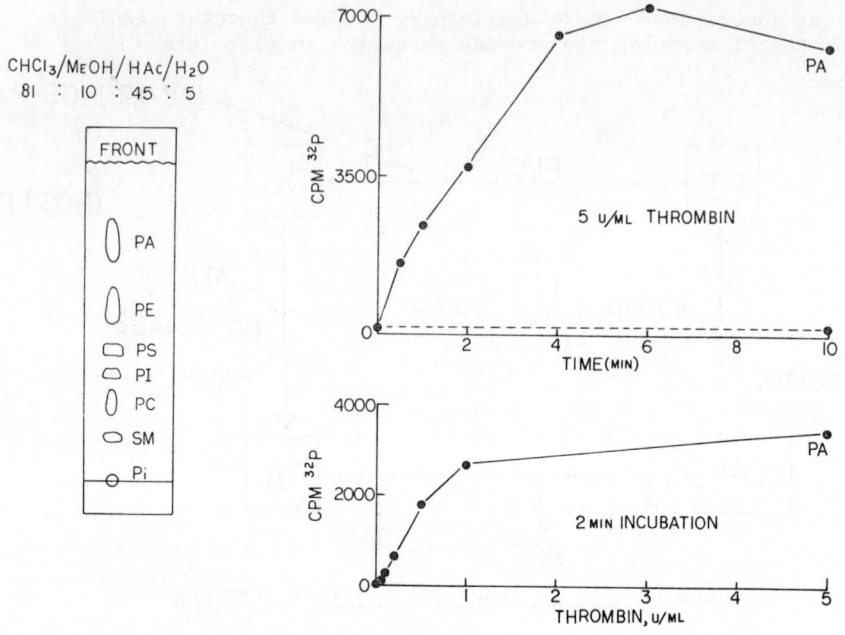

Figure 3. Incorporation of ^{32}P in Phosphatidic acid (PA) in GFP

PRP was incubated with ^{32}P orthophosphate, gel filtered (Table II) and incubated with thrombin as shown in the right panels. At the times given, aliquots were extracted according to Lapetina & Cuetricases (1979) and separation in the TLC system shown in the left panel.

This work was supported by DHEW SPI 7 HHL 14127-08 and was done under a tenure of an Established Investigatorship of the American Heart Association.

REFERENCES

Adelstein, R.S. and Conti, M.A., 1972. Phosphorylation of platelet myosin increases actin-activated myosin ATPase activity. Nature 256, 597-598.

Akkerman, J.W.N., Holmsen, H. and Driver, H.A., 1979. Platelet aggregation and Ca^{2+} secretion are independent of simultaneous ATP production. FEBS Lett, 100, 286-290.

Antoniades, H.N. and Scher, C.D., 1977. Radioimmunoassay of human serum growth factor for Balb/c - 3T3 cells: Derivation from platelets. Proc.Nat.Acad.Sci., USA, 74, 1973-1977.

Brot, F.E., Glaser, J.H., Roosen, K.J., Sly, W.H., and Stahl, P.D., 1974. In vitro correction of deficient human fibroblasts by β-glucuronidase from different human sources. Biochem.Biophys.Res.Comm. 57, 1-6.

Charo, T., Feinman, R.D. and Detwiler, T.C., 1977. Interrelations of platelet aggregation and secretion. J.Clin.Invest. 60, 866-873.

Claesson, H.E. and Malmsten, C., 1977. On the interrelations of prostaglandin endoperoxide G_2 and cyclic nucleotides in platelet function. Eur.J.Biochem. 76, 277-283.

Costa, F.L. and Murphy, D.L., 1975. Platelet 5HT uptake and release is stopped rapidly by formaldehyde. Nature, 255, 407-410.

Daniel, J.L., Holmsen, H. and Adelstein, R.S., 1977. Thrombin-stimulated myosin phosphorylation in intact platelets and its possible involvement in secretion. Thrombosis and Haemostasis 38, 984-989.

Daniel, J.L., Molish, I. and Holmsen, H., 1980. Radiolabeling of purine nucleotide pool of cells as a method to distinguish among intracellular compartments: Studies on human platelets. Biochim.Biophys.Acta., In press.

Dangelmaier, C.A. and Holmsen, H., 1980. Determination of acid hydrolases in human platelets. Anal.Biochem., in press.

Davey, M.G. and Luscher, E.F., 196 . Release reactions of human platelets induced by thrombin and other agents. Biochim.Biophys.Acta., 165, 490-506.

Doolittle, R.F., Takaji, T. and Cottrell, B.A., 1974. Platelet and plasma fibrinogens are identical gene products. Science, 185,

Fukami, M.H., Dangelmaier, C.A., Bauer, J. and Holmsen, H., 1980. Metabolic status, subcellular localization and secretion characteristics of platelet inorganic pyrophosphate, a major constituent of the anine-steering granules. Biochem.J. In press.

Fukami, M.H., Holmsen, H. Salganicoff, L., 1976. Adenine nucleotide metabolism of blood platelets. IX. Time course of secretion and changes in metabolism in thrombin-treated platelets. Biochim.Biophys.Acta., 444, 633-643.

Haslam, R.J. and Lynham, J.A., 1978. Relationship between phosphorylation of blood platelet proteins and secretion of granule constituents. Thromb.Res. 12, 619-625.

Hathaway, D.R. and Adelstein, R.S., 1979. Human platelet myosin light chain kinase requires the calcium-binding protein calmodulin for activity. Proc.Nat.Acad. of Sci. USA, 76, 1655-1657.

Holme, R., Sixma, F.F., Murer, E.H. and Houig, T., 1973. Demonstration of platelet fibrinogen secretion via the surface connecting system. Thromb.Res., 3, 347-352.

Holmsen, H., 1974. Are platelet shape change, aggregation and release reaction tangible manifestations of one basic function? In <u>Platelets: Production, Function, Transfusion and Storage</u> (eds., Baldwin and Ebbe). Grune & Stratton, New York.

Holmsen, H., 1976. Classification and possible mechanisms of action of some drugs that inhibit platelet aggregation. <u>Series Haematologica</u>, 8, 50-80.

Holmsen, H., 1977. Prostaglandin endoperoxide-thromboxane synthesis and dense granule secretion as positive feedback loops in the propagation of platelet responses during "the basic platelet reaction". <u>Thromb. et Haemost.</u> 38, 1030-1041.

Holmsen, H., 1978. Platelet secretion (release reaction) mechanism and pharmacology. <u>Advances in Pharmacology and Therapeutics</u>.

Holmsen, H. and Akkerman, J.W.N., 1980. On the requirement for ATP availability in platelet responses - a quantitative approach. In <u>The regulation of coagulation</u> (eds. Mann and Taylor) pp. 409-417, Elsevier, North Holland Press, New York.

Holmsen, H., Day, H.J. and Setkowsky, C.A., 1972. Secretory mechanisms. Behavior of adenine nucleotides during the platelet release reaction induced by adenosine diphosphate and adrenaline. <u>Biochem.J.</u> 129, 67-82.

Holmsen, H., Robkin, L. and Day, H.J., 1980. Effects of antimycin A and 2-deoxyglucose are secretion in luman platelets. Differential inhibition of the secretion of acid hydrolases and adenine nucleotides. <u>Biochem.J.</u> 182, 413-419.

Holmsen, H. and Setkowsky-Dangelmaier, C.A., 1977. Adenine nucleotide metabolism of blood platelets. X. Formaldehyde stops centrifugation-induced secretion after A 23187 stimulation and causes breakdown of metabolic ATP. <u>Biochim.Biophys.Acta.</u>, 497, 46-61.

Holmsen, H. and Weiss, H.J., 1979. Secretable storage pools in platelets. <u>Annual Review of Medicine</u>, 30, 119-134.

Holmsen, H., Østvold, A.-C. and Day, H.J., 1973. Behaviour of endogenous and newly absorbed serotonin in the platelet release reaction. <u>Biochem.Pharmacol</u>. 22, 2599-2608.

Kinlough-Rathbone, R.L., Packham, M.A., Reivers, H.J., Cazenave, J.P. and Mustard, J.F., 1977. Mechanisms of platelets shape change, aggregation and release induced by collagen, thrombin or A 23187. <u>J.Lab.Clin.Med.</u> 90, 707-720.

Kinlough-Rathbone, R.L., Reimers, H.J., Mustard, J.F. and Packham, M.A., 1976. Sodium arachidonate can induce platelet shape change and aggregation which are independent of the release reaction. <u>Science</u> 192, 1011-1013.

Lages, B., Scrutton, M.C. and Holmsen, H., 1975. Studies on gel filtered human platelets: Isolation and characterization in a medium containing no added Ca^{2+}, Mg^{2+} and K^+. J.Lab.Clin.Med. 85, 811-825.

Lapetina, E.G. and Cuatrecasas, P., 1979. Stimulation of phosphatidic acid production in platelets precedes the formation of arachidonate and parallels the release of serotonin. <u>Biochim. Biophys.Acta.</u>, 573, 394-402.

Lawler, J.W., Slayter, H.S. and Coligan, J.E., 1978. Isolation and characterization of a high molecular weight glycoprotein from human blood platelets. <u>J.Biol.Chem</u>. 253, 8609-8616.

Lebowitz, E.A. and Cooke, R., 1978. Contractile properties of actomyosin from human blood platelets. J.Biol.Chem. 253, 5443-5447.

Leung, N.L., Kinlough-Rathbone, R.L. and Mustard, J.F., 1977. Incorporation of $^{32}PO_4$ into phospholipids of blood platelets. Brit.J.Haematol. 36, 417-425.

Lloyd, J.V. and Mustard, J.F., 1974. Changes in ^{32}P-content of phosphatidic acid and the phosphoinositides of rabbit platelets during aggregation induced by collagen and thrombin. Brit.J. Haematol. 26, 243-253.

Lloyd, J.V., Nishizawa, E.E. and Mustard, J.F., 1973. Effect of ADP-induced shape change on incorporation of ^{32}P into platelet phosphatidic acid and mono, -di-and triphosphatidyl inositol. Brit. J.Haematol. 25, 77-99.

Lyons, R.M., Stanford, N. and Majerus, P.W., 1975. Thrombin-induced protein phosphorylation in human platelets. J.Clin.Invest. 56, 924-933.

Meyers, K.M., Holmsen, H., Seachord, C.L. Hopkins, G.E., Borchard, R.E. and Padgett, G.A., 1979. Storage pool deficiency in platelets from Cchediak-Higashi cattle. Am.J.Physiol. 237, R239-R248.

Meyers, K.M., Holmsen, H., Smith, F.B. and Prieur, D., 1979. The dominant role of thromboxane formation in secondary aggregation of platelets. Nature, 282, 331-333.

Michell, R., 1975. Inosine phospholipids and cell surface receptor function. Biochim.Biophys.Acta., 415, 81-123.

Nachman, R., Levine, R. and Jaffe, E., 1978. Synthesis of actin by cultured guinea pig megakaryocytes. Biochim.Biophys.Acta., 531, 91-101.

Murer, E.H. and Stewart, G.J., 1977. Insights into the mechanism of platelet action through studies at pH 5.3. Thromb.Haemost. 38, 1018-1029.

White, F.G., 1971. Platelet morphology, in The Circulating Platelet (ed. S.A. Johnson) pp 44-76, Acad. Press, New York.

Zucker, M.B.,1980. Observations on the release reaction, in The Regulation of Coagulation (eds. Mann and Taylor), pp 385-391. Elsevier North Holland, Inc. New York.

Zucker, M.B., Mosesson, M.W., Broekman, M.J. and Kaplan, K.L., 1979. Release of platelet fibronectin (cold-insoluble globulin) from alpha granules induced by thrombin and collagen; lack of requirement for plasma fibronectin in ADP-induced platelet aggregation. Blood, 54, 8-12.

Platelet Pharmacology

Platelet pharmacology is highly complex and only a few aspects are dealt with. The main emphasis is on the involvement of biogenic amines with platelet. Platelets resemble neurons in several respects, for example the active uptake of serotonin, inhibition of uptake by drugs and storage and release of this amine show many similarities. Platelets also contain a monoamine oxidase similar in its properties to the brain enzyme. Due to this similarity, platelets have come to be studied not only for themselves but also as a model for the neuron. The justification and limitations of this model system are discussed.

The suitability of platelets as a model in the study of psychiatric disorders in humans is a related question of great importance. The effect of drugs on the uptake of serotonin and the response of platelet to such agents must be related to the function of platelet serotonin. Serotonin is a natural amine stored in platelets but amines, such as catecholamines and histamine, can also be stored. The specificity of this storage, its purpose and the question of the storage pools involved are questions of fundamental significance.

Platelet Pharmacology

USE AND LIMITATIONS OF PLATELETS AS MODELS FOR
NEURONS: AMINE RELEASE AND SHAPE CHANGE REACTION

A. Pletscher and A. Laubscher

Research Department of the University Clinics and
Institutes, Cantonal Hospital Basel, Switzerland

ABSTRACT

In platelets and neurons release of catecholamines and 5HT can be brought about in 3 ways: by exocytosis, by reserpine-like drugs and by arylalkylamines. In both types of cell, the reserpine-like benzoquinolizine Ro 4-1284 acts exclusively on granular stores whereas arylalkylamines seem to affect both granular and extragranular sites. There are also differences between neurons and platelets, for instance the physiological stimulus necessary for exocytosis (electrical stimulation in neurons, thrombin in platelets) the relative amounts of granular 5HT and catecholamines released by the drugs, their quantitative action on extragranular stores etc. The 5HT receptor of platelets, as characterized by the shape change reaction, has a pharmacological profile similar to that of the 5HT receptors of certain areas of the central nervous system (CNS) e.g. the cortex and the spinal cord. Furthermore, the non receptor-mediated shape change induced by basic proteins seems to provide a relatively simple model for detecting those basic proteins which cause neuronal depolarization.

INTRODUCTION

Platelets resemble monoaminergic neurons in several respects, i.e. the uptake of 5-hydroxytryptamine (5HT) and its inhibition at the plasma membrane, the subcellular storage and release of 5HT, and the metabolism of aromatic amines brought about by monoamine oxidase. However, there are also some differences between the two cell types for instance in the uptake kinetics of catecholamines at the plasma membrane and in the biosynthesis and turnover of 5HT and other amines.

This paper deals with two aspects of platelet dynamics whose usefulness as models for functional changes in neurons has not yet been systematically investigated: the release of catecholamines and the shape change reaction.

RELEASE OF AMINES

In monoaminergic neurons amines can be released by exocytosis, by reserpine-like drugs and by arylalkylamines. In platelets these three types of release (whose mechanisms are different) are known to exist for 5HT, whereas little is known about the liberation of catecholamines.

For the following release experiments platelet-rich plasma (PRP) of guinea pigs was incubated with ^{14}C-5HT plus ^{3}H-dopamine (^{3}H-DA) or with ^{14}C-5HT plus ^{3}H-noradrenaline (^{3}H-NA), with or without 2×10^{-6}M reserpine. After two successive passages of the PRP through dextran-T_{10} gradients, the isolated, double labelled platelets were resuspended in tris-buffer for use in the experiments (Graf, Laubscher, Richards and Pletscher, 1979). Previous experiments have shown that in platelets the subcellular distributions of endogenous and exogenous catecholamines are similar to those of 5HT (Da Prada and Pletscher, 1969; Da Prada and Picotti, 1979).

Exocytosis. Thrombin is a substance thought to act by exocytosis (extrusion of the whole content of the 5HT granules without affecting other 5HT-pools) in platelets. Fig. 1 demonstrates that this agent, in the presence of Ca^{++} caused marked decreases of ^{14}C-5HT, ^{3}H-DA and ^{3}H-NA in these cells. The diminutions of ^{3}H-DA and ^{3}H-NA showed identical time curves whereas the initial decrease of ^{14}C-5HT was followed by a partial recovery. This was caused by reuptake of the amine, as indicated by experiments with imipramine, which blocked the ^{14}C-5HT recovery.

The thrombin-induced initial decreases in all the three amines were dependent on concentration in a similar way. Preliminary experiments indicate that in reserpinized platelets (in which the granular storage is abolished although, in contrast to exocytosis the storage vesicles remain intact) thrombin in the presence of Ca^{++} caused a considerably less marked absolute and percentage decrease of the labelled amines than in normal platelets.

These findings indicate that in platelets catecholamines, like 5HT, can be released by exocytosis and they confirm that the greater part of the labelled amines is located in granular storage organelles. Therefore, with regard to exocytotic release of catecholamines platelets may be used as models for both 5HT- and for catecholamine-neurons although the physiological stimuli leading to exocytosis are usually different (electrical in neurons, thrombin in platelets).

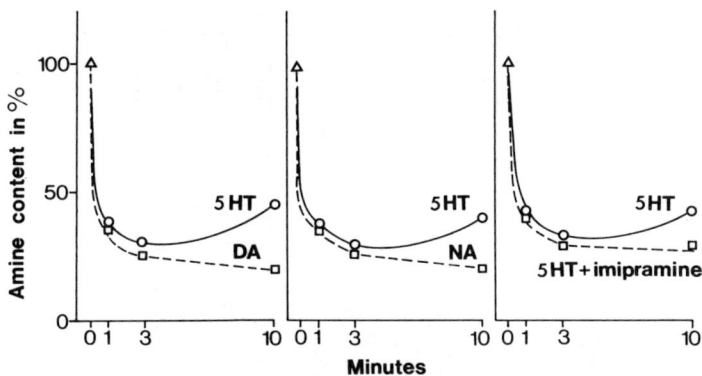

Fig. 1. Effect of 1 i.u./ml thrombin in the presence of 3×10^{-3}M Ca^{++} on the contents of labelled amines in platelets of guinea pigs. Imipramine (10^{-6}M) was added to the platelet suspension 15 minutes before thrombin.

Benzoquinolizine Ro 4-1284. This reserpine-like drug (Ro 4-1284 = 2-hydroxy-2-ethyl-3-isobutyl-9,10-dimethoxy-1,2,3,4,6,7-hexahydro-11-bH-benzo{a}quinolizin) caused a progressive decrease of all the three labelled amines in normal platelets. ^{3}H-DA was more markedly diminished than ^{14}C-5HT and ^{3}H-NA less. In reserpinized platelets Ro 4-1284 did not induce a decrease in any of the amines.

These results indicate that Ro 4-1284 releases catecholamines as well as 5HT and that the release is from the granular stores. The difference in the release of ^{14}C-5HT and ^{3}H-DA cannot be due to reuptake of ^{14}C-5HT since imipramine did not affect the release pattern.

In monoamine neurons Ro 4-1284 also causes a release of 5HT, DA and NA and this release is thought to occur by interfering exclusively with the granular storage. However 5HT and NA seem to be about equally affected in neurons which is not so in platelets. Therefore, with regard to the drug-induced release of granular amines, platelets seem to be only partially similar to monoaminergic neurons. However, differences in the experimental conditions have to be considered (in vivo experiments with neuronal tissue, in vitro experiments with platelets).

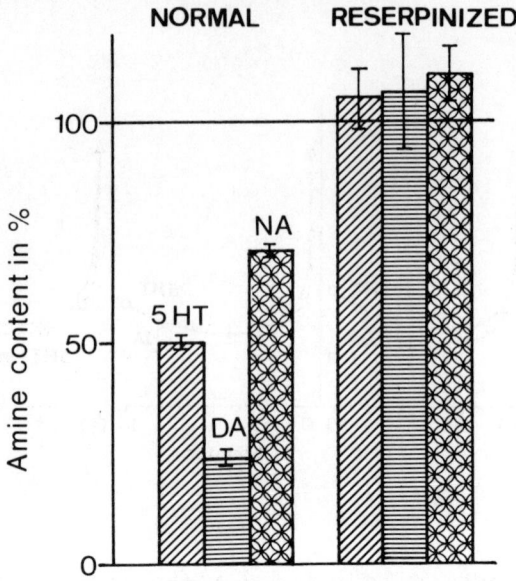

Fig. 2. Effect of 10^{-6}M Ro 4-1284 on the contents of labelled amines in normal and reserpinized platelets of guinea pigs. The contents of labelled amines 2 hours after incubation with the drug are indicated in percent of labelled amines present in the platelets 2 hours after incubation without the drug. Averages with s.e.m. of 3 (^{3}H-DA and ^{3}H-NA) and 6 (^{14}C-5HT) experiments.

<u>Arylalkylamines.</u> In normal platelets both tyramine and p-chlormethamphetamine (PCMA) caused concentration-dependent decrease of ^{14}C-5HT, ^{3}H-DA and ^{3}H-NA. Both drugs had a more marked effect on ^{3}H-DA than on ^{14}C-5HT and a less marked one on ^{3}H-NA than on ^{14}C-5HT.

In reserpinized platelets tyramine and PCMA still decreased ^{14}C-5HT and ^{3}H-DA but no longer affected ^{3}H-NA. Also, the action of the drugs on ^{14}C-5HT was more marked than on ^{3}H-DA.

These results show that tyramine and PCMA, in contrast to Ro 4-1284 cause a release of ^{14}C-5HT and ^{3}H-DA from extragranular stores in reserpinized platelets. These stores probably contain a relatively large proportion of the intracellular amines because the granular store has been abolished. However, the drugs also affected the granular amines; this is indicated by their marked lowering action on the contents of ^{14}C-5HT and ^3H-DA in normal platelets, whose intracellular amines are mainly localized at granular sites. On the other hand, the ^3H-NA was released from granular stores only since in this case the drugs were not effective in reserpinized platelets.

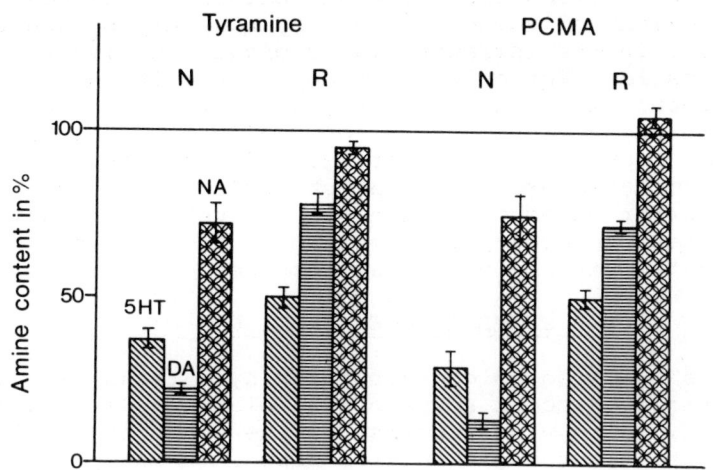

Fig. 3. Effect of $10^{-3}M$ tyramine and $10^{-3}M$ p-chlormethamphetamine on the contents of labelled amines in normal and reserpinized platelets of guinea pigs. The contents of labelled amines 1 hour after incubation with drugs are indicated in percent of the labelled amines present in the platelets 1 hour after incubation without the drugs. Averages with s.e.m. of 3 (^3H-DA and ^3H-NA) and 6 (^{14}C-5HT) experiments.

In normal and reserpinized brain synaptosomes arylalkylamines such as PCMA have been found to exert a releasing effect on the 5HT and DA of extravesicular sites but not on the NA (Ross, 1979). This is in agreement with the present findings in platelets. On the other hand, tyramine, which, as shown above, had a similar effect to PCMA in platelets, did not affect extragranular NA, 5HT or DA in brain synaptosomes. In addition, PCMA caused a more marked release of 5HT than of DA in neuronal tissue of guinea pigs in vivo (Pletscher, Bartholini, Bruderer, Burkard and Gey, 1964), whereas in platelets the reverse was the case. Therefore, platelets seem to be only partly similar to neurons with regard to the amine releasing action of arylalkylamines.

Discussion. In the central nervous system (CNS) most of the 5HT, DA and NA is probably stored in different neuronal populations, which may differ from each other in various functional properties e.g. in the transport of drugs across the plasma membrane. In platelets all the amines are stored in the same cell type. Therefore the discrepancies between platelets and catecholamine-neurons in drug-induced amine release may not only be due to differences in the intragranular storage but also to differences in other cell functions. Since in the platelets the catecholamines are probably co-stored with 5HT in the same organelles (the 5HT organelles) platelets might be more accurate models for those 5HT neurons which have accumulated exogenous catecholamines as false transmitters than for catecholamine-neurons. Such accumulations seem in fact to occur e.g. in animals and possibly humans treated with L-Dopa, the precursor of DA.

THE SHAPE CHANGE REACTION

This reaction is characterized by a transition of the normally discoid shape of the platelets into a spheroid form, whereby an increase of the light absorption of the platelet suspensions takes place. In the present experiments the shape change reaction has been measured in rabbit and human platelets isolated by centrifugation on a dextran-T_{10} gradient and resuspended in tris-buffer. Under these conditions no aggregation of the platelets and virtually no protein-binding of drugs occurred (Graf, Laubscher, Richards and Pletscher, 1979).

Receptor-mediated shape change. Various biogenic amines (e.g. 5HT, DA, NA, adrenaline, tryptamine, histamin) and their precursors and metabolites were tested, but only 5HT (Fig. 4) and tryptamine caused a reversible shape change reaction in rabbit and human platelets. This reaction was antagonized by very low concentrations of 5HT antagonists such as methysergide, cyproheptadine, methiothepine and spiroperidol. Butaclamol, which also counteracted the 5HT-induced shape change reaction, showed a high stereoselectivity. Only those compounds known to be 5HT-agonists in other tissues caused a shape change reaction which was antagonized by methysergide. Some of them were mixed 5HT agonists/antagonists, e.g. LSD, which also showed high stereoselectivity (table 1) (Laubscher and Pletscher, 1979).

TABLE 1

Substance	Agonist action EC_{50}	Antagonist action IC_{50}
5HT	$1.4\pm0.5\times10^{-7}$	
Psilocin	$9.9\pm1.2\times10^{-9}$	
Tryptamine	$1.4\pm0.3\times10^{-6}$	
Quipazine	$2.0\pm0.3\times10^{-6}*$	
Mezcaline	$2.0\pm0.5\times10^{-5}$	
Spiroperidol		$2.2\pm0.4\times10^{-9}$
Mianserin		$3.9\pm0.3\times10^{-9}*$
Methiothepin		$4.1\pm0.2\times10^{-9}$
Methysergide		$1.4\pm0.1\times10^{-8}$
D-Butaclamol		$1.7\pm0.3\times10^{-8}$
Cinanserin		$4.8\pm1.1\times10^{-8}$
L-Butaclamol		$3.2\pm0.4\times10^{-6}$
D-LSD	$9.9\pm1.2\times10^{-9}$	$4.3\pm0.4\times10^{-9}$
N,N'-Dimethyltrypt.	$2.0\pm0.9\times10^{-6}$	$2.0\pm1.1\times10^{-6}$
L-LSD	>10	$1.9\pm0.3\times10^{-5}$
Prostaglandin E_1		$5.4\pm0.2\times10^{-9}*$

EC_{50} (concentration causing half maximal shape change) and IC_{50} (concentration causing 50% inhibition of shape change induced by $10^{-6}M$ 5HT) in human platelets. * rabbit platelets

These findings strongly indicate that the shape change reaction induced by 5HT and 5HT-agonists is mediated by a stimulation of 5HT receptors at the plasma membrane.

It is of interest that prostaglandin E_1 was a strong inhibitor of the 5HT-induced shape change reaction and of other receptor-mediated shape change reactions, e.g. that due to ADP. Furthermore, treatment of platelets with 3% butanol, which removes superficial proteins from the plasma membrane, blocked the 5HT-induced shape change reaction.

In general, those substances thought to act as neuronal 5HT receptor agonists in the CNS (tryptamine- and 5HT-derivatives, D-LSD, quipazine, mezcaline) also acted on platelets as 5HT agonists or mixed agonists/antagonists. With regard to the effect of 5HT-antagonists on the 5HT-induced changes of the electrical activity of 5HT-neurons there seem to be regional differences in the CNS. The 5HT recptors in areas like the cortex and the spinal cord, in contrast to those of other regions, show close analogies to the platelet receptor. In fact, in these areas the neuronal 5HT receptors have been shown to react to the same antagonists as the platelet receptor, and the order of potency of the antagonists was similar in both types of receptors (Laubscher and Pletscher, 1979). Therefore, with respect to the action of drugs the 5HT receptor of platelets seems to be a reasonable model for the neuronal receptor in certain areas of the CNS.

Non receptor-mediated shape change. Various basic proteins, includings myelin basic protein, caused a concentration-dependent shape change reaction in platelets which

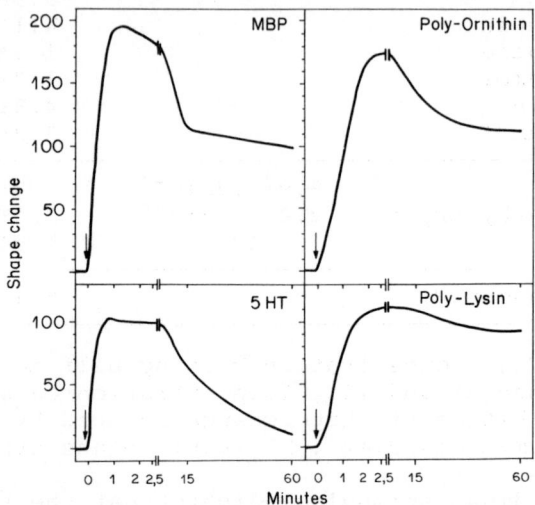

Fig. 4. Shape change induced by 10^{-6}M myelin basic protein (MBP), 10^{-7}M polyornithine 40,000, 10^{-6}M 5HT and 3×10^{-6}M polylysin in human platelets. The ordinate indicates the shape change in percent of that induced by 10^{-6}M 5HT (= 100).

was not counteracted by antagonists of 5HT-, DA- and NA-receptors, by prostaglandin E_1 or by washing of the platelets with 3% butanol. However, the acid mucopolysaccharide heparin antagonized this type of shape change. These results indicate that the shape change reaction induced by basic proteins is probably not mediated by specific receptors. According to previous findings (see Laubscher, Pletscher, Honegger and Richards, 1979), the basic proteins, which have a positive charge, probably interact with the negatively charged plasma membrane by electrostatic forces thus triggering off functional changes, e.g. the shape change reaction. This would also explain why the negatively charged heparin interferes with this type of shape change.

In spite of this rather unspecific action not all basic proteins caused a shape change reaction. Their effect depended on the molecular size and conformation. Thus, low molecular weight polyornithine (M.W. 4000), in contrast to polyornithine 40,000, did not induce a shape change reaction, although the isoelectric point of the two peptides is the same. Also, the basic protein cytochrome C, a non random-coil protein, was not a shape change inducer, whereas protamine, a random-coil protein of similar size was effective (Laubscher, Pletscher, Honegger and Richards, 1979).

In neurons of the CNS (e.g. of spinal cord in situ and in cerebellar neuronal cultures) basic proteins have been shown to cause depolarization (Honegger, Gähwiler and Isler, 1977; Gähwiler and Honegger, 1979). Only those proteins which caused a shape change reaction in platelets had this action in neurons and the depolarizing effect was not antagonized by specific receptor antagonists. Therefore, the shape change reaction of platelets is probably a relatively simple model system for detecting those basic proteins which cause neuronal depolarization. Furthermore, the shape change reaction of platelets may be of interest for demyelinating disorders e.g. multiple sclerosis, in which basic proteins are liberated from neuronal tissues.

REFERENCES

Da Prada, M., and Pletscher A., 1969. Storage of exogenous monoamines and reserpine in 5-hydroxytryptamine organelles of blood platelets. Europ. J. Pharmacol. 7, 45-48.
Da Prada, M., and Picotti, G.B., 1979. Content and subcellular localization of catecholamines and 5-hydroxytryptamine in human and animal blood platelets: monoamine distribution between platelets and plasma. Br. J. Pharmacol. 65, 653-662.
Gähwiler, B.H., and Honegger, C.G., 1979. Myelin basic protein depolarizes neuronal membranes. Neurosci. Lett. 11, 317-321.
Graf, M., Laubscher, A., Richards, J.G., and Pletscher, A., 1979. Blood platelets isolated by polysaccharide gradients: reaction to 5-hydroxytryptamine. J. Lab. Clin. Med. 93, 257-265.
Honegger, C.G., Gähwiler, B.H., and Isler, H., 1977. The effect of myelin basic protein (MBP) on the bioelectric activity of spinal cord and cerebellar neurons.

Neurosci. Lett. 4, 303-307.

Laubscher, A., and Pletscher, A., 1979. Shape change and uptake of 5-hydroxytryptamine in human blood platelets: action of neuropsychotropic drugs. Life Sci. 24, 1833-1840.

Laubscher, A., Pletscher, A., Honegger, C.G., and Richards, J.G., 1979. Shape change of blood platelets brought about by myelin basic protein and other basic polypeptides. Arch. Pharm. 310, 87-92.

Pletscher, A., Bartholini, G., Bruderer, H., Burkard, W.P., and Gey, K.F., 1964. Chlorinated arylalkylamines affecting the cerebral metabolism of 5-hydroxytryptamine. J. Pharmacol. Exp. Ther. 145, 344-350.

Ross, S.B., 1979. Interactions between reserpine and various compounds on the accumulation of ^{14}C-5 hydroxytryptamine and ^{3}H-noradrenaline in homogenates from hypothalamus. Biochem. Pharmacol. 28, 1085-1088.

SEROTONIN, HISTAMINE, CATECHOLAMINES, NORMETANEPHRINE
AND OCTOPAMINE IN BLOOD PLATELETS.

M. Da Prada, G.B. Picotti[*], R. Kettler and J.M. Launay[1]

F. Hoffmann-La Roche & Co., Ltd., Pharmaceutical Research
Department, CH-4002 Basle, Switzerland

[*] Institute of Pharmacology, School of Medicine,
University of Milan, 20129 Milan, Italy

ABSTRACT

Human and animal blood platelets store in their dense bodies the majority of the monoamines that occur in plasma, i.e. serotonin (5-HT), histamine, catecholamines (CA), normetanephrine (NMN) and p-octopamine. Storage pool deficient platelets of rodents show impaired storage mechanisms not only for 5'-phosphonucleotides and 5-HT but also for CA and histamine and possibly for NMN and p-octopamine. In human but not in rabbit, rat and guinea-pig platelets 5-HT, CA and NMN are present in sulphoconjugated form.

INTRODUCTION

Recently improved radioenzymatic techniques of high specificity and sensitivity have permitted the measurement of different biogenic amines in small aliquots of tissues and plasma extracts. In the present experiments precise radioenzymatic assays of serotonin (5-hydroxytryptamine, 5-HT), histamine, adrenaline (A), noradrenaline (NA), dopamine (DA), normetanephrine (NMN) as well as p-octopamine were performed in minute platelet (1 to 5 ml platelet-rich plasma) and plasma samples ($<$ 1 ml) of human and different animal species. In order to ascertain similarities and differences in the storage (subcellular localization) of various amines in respect to 5-HT, the concentration of various endogenous amines was measured in platelets with pharmacologically impaired 5-HT storing capacity viz. after reserpine injection, and in platelets of rodents with inherited storage pool deficiencies (SPD). Moreover, the subcellular distribution of various endogenous amines was studied in rabbit platelet homogenates submitted to density gradient centrifugation.

Since amine conjugation by platelets could represent a process relevant to their distribution between platelets and plasma, the relative concentrations of unconjugated (free) and conjugated amines in platelets and plasma were also determined.

[1] Present address: Laboratoire de Biochimie, Hôpital
St. Louis, Paris.

Finally, some comparative data concerning the effect of reserpine on the in vitro accumulation of labelled amines by human and rabbit platelets will be presented.

MATERIALS AND METHODS

Blood collection in EDTA (1% v/v) and platelet isolation was performed as previously described (Da Prada and Picotti, 1979). In platelets and plasma unconjugated DA, A and NA were measured by a catechol-O-methyltransferase (COMT) radioenzymatic method (Da Prada and Zürcher, 1976; Da Prada and Zürcher, 1979) whereas NMN, m- and p-octopamine were assayed simultaneously by a modified phenylethanolamine-N-methyltransferase (PNMT) single isotopic radioenzymatic technique (Zürcher and Da Prada, in preparation). The assay of 5-HT and histamine was also performed radioenzymatically (Saavedra et al., 1973; Taylor and Snyder, 1972).

Measurements of total (conjugated plus unconjugated) 5-HT, CA, NMN and p-octopamine were made submitting platelets and plasma perchloric acid extracts to hydrolysis for 20 min at $100^{\circ}C$. (Da Prada and Picotti, 1979; Da Prada and Zürcher, 1979). The subcellular distribution of the endogenous amines was studied submitting rabbit platelet homogenates to Urografin ® density gradient ultracentrifugation (Da Prada, von Berlepsch and Pletscher, 1972). Proteins were measured colorimetrically (Lowry, Rosebrough, Farr and Randall, 1951). Uptake of labelled amines was performed in platelet-rich plasma (PRP) as previously described (Picotti, Da Prada and Pletscher, 1976; Picotti, Carruba, Zambotti and Mantegazza, 1977). Chemicals used and their respective sources were: reserpine (Serpasil, Ciba-Geigy; Urografin, Schering). All other reagents used were Analytical Grade and obtained from commercial sources. ^{14}C-labelled 5-HT, DA, A, NA and histamine (50 - 60 mCi/mmol) were obtained from the Radiochemical Center, Amersham; ^{14}C-NMN (53 mCi/mmol) and p-octopamine (57 mCi/mmol) from CEA, Gif-sur-Yvette.

Albino SPF rats of Wistar origin, Fawn-hooded rats, Burgundian rabbits as well as guinea-pigs of the Füllinsdorf strain were used. In some experiments black mice (strain C 57 BL / 6 J) and beige mice (strain C 57 BL / 6 J - bg/bg, Jackson Laboratory), were used.

RESULTS

Content of free monoamines in human and animal platelets. Table 1 shows that platelets from all mammalian species so far investigated contain variable amounts of 5-HT, histamine and CA, rabbit platelets being very rich in both 5-HT and histamine (see also Da Prada and Picotti, 1979). In general, except for guinea-pigs, platelets contain more 5-HT than histamine. On the other hand the platelet CA content is several thousand times lower than that of 5-HT, NA being the prevailing CA (Da Prada and Picotti, 1979).

TABLE 1. Content of free serotonin, histamine, dopamine, adrenaline, noradrenaline, normetanephrine and p-octopamine in platelets of different animal species.

Amine	Man	Rabbit	Rat	Guinea-pig
serotonin	2,200	86,000	9,000	820
histamine	1.4	52,200	394	5,850
dopamine	0.10	1.70	0.20	0.26
adrenaline	0.05	2.50	0.05	0.27
noradrenaline	2.00	6.70	0.35	1.39
normetanephrine	2.10	10.76	0.76	26.05
p-octopamine	0.15	0.28	0.19	0.05

Mean values in pmol/mg protein, n=3-9

Among the animal species studied rabbit and cat platelets contain relatively high amounts of CA (Da Prada and Picotti, 1979). The findings presented in Table 1 show also that free NMN and p-octopamine are consistently detected in human as well as in animal platelets.

Content of conjugated monoamines in human and animal platelets. The enzyme phenol sulphotransferase (EC 2.8.2.1) has been recently demonstrated in human platelets (Hart, Resnkers, Nelson and Roth,1979). In order to assess whether platelets contain sulphoconjugated amines, free and total 5-HT, CA and NMN were measured in human and animal platelet extracts. Apparently, following acid hydrolysis only sulphoconjugated derivatives are hydrolyzed, glucuronoconjugates being acid resistant (Weil-Malherbe, 1971). In human platelets (six healthy subjects) conjugated 5-HT, DA, A, NA and NMN corresponded to 10, 93, 69, 57 and 76%, respectively. Only trace amounts (1-5%) of these amines were found in conjugated form in rabbit, rat and guinea-pig platelets. In accordance, among the different mammalian platelets investigated (cat, rat, dog, pig, guinea-pig, monkey, rabbit), only human platelets showed very high phenol sulphotransferase activity.

Preliminary experiments indicated that 5-HT, CA and their methoxy-derivatives are better phenol sulphotransferase substrates than p-octopamine (data not presented).

Content of serotonin and histamine in healthy vs storage pool disease platelets. The findings presented in Table 2 show that rabbit platelets and plasma have a histamine content several times higher than that found in human, guinea-pig, or rat. Among the species analyzed so far, human plasma and platelets show the lowest histamine level. Rodents with SPD such as Fawn-hooded rats and beige mice have much less 5-HT and histamine in their platelets than those from control animals. (Table 3).

Distribution of free and conjugated catecholamines and normetanephrine between human platelets and plasma: As previously shown, free 5-HT and CA are more concentrated in platelets than in plasma (Da Prada and Picotti, 1979). In humans the concentration-ratio platelet

TABLE 2. Histamine level in platelets and plasma of man and animals.

Species	Platelets (pmol/mg prot.)	Plasma (pmol/ml)
Rabbit	52,200 ± 3,000	1,354 ± 372
Guinea-pig	5,850 ± 400	229 ± 56
Rat (Wistar)	394 ± 49	167 ± 40
Man	1.4 ± 0.2	40 ± 2

Values are means ± SEM; n=3-8

TABLE 3. Content of serotonin and histamine in normal (N) and storage pool deficient (SPD) rodents

| Amine | Rat | | Mouse | |
	Wistar albino (N)	Fawn-hooded (SPD)	Black (N)	Beige (SPD)
Serotonin	10,200 ± 700	3,700 ± 700	21,200 ± 1,800	traces
Histamine	436 ± 73	35 ± 10	340 ± 20	traces

Values in pmol/mg protein are means ± SEM, n=6-12

/plasma is about 40 times higher for 5-HT than for NA indicating that 5-HT but not CA are most likely transported in the platelets by a high affinity uptake process. The findings in Table 4 show that free as well as conjugated CA and NMN are more concentrated in platelets than in plasma. NMN-SO$_4$, which in human platelets attains a concentration-ratio platelet/plasma of about 350 is the sulphoconjugated catechol-derivative present in the platelets in the highest absolute concentration.

Distribution of free-serotonin, histamine and catecholamines between rabbit platelets and plasma. It was previously reported that rabbit platelets contain relevant amounts of 5-HT and histamine. (Solatunturi and Paasonen, 1966; Da Prada et al., 1967). In rabbits, the data presented in Table 5 show that 5-HT is about 25,000 times more concentrated in platelets than in plasma. On the other hand, histamine is concentrated about 10,000 times and CA at best are concentrated 800 times more in platelets than in plasma.

Serotonin, histamine, catecholamines and octopamines in the subcellular structures isolated from rabbit platelet. The localization of 5-HT, histamine, A, NA, DA, m- and p-octopamine in rabbit platelet homogenates was assessed after isolation of the subcellular structures of the platelets by density gradient ultracentrifugation.

TABLE 4. Distribution of free and conjugated CA and NMN between human platelets and plasma

Amine		Platelets (pmol/ml)	Plasma (pmol/ml)	Platelets/Plasma
Dopamine	free	33	0.30	110
	conj.	193	12	16
Adrenaline	free	103	0.41	251
	conj.	136	1.10	123
Noradrenaline	free	1,701	3.57	476
	conj.	1,179	7.18	164
Normetanephrine	free	930	5.80	160
	conj.	3,334	9.60	347

Values are means of three experiments. (Da Prada and Picotti, 1979)

TABLE 5. Distribution of serotonin, histamine and CA between rabbit platelets and plasma

Amine	Platelets (pmol/ml)	Plasma (pmol/ml)	Platelets/Plasma
Serotonin	26,832,000	971	27,633
Histamine	12,672,000	1,354	9,360
Dopamine	355	1.41	251
Adrenaline	739	0.91	815
Noradrenaline	1,632	2.32	703

Values are means of 3-6 experiments. (Da Prada and Picotti, 1979)

5-HT, taken as a biochemical marker of the 5-HT organelles, as well as all the other amines were measured radioenzymatically in the particulate matter sedimented from the 7 fractions of the density gradient and in the pellet consisting of pure 5-HT organelles (fraction 8).

Typical patterns of the subcellular distribution of these seven monoamines are shown in Fig. 1 and 2. The relative specific concentrations (% amine/% protein per fraction) for 5-HT, histamine, A, NA, DA, m- and p-octopamine were by far the highest in the 5-HT organelle fraction. The content of these amines was up to several hundred times higher in the 5-HT organelle fraction than in any other one.

The degree of accumulation of several endogenous monoamines in isolated 5-HT organelles compared to intact rabbit platelets does not markedly differ from that of 5-HT (Table 6). Thus, the content of the organelles in 5-HT is about 200 times superior to that of the whole platelets and the concentration of histamine, A, p- and m-octopamine is also about 200 times higher in the organelles than in

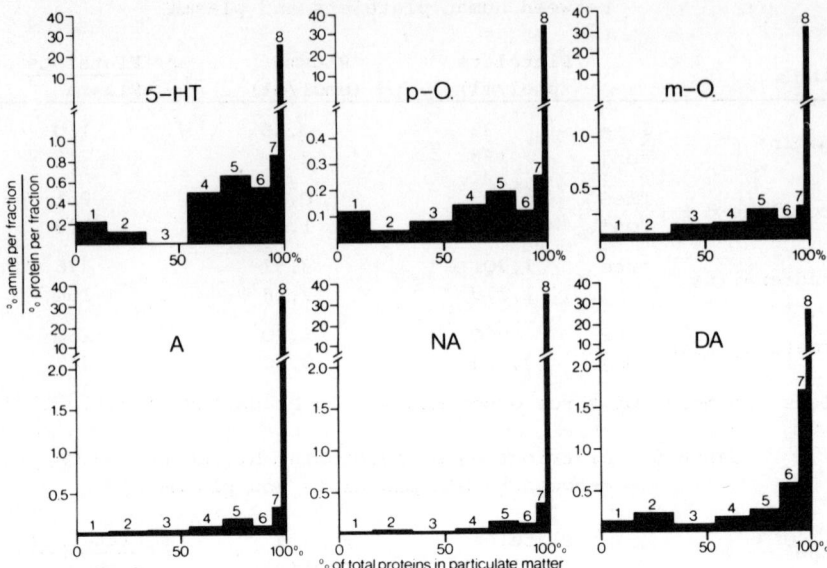

Fig. 1: Subcellular distribution of serotonin (5-HT), p-octopamine (p-O), m-octopamine (m-O), adrenaline (A), noradrenaline (NA) and dopamine (DA) in the particulate matter of rabbit platelet homogenates submitted to density gradient centrifugation.

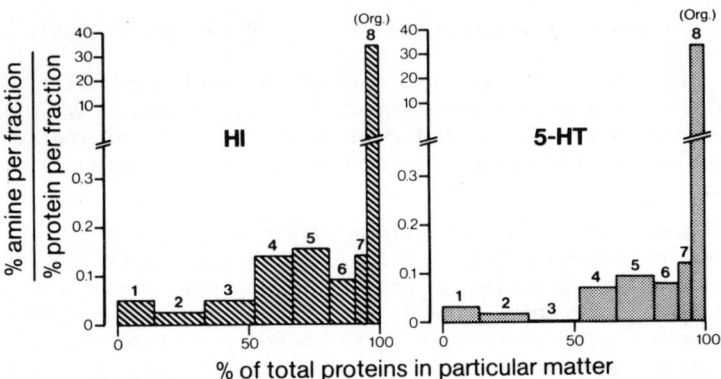

Fig. 2.: Subcellular distribution of histamine (HI) and serotonin (5-HT) in the particulate matter of rabbit platelet homogenates submitted to density gradient centrifugation.

the platelets. However, the concentrations of NA, DA and NMN are only about 110 - 160 times higher in the 5-HT organelles than in the intact platelets. (Table 6).

TABLE 6. Content of endogenous monoamines in isolated 5-HT organelles and intact blood platelets of rabbits

Amine	5-HT organelles (nmol/mg protein)	platelets (pmol/mg protein)	organelles / platelets
Serotonin	21,000	86,000	244
Histamine	8,800	42,200	209
Adrenaline	0.48	2.50	192
Noradrenaline	0.86	6.70	128
Dopamine	0.19	1.70	113
Normetanephrine	1.76	10.76	163
p-Octopamine	0.08	0.35	229
m-Octopamine	0.05	0.24	208

Values are means of two experiments.

Effect of reserpine on the content of serotonin, histamine, catecholamines, p-octopamine and normetanephrine of guinea-pig platelets. It was previously reported that reserpine depleted 5-HT, CA and histamine from rabbit platelets (Da Prada, Pletscher, Tranzer and Knuchel, 1968; Da Prada and Picotti, 1979). In in vivo experiments in guinea-pig (data not shown) reserpine caused a marked decrease of 5-HT and a less pronounced depletion (about 40%) of histamine, normetanephrine and NA.

Effect of reserpine in vitro on the uptake of ^{14}C-5-HT and other ^{14}C-labelled amines by isolated human and rabbit platelets. The amount of ^{14}C-5-HT and ^{14}C-CA taken up by human and rabbit platelets incubated 30 min at 37°C in plasma, containing equimolar concentrations of the amines (10^{-6} M), did not markedly differ in the two species (Table 7).

In contrast, the uptake of labelled NMN and p-octopamine was about 3 times higher in human than in rabbit platelets (Table 7). Histamine and NA accumulated only in minor amounts in the platelets. In rabbit platelets suspended in plasma, reserpine strongly inhibited the uptake of all the labelled amines under study (Table 7) with the exception of histamine, whose uptake was resistant to reserpine.

In contrast, in human platelets the alkaloid blocked effectively the uptake of 5-HT and p-octopamine whereas the uptake of labelled CA and NMN was only partially inhibited (20 - 40 %) (Table 7).

TABLE 7. Effect of reserpine on the uptake of various ^{14}C-labelled amines by human and rabbit platelets in plasma (pmol/mg protein).

^{14}C-amine	Human			Rabbit		
	Control	Reserpine	(% of contr.)	Control	Reserpine	(% of contr.)
Serotonin	832	211	(25)	714	192	(27)
Dopamine	221	136	(61)	181	28	(15)
Adrenaline	40	31	(76)	51	4	(8)
Noradrenaline	24	17	(72)	30	5	(15)
Normetanephrine	305	245	(80)	91	38	(42)
p-Octopamine	231	42	(18)	82	17	(21)
Histamine	ND	ND	—	19	15	(80)

Platelets (0.5 ml of EDTA-PRP plus pargyline 10^{-4} M) were incubated 10 min at $37^{\circ}C$ with or without (controls) reserpine (10^{-5} M). The incubation continued for 30 min in the presence of ^{14}C-amines (10^{-6} M). Human and rabbit plasma containing 2.75×10^8 platelets/ml and 5.22×10^8 platelets/ml respectively were used. Values are means of one experiment in triplicate.

DISCUSSION

In the present study the utilization of highly sensitive and specific radioenzymatic techniques has permitted the measurement of eight different amines in pellets from reasonably small amounts of plasma (<5 ml) or in the various sediments obtained from density gradient fractions. By means of a recently improved single isotope radioenzymatic method, permitting the concomitant determination of femtomole amounts of free and conjugated NMN, m- and p-octopamine, reliable measurements of these "trace" amines were performed in normal human and animal platelets.

Platelets as multitransmitter storage sites. The present accurate radioenzymatic measurements confirm and extend the notion that blood platelets behave as a multitransmitter storage site (Da Prada and Picotti, 1979; Da Prada, Richards and Lorez, 1978). Thus, according to our findings human and animal platelets have the ability to store several transmitter substances such as 5-HT, histamine, CA, octopamine and the NA metabolite NMN. Therefore, platelets challenge the validity of "Dale's principle" (Osborne, 1979), at least for nonneuronal cells. A large number of studies indicate that unconjugated plasma monoamines cross the outer platelet membrane by active and/or passive transport mechanisms (Pletscher, 1978). However, an essential prerequisite for the formation and the maintenance of a concentration gradient for the amines is the presence, in the platelets, of intact 5-HT storage sites. Biochemical and cytochemical experiments have demonstrated that human and animal SPD platelets frequently contain atypical 5-HT organelles. These atypical structures have a reduced capacity for storing 5'-phosphonucleotides, bivalent metals, 5-HT (Richards and Da Prada, 1977; Da Prada, Richards and Lorez, 1978; Weiss et al., 1979) as well as CA and the fluorescent probe, mepacrine (Lorez et al., 1979). The present data show that SPD platelets have an impaired storage mechanism for histamine, too. Compared to normal platelets, those of Fawn-hooded rats and beige mice contain only trace amounts of this amine. The low level of histamine found in SPD platelets, the subcellular fractionation experiments with rabbit platelets and the liberation of histamine from guinea-pig platelets after reserpine, indicate that at least for rat, mouse and rabbit the bulk of the platelet histamine is stored in the 5-HT organelles. However, our uptake experiments in rabbit platelets incubated with reserpine and labelled histamine point to the existence of extragranular and reserpine-resistant pools of this amine. In the human and guinea-pig, histamine appears to be losely bound to the platelets and only in part stored in the 5-HT organelles. Accordingly, both human and guinea-pig platelets contain significantly higher amounts of histamine when the cells are separated by means of Stractan gradients (mild isolation technique), than when sedimented and washed by differential centrifugation.

<u>Free and sulphoconjugated amines in platelets and plasma</u>. Our study documents for the first time the regular occurrence of free p-octopamine and NMN in human, rabbit, rat and guinea-pig platelets. The levels of these two amines are low in comparison to the high concentrations of 5-HT in these cells but are of the same order of magnitude as the concentrations of platelet CA. On the other hand, the histamine level differs considerably among platelets from different animal species. Rabbit platelets are very rich in this amine, whereas rat and, particularly, human platelets contain relatively low amounts of histamine. Guinea-pig platelets are the only platelets in which the histamine concentration is higher than that of 5-HT. Interestingly enough the concentration of histamine in plasma parallels its level in the platelets. Thus, rabbits are the animals with the highest amount of histamine both in plasma and platelets. According to our data (Da Prada and Picotti, 1979) the concentration-ratio between platelets and plasma CA in man and rabbit attains, at best, a value of about 800 which is at least 10 and 30 times lower than that for histamine (rabbit platelets) and 5-HT, respectively. Therefore, it is reasonable to assume that the platelets take up from the plasma <u>in vivo</u> circulating 5-HT more efficiently than histamine or CA. Detectable amounts of sulphoconjugated CA and NMN could be measured in our laboratories in human but not in cat, rat, dog, pig, guinea-pig, monkey and rabbit platelets (data not shown). As to be expected, in preliminary experiments, human but not animal platelets showed a relevant sulphotranferase activity for NMN and CA. Since high concentrations of sulphoconjugated CA in plasma have

been detected also in animals (Tyce et al., 1980) it is reasonable to assume that the high levels of conjugated NMN and NA found in human platelets originate from in situ sulphation of the parent amines rather than from direct accumulation in the platelet of the sulphoconjugates present in plasma (Da Prada and Zürcher, 1979). Human platelets, therefore, differ substantially from animal platelets, since they apparently have an extragranular cytoplasmic pool of sulphoconjugated CA, NMN and 5-HT. Presumably the conjugated amines are in dynamic equilibrium with an additional pool of free amines within the cytoplasmic compartment (Reimers et al., 1975; Costa, Murphy and Reveille, 1977) and with the bulk of the free amines stored in the 5-HT organelles, suggesting that, at least for human platelets, the dynamics of the uptake and storage system are quite complex.

Subcellular localization of serotonin, histamine, catecholamine, normetanephrine and octopamine in rabbit platelets. The subcellular distribution of the various endogenous amines measured radioenzymatically in the different fractions isolated from rabbit platelet homogenates by density gradient centrifugation, directly demonstrate that 5-HT organelles are also the storage sites of the platelet histamine, CA, m- and p-octopamine. NMN, too, had a similar distribution (data not shown). In the isolated 5-HT organelles the various amines stored together with the 5'-phosphonucleotides within these subcellular structures, are about 200 times more concentrated in the 5-HT organelles than in the whole platelets. Reserpine, injected in vivo to guinea-pigs, depleted not only 5-HT but also histamine, NA and NMN, confirming the opinion that the bulk of the endogenous monoamines of the platelets is stored in the 5-HT organelles.

Effect of reserpine in vitro. Comparing the effects of reserpine on the uptake of various labelled amines in human and rabbit platelets, it appears that in man CA and NMN, which are preferred substrates for the sulphotransferase, are also relatively insensitive to reserpine. Moreover, in accordance with previous findings in man (Murphy, Cahan, Molinoff, 1975) in our experiments, too, it is clearly shown that reserpine has an inhibitory effect on the accumulation of labelled p-octopamine in human as well as in rabbit platelets. Thus, it is likely that both in human and rabbit platelets, p-octopamine, which is not a preferred substrate for the sulphotransferase (unpublished results) enters the amine storage vesicles and is stored within them.

In conclusion, the experiments described here focus on the comparison of the concentration, intracellular distribution and uptake of 5-HT and several other biogenic amines in human and animal platelets. In the light of our data, the circulating platelet shows new interesting biochemical features which indicate that platelets should be utilized more extensively in human, pharmacological and pathological studies. Since platelets constitute an easily accessible biochemical compartment, they should be utilized also for the assessment of the functionality of the peripheral sympathetic nervous system. The high sulphotransferase activity present in human platelets could constitute an important pharmaco-metabolic compartment in human blood.

REFERENCES

Buu, N.T., and Kuchel, O., 1979. The direct conversion of dopamine 3-O-sulfate to norepinephrine by dopamine-β-hydroxylase. Life Sci., 24, 783-790.

Costa, J.L., Murphy, D.L., and Reveille, J., 1977. Evaluation of the uptake of various amines into storage vesicles of intact human platelets. Br. J. Pharmac., 61, 223-228.

Da Prada, M., Pletscher, A., Tranzer, J.P., and Knuchel, H., 1968. Action of reserpine on subcellular 5-hydroxytryptamine organelles of blood platelets. Life Sci., 7, 477-480.

Da Prada, M., Richards, J.G., and Lorez, H.P., 1978. Blood platelets and biogenic monoamines: biochemical, pharmacological and morphological studies, in Platelets: a Multidisciplinary Approach (Eds. de Gaetano and Garattini), pp 331-353. Raven Press, New York.

Da Prada, M., and Zürcher, G., 1976. Simultaneous radioenzymatic determination of plasma and tissue adrenaline, noradrenaline, and dopamine within the femtomole range. Life Sci., 19, 1161-1174.

Da Prada, M., and Zürcher, G., 1979. Radioenzymatic assay of plasma and urinary catecholamines in man and various animal species: physiological and pharmacological applications, in Radioimmunoassay of drugs and hormones in cardiovascular medicine (Eds. Albertini, Da Prada and Peskar), pp 175-198. Elsevier, Amsterdam.

Da Prada, M., and Picotti, G.B., 1979. Content and subcellular localization of catecholamines and 5-hydroxytryptamine in human and animal blood platelets: monoamine distribution between platelets and plasma. Br. J. Pharmac., 65, 653-662.

Da Prada, M., Pletscher, A., Tranzer, J.P., and Knuchel, H., 1967. Subcellular localization of 5-hydroxytryptamine and histamine in blood platelets. Nature, 216, 1315-1317.

Hart, R.F., Renskers, K.J., Nelson, E.B., and Roth, J.A., 1979. Localization and characterization of phenol sulphotransferase in human platelets. Life Sci., 24, 125-130.

Lorez, H.P., Richards, J.G., Da Prada, M., Picotti, G.B., Pareti, F.I., Capitanio, A., and Mannucci, P.M., 1979. Storage pool disease: comparative fluorescence microscopical, cytochemical and biochemical studies on amine-storing organelles of human blood platelets. Brit. J. Haematol., 43, 297-305.

Lowry, O.H., Rosebrough, N.J., Farr, A.L., and Randall, R.J., 1951. Protein measurement with the folin phenol reagent. J. Biol. Chem., 193, 265-275.

Merits, I., 1976. Formation and metabolism of ^{14}C-dopamine 3-O-sulfate in dog, rat and guinea-pig. Biochem. Pharmacol., 25, 829-833.

Murphy, D.L., Cahan, D.H., and Molinoff, P.B., 1975. Occurrence, transport and storage of octopamine in human thrombocytes. Clin. Pharmacol. Therap., 18, 587-593.

Osborne, N.N., 1979. Is Dale's principle valid? Trends in Neurosciences, 2, 73-75.

Paulus, J.-M., 1975. Platelet size in man. Blood, 46, 321-336.

Picotti, G.B., Carruba, M.O., Zambotti, F., and Mantegazza, P., 1977. Effects of mazindol and d-fenfluramine on 5-hydroxytryptamine uptake, storage and metabolism in blood platelets. Eur. J. Pharmacol., 42, 217-224.

Picotti, G.B., Da Prada, M., and Pletscher, A., 1976. Uptake and liberation of mepacrine in blood platelets. Arch. Pharmacol., 292, 127-131.

Pletscher, A., 1978. Platelets as models for monoaminergic neurons, in Essays in Neurochemistry and Neuropharmacology, Volume 3 (Ed. Youdim), pp 49-101. Wiley, London.

Reimers, H.J., Allen, D.J., Feuerstein, I.A., and Mustard, J.F., 1975. Transport and storage of serotonin by thrombin-treated platelets. J. Cell Biol., 65, 359-372.

Richards, J.G., and Da Prada, M., 1977. Uranaffin reaction: a new cytochemical technique for the localization of adenine nucleotides in organelles storing biogenic amines. J. Histochem. Cytochem., 25, 1322-1336.

Richards, J.G., and Da Prada, M., 1980. Cytochemical investigations on subcellular organelles storing biogenic amines in peripheral adrenergic neurons, in Histochemistry and Cell Biology of Autonomic Neurons, SIF Cells and Paraneurons (Eds. Eränkö et al.), in press. Raven Press, New York.

Saavedra, J.M., Brownstein, M., and Axelrod, J., 1973. A specific and sensitive enzymatic isotopic microassay for serotonin in tissues. J. Pharmacol. Exp. Ther., 186, 508-515.

Solatunturi, E., and Paasonen, M.K., 1966. Intracellular distribution of monoamine oxidase, 5-hydroxytryptamine and histamine in blood platelets of rabbit. Ann. Med. exp. Fenn., 44, 427-430.

Taylor, K.M., and Snyder, S.H., 1972. Isotopic microassay of histamine, histidine, histidine decarboxylase and histamine methyltransferase in brain tissue. J. Neurochem., 19, 1343-1358.

Tyce, G.M., Sharpless, N.S., Kerr, F.W.L., and Muenter, M.D., 1980. Dopamine conjugate in cerebrospinal fluid. J. Neurochem., 34, 210-212.

Weil-Malherbe, H., 1971. Analysis of biogenic amines and their related enzymes, in Methods of Biochemical Analysis, Suppl. Vol. Ed. Glick), pp 119-152. Interscience Publishers, New York.

Weiss, H.J., Witte, L.D., Kaplan, K.L., Lages, B.A., Chernoff, A., Nossel, H.L., Goodman, D.W.S., and Baumgartner, H.R., 1979. Heterogeneity in storage pool deficiency: studies on granule-bound substances in 18 patients including variants deficient in α-granules, platelet factor 4, β-thromboglobulin, and platelet-derived growth factor. Blood, 54, 1296-1319.

PLATELET FUNCTION AND MONOAMINE OXIDASE
ACTIVITY IN PSYCHIATRIC DISORDERS.

M.B.H. Youdim and A. Hefez

Technion, Departments of Pharmacology and Psychiatry,
Faculty of Medicine,
Haifa, Israel.

ABSTRACT

The human blood platelet displays a great similarity to nerve ending with regard to monoamine uptake, metabolism and release. Despite its complexity, exhibiting both pre-synaptic and post-synaptic function, as compared to synaptosomes, it is unique in providing a human system in which the 5-hydroxytryptamine (5-HT), epinephrine (E) and nor-epinephrine (NE) receptors per se can be studied in the periphery. The platelets aggregate in the presence of several agents including the above neurotransmitters and ADP. These responses are mediated by specific receptors. Boullin et al.(1978a) suggested that the enhanced platelet aggregation responses (PAR) to 5-HT and dopamine (DA) can be used as a predictor of the clinical response to the chlorpromazine (CPZ) and fluphenazine, which block the receptors of amine neurotransmitters in the brain. PAR to 5-HT, DA, E and ADP and the clinical status were determined in a group of 42 schizophrenic patients having their first psychotic episode. The present study has shown that 2-3 weeks after the start of CPZ treatment, patients can be divided into clinical responders and non-responders, with the responders showing enhanced PAR only to 5-HT. We could not confirm PAR to DA. Similar results were obtained with the nucleotide adenylyl-imidodiphosphate (AIP) which mimics the platelet aggregation inducing property of 5-HT. The enhanced PAR to 5-HT and AIP are a property of platelets and no due to a metabolite of CPZ. The results suggest that a nucleotide may be involved in the receptor responsible for 5-HT induced aggregation and the enhanced PAR to 5-HT and AIP could be a useful indication of efficacy of CPZ.

In addition the platelet contains mitochondrial monoamine oxidase (MAO) type B, which preferentially deaminates type B monoamine substrates to the corresponding aldehyde, a property closely shared by the human brain enzyme. On numerous occasions it has been reported that platelet MAO activity is lower in schizophrenics. Results will be presented to support the view that lowered platelet MAO activity could be explained on the basis of long term treatment with the neuroleptics, since CPZ and its metabolites inhibit platelet MAO in vitro. The use of platelet MAO activity as a marker for the CNS enzyme in the treatment of depression and Parkinson's disease with irreversible MAO inhibitors is discussed.

1. INTRODUCTION

Human blood platelets have been considered for some time as a peripheral model for monoaminergic neurons, both as an isolated system for in vitro investigation and for the study of the effect of neuroleptics and anti-depressants in vivo (see Pletscher, this volume and Pletscher, 1978). Blood platelets display a great similarity to nerve endings with regard to monoamine uptake, metabolism and release. They contain osmiphillic dense granules in which 5-hydroxytryptamine (5-HT) is stored; the neurotransmitter is taken up by platelets into storage vesicles and is released by exocytosis upon stimulus by a releasing agent or an aggregation inducer. In addition, they contain mitochondrial monoamine oxidase (MAO), solely of type B, which catabolises monoamines to the corresponding aldehyde in vitro, a similarity shared by human brain MAO (Murphy & Donnelly, 1974; Youdim et al., 1976; Riederer et al., 1978). The platelets aggregate in the presence of several types of inducers, including the neurotransmitters 5-HT, epinephrine (E), norepinephrine (NE) and also ADP, all at very low concentrations (1-10 uM). At saturating concentrations, only the response to 5-HT is reversible and after the platelets reach a certain degree of aggregation they disaggregate again. The platelet aggregation response (PAR) to E, NE and ADP are irreversible and concentration dependent, but differ in kinetic behaviour from each other. It is certain that the receptor for ADP is entirely different from that of 5-HT, and there are data indicating that a separate adrenergic receptor is present on the platelet surface (Born & Michal, 1975; Boullin et al., 1978b).

Despite the complexity of the platelets system (exhibiting both pre-synaptic and post-synaptic function) as compared to synaptosomes, it is unique in providing a human system in which the 5-HT, NE, E and ADP receptors and MAO and uptake per se can be studied in the periphery (Pletscher, 1978; Youdim, 1979; Youdim et al., 1980a). This is important when examining platelet function in normal and abnormal conditions and for purposes of monitoring the effects of psychotropic drugs.

The aim of the present investigation has been to use the platelets namely platelet aggregation response (PAR) and MAO as a biological model to monitor the action of neuroleptics and MAO inhibitor anti-depressants respectively in schizophrenic and depressed patients.

II. PLATELET AGGREGATION RESPONSE (PAR) AND NEUROLEPTICS

The importance of detecting subgroups of schizophrenic drug responders has been repeatedly stressed and attempts have been made to define the clinical and biological characteristics of good responders as contrasted to non-responders (May & Goldberg, 1978). Such attempts, when successful, lead to refinement of diagnostic subgrouping, better understanding of underlying pathology and consequently more accurate prescription of treatment. This issue is of prime importance in schizophrenia, which is usually considered as a group of clinical syndromes with various course and prognosis.

The validity of the few predictors of schizophrenics' response to
chlorpromazine (CPZ) and other neuroleptics have not been demonstrated (May & Goldberg, 1978; Hefez et al., 1980; Boullin et al.,
1978a). Therefore, a biological assay to predict drug efficacy
will be of great assistance. The aggregation responses of amines
such as 5-HT and NE are probably mediated by a specific receptor on
the platelet membrane (Born & Michal, 1975; Boullin et al., 1978b).
In vitro studies have shown the neuroleptics can block the
aggregation responses to the amines (Mills & Roberts, 1967a) while
platelets from patients receiving the neuroleptics chlorpromazine
(CPZ) or fluphenazine show enhanced irreversible aggregation
response to 5-HT (Boullin et al., 1975a; 1975b; Orr & Boullin,
1976; Hefez et al., 1979; Hefez et al., 1980). This enhancement
is seen only in the responder patients and Boullin et al. (1978a)
has suggested that the PAR to 5-HT and DA could be used as a predictor of schizophrenic patients' response to CPZ and other neuroleptics.

(A) Patients selection and clinical assessment.

Every adult admitted to the Department of Psychiatry, Rambam
Hospital, and suspected of having a functional psychotic episode
using the exclusion criteria of Research Diagnostic Criteria (RDC)
(Sudilovsky et al., 1975) were included. These included only
patients having their first or with one previous psychotic breakdown at least two years before the present one. The patients must
not have received anti-psychotic medication before admission and in
case such medication was given a wash out period of eight days was
introduced. During this period the patients received only diazepan.
The clincal assessment was made from a check-list which included
Bleuler's (1950), Schneider's (1959) and Feighner's (1972) criteria
for schizophrenia. The degree of pathology was assessed using the
Hopkins Psychiatric Rating Scale (HPRS). Four subscales chosen as
our clinical parameters for degree of pathology are: the Global
Pathology Score, Psychoticism, Conceptual Dysfunction and Paranoid
Ideation. The scales are 7 points with anchoring definition and
satisfactory reliability. A decrease of at least two points on the
Global Pathology Score, provided that by the end of 6 weeks the
score is not higher than 3, is considered a responder. A score of
3 on HPRS indicates a mild degree of dysfunction, mainly subjective.
Since our main aim was to compare schizophrenic CPZ-responders to
non-responders, only patients who satisfy the criteria of schizo-
prenia according to one of the above mentioned systems were considered. However, occasionally we included a non-schizophrenic
patient or schizophrenic patients under other forms of drug treatment for the purpose of comparison and control. The patients
studied followed a standardized treatment plan with CPZ as the only
anti-psychotic medication administered on a flexible dose design and
Trihexyphenidyl HCl (anti-cholinergic drugs) up to 10 mg a day to
counteract extrapyramidal side-effects, if such symptoms appeared.

(B) Clinical and biochemical studies.

The clinical status and platelet aggregation response (PAR)

(Baumgartner & Born, 1968) were assessed on the day of hospitalization, day 3 and weekly intervals up to 3 months. For the purpose of control, blood samples were drawn from 40 healthy subjects not receiving any form of medication and PAR to 5-HT, E, dopamine (DA) and ADP determined. For kinetic analyses, initial rates of aggregation were measured and in order to normalize the values from various blood samples the ratios of 5-HT/ADP and E/ADP are determined for each individual. In addition, the total changes in the optical density (areas under the curves) of the responses to 5-HT/ADP and E were determined.

(C) Results and Discussion.

The observation that schizophrenic patients receiving chlorpromazine of fluphenazine show an enhanced (irreversible) PAR to 5-HT (Boullin et al., 1975a; Orr & Boullin, 1976) led us to start an investigation with the aim of detecting a possible relation between platelet aggregation responses (PAR) to 5-HT and clinical response of schizophrenic patients to CPZ treatment.

In a double blind study we have examined PAR in 42 patients (age 19-40; 29 males and 13 females) admitted to the Psychiatry Department and having their first suspected schizophrenic. 33 patients satisfied the clinical criteria for schizophrenia and had a reversible PAR to 5-HT before treatment started. 12 patients (Group A) developed an irreversible PAR with a second phase of aggregation to 5-HT, similar to ADP, two to three weeks after the start of CPZ treatment (Fig. 1 and 2). However, the remaining 21 patients (Group B) showed no change in the PAR to 5-HT during CPZ treatment (Fig. 2), but only 11 of these patients showed clinical improvement during the experimental period. The remaining patients did not show an improvement.

The demographic and symptom profile of these two groups were similar. We found no significant difference as to general predictors, e.g. onset, duration, premorbid personality, precipitation, age, etc. However, their clinical response to CPZ was significantly different. Group A showed irreversible PAR and improved condition within two to three weeks of treatment. In contrast, none of Group B patients showed any significant improvement before the 12th week of CPZ treatment (Fig. 3).

Comparison of the Global Pathology Score, Conceptual Dysfunction and Psychoticism indecies of these two subgroups shows that Group A fared better during the 16 weeks of treatment (Fig. 3). However, using the criterion for improvement mentioned, we found that not every improved patient had an irreversible PAR to 5-HT. The parallelism between improvement and irreversible PAR is much better when Feighner's criteria are used for diagnosis. Moreover, contrary to Boullin et al. (1978a) we had no patient with irreversible PAR to 5-HT who did not improve.

It is important to note that both the change in PAR and clinical improvement coincide roughly in time, occurring at the end of the

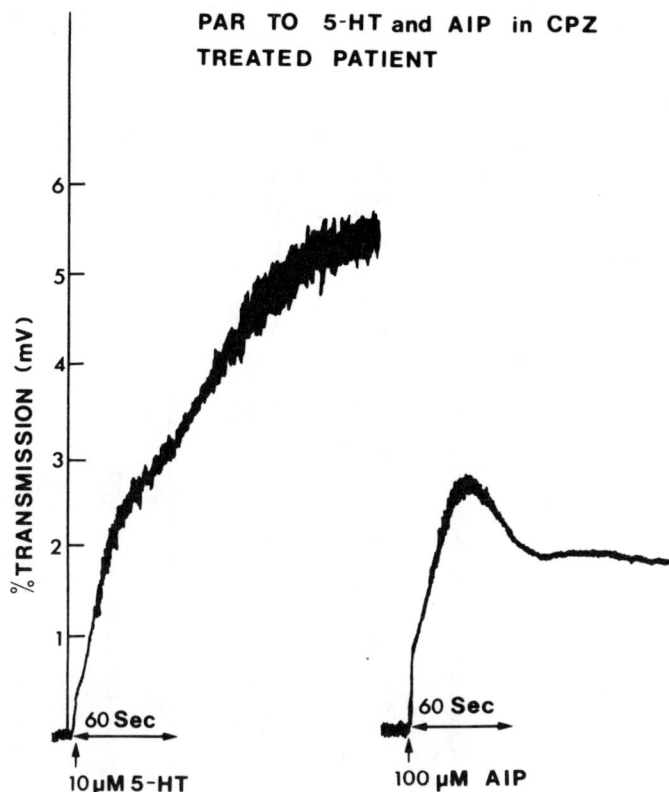

Fig. 1. Potentiation of platelet aggregation responses to (A) serotonin and (B) adenylylimidodiphosphate (AIP) in one schizophrenic patient (B.H., female, age 21) who showed clinical improvement to chlorpromazine within three weeks of treatment (Hefez et al., 1980). Note that aggregation response to serotonin is irreversible while to AIP is reversible. AIP is also a potent inhibitor of second phase aggregation (Oppenheim and Youdim 1979).

second to third week (Fig. 2 and 3). On the otherhand, we found no correlation between CPZ dosage and platelets response to 5-HT in these patients (Hefez et al. 1980).

There are no universally accepted criteria that have utility for planning treatment or schizophrenia. Therefore, a method by which one can distinguish at an early stage between drug responders and non-responders is of great practical theoretical importance.

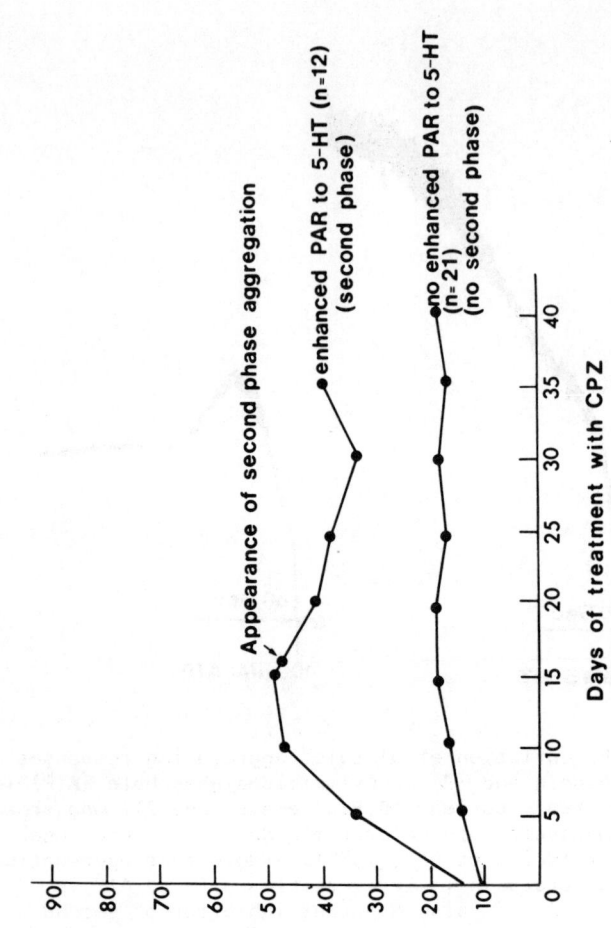

Fig. 2. The change in platelet aggregation response to serotonin in acute schizophrenic patients receiving only chlorpromazine. The results are expressed as the ratio of area under PAR curve of serotonin: ADP. The ± S.E.M. are not included for sake of clarity. The two curves differ significantly ($P<0.01$).

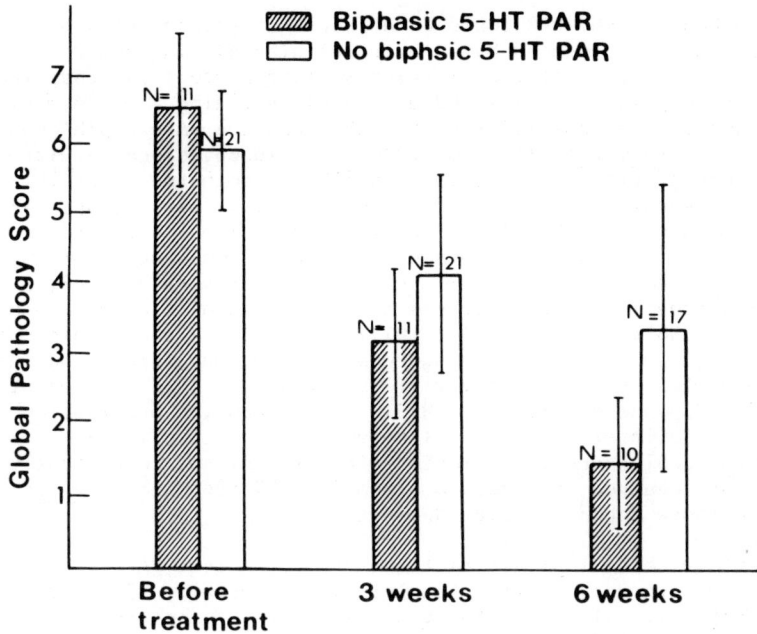

Fig. 3. The clinical improvement of acute schizophrenic patients with (Group A) and without (Group B) a biphasic PAR to 5-HT during treatment with CPZ. Note that the Group B (no biphasic 5-HT PAR) includes patients that clinically improved (N = 11) by the 12th week (P<0.05) and not improved (N = 10) by the 16th week of therapy. The Global Pathology Score of Group A (biphasic 5-HT PAR) was significantly lower at third (P<0.05) and sixth (P<0.01) week of CPZ therapy.

Our preliminary studies with 42 patients indicate that irreversible PAR to 5-HT may prove to be a reliable predictor of the efficacy of CPZ treatment and might eventually help to delineate a subgroup of schizophrenics having special biochemical correlates. Thus the appearance of a second phase in PAR to 5-HT has been found only in those schizophrenic patients who clinically improved on CPZ. So far such a response has not been seen in CPZ treated patients with organic brain syndrome, affective disorders, or in schizophrenics on haloperidol therapy. More data, however, are required to be able to draw definitive conclusions. A recent attempt by Boullin et al. (1978c) to replicate earlier data with a group of chronic patients treated with CPZ for over two years failed to show any enhanced 5-HT

PAR is indeed a property unique to patients having their first psychotic episode and of predictive value.

The enhanced 5-HT PAR could be a result of several possible causes:
1) a change introduced by an extracellular plasma factor;
2) a modification of the platelet surface properties rendering them more susceptible to 5-HT and ultimately yielding a maximum biphasic response. The possibility that the enhanced PAR to 5-HT could be due to an in vitro effect of CPZ was excluded, since in vitro CPZ and some of its major metabolites inhibit both the reversible and the irreversible 5-HT PAR (Boullin et al., 1975a; 1975b; 1975c; Mills & Roberts, 1967a). Phenothiazines also inhibit PAR to E but have no effect on ADP response. E and NE are capable of enhancing in vitro the reversible 5-HT PAR into an irreversible PAR, at low, non-aggregating concentrations and in a synergistic manner (Mills & Robert, 1967b; Ball et al., 1977). Similarly they enhance the responses to several other aggregating and non-aggregating inducers such as ADP, ATP and adenylylimidodiphosphate (AIP) (Hefez et al., 1979; Oppenheim & Youdim, 1979). Although the observation is of scientific interest it is unlikely to be the case in CPZ treated schizophrenic patients, since the plasma concentrations of E or NE required to induce a biphasic 5-HT response in vitro are far above those found in human subjects.

Recent evidence indicate that the change in 5-HT PAR is due to a modified property of the platelets (Hefez et al., 1979; Boullin et al., 1975c). It is postulated that in vivo exposure of circulating platelets to CPZ or its derivatives in schizophrenic patients, may lead to changes in the platelet amine receptor function (as reflected by PAR) which may parallel changes occurring at post-synaptic receptors within the C.N.S. neurons (Heal et al., 1976).

We have demonstrated a 5-HT-like PAR caused by the nucleotide derivative AIP (Oppenheim & Youdim, 1979). Drugs that interfere with PAR to 5-HT affect similarly the PAR to AIP. Enhancement of AIP PAR in schizophrenic patients with an irreversible 5-HT PAR have been observed in several patients (Fig. 1), but needs to be regularly and systematically determined in such patients, in order to establish the similarity between AIP and 5-HT effects, and to examine the possibility that a nucleotide is involved in 5-HT receptor function. These observations may open up a way of examining receptor function and its modification during CPZ therapy. Finally, unlike Boullin et al. (1978a), we have not observed PAR to DA in 200 control subjects or 54 patients receiving CPZ. Our results suggest that platelets do not aggregate in the presence of DA. We have no answers for this discrepancy.

III.   HUMAN PLATELET VERSUS C.N.S. MAO ACTIVITY

Platelets which provide the most readily accessible source of mitochondrial MAO in man has been used as a peripheral marker of the C.N.S. enzyme in a number of pathological and physiological and drug therapy conditions (Murphy & Donnelly, 1974; Youdim & Holzbauer, 1976a; Youdim et al., 1976; Youdim et al., 1980a) (see Table 1).

TABLE 1. Platelet MAO Activity Changes in Physiological and Pathological Conditions*

Schizophrenia

Depressive illness

Migraine

Iron deficiency anaemia

Alcoholism

Hyperthyroidism

Autism

Pregnancy

Menstrual cycle

Age

*Taken from Youdim & Holzbauer (1976b) and Boullin (1978).

Based on substrate specificities (Table 2) and inhibitor sensitivity to clorgyline and deprenyl, the blood platelets MAO can be considered to be B type MAO and similar to the major components of the enzyme found in the human brain (Youdim, 1980) and beef liver (Salach et al., 1979) (Fig. 4). MAO type B deaminates B substrates (benzylamine and phenylethylamine) and AB substrates (dopamine and tyramine) well and A substrates (5-HT, epinephrine and norepinephrine) poorly (Table 2). It is selectively inhibited by the acetylenic inhibitor, deprenyl (Fig. 4) (Murphy & Donnelly, 1974; Youdim et al., 1976; Houslay et al., 1976; Tipton et al., 1976; Salach et al., 1979; Fowler et al., 1978). Murphy & Wyatt (1972) and Wyatt et al. (1973) reported that lowered platelet MAO activity found in schizophrenic subjects may be a genetic marker for vulnerability to schizophrenia. There are many reports for and against schizophrenic patients having lower platelet MAO activity (see Youdim, 1979, for review, Brockington et al., 1976; Agarwal et al., 1980; Oreland, 1980). A reduced brain enzyme activity could be a logical consequence of the disease. However, it should be stressed, unlike the controversy surrounding the platelet MAO activity in schizophrenics, brains obtained at autopsy from such patients show normal MAO activity (see Youdim & Holzbauer, 1976b, and Oreland, 1980) as compared to matched controls. The results of platelet studies are contradictory and in any attempt to seek a link between schizophrenia and reduced MAO activity in blood platelets and brains many factors have to be taken into account. They include choice of patients and matched control,

TABLE 2. Deamination of Substrates by MAO Type B.

		Relative Rate		
Substrate	Type	Platelet	Human Brain	Beef Liver
Benzylamine	B	100	100	100
Tyramine	A and B	105	110	85
Tryptamine	B	-	-	45
2-Phenylethylamine	B	51	52	45
Dopamine	A and B	48	54	44
5-Hydroxytryptamine	A	16	14	19
Epinephrine	A	14	12	9
Norepinephrine	A	-	-	4

MAO activity was assayed using the above substrates according to the radiosotopic method of Tipton and Youdim (1976). All substrate concentrations were 1 mM with the exception of phenylethylamine which was 20 μM. All activities are expressed relative to benzylamine (100%)(Youdim, 1980).

age, sex, duration of drug treatment with neuroleptics (e.g. phenothiazines), drug wash out period, a possible history of other pathological and physiological conditions listed in Table 1, time at which blood platelets or brain tissues were obtained and substrates used for MAO activity.

(A) Platelet MAO activity in schizophrenic patients.

We have investigated platelet MAO activity in drug-free patients having their first or withone previous psychotic breakdown at least two years before as described in the section on platelet aggregation studies and compared them to age and sex matched controls. The mean (±SEM) platelet MAO activities of schizophrenics with 5-hydroxytryptamine (5-HT) and phenylethylamine (PEA), the selective substrates of MAO type A (Johnston, 1968) and type B (Yang & Neff, 1973) respectively, were not significantly different from controls when assessed on the basis of sex and age and other pathological and physiological conditions (Fig. 5) prior to treatment with CPZ. Weekly measurement of MAO activity in controls and CPZ treated

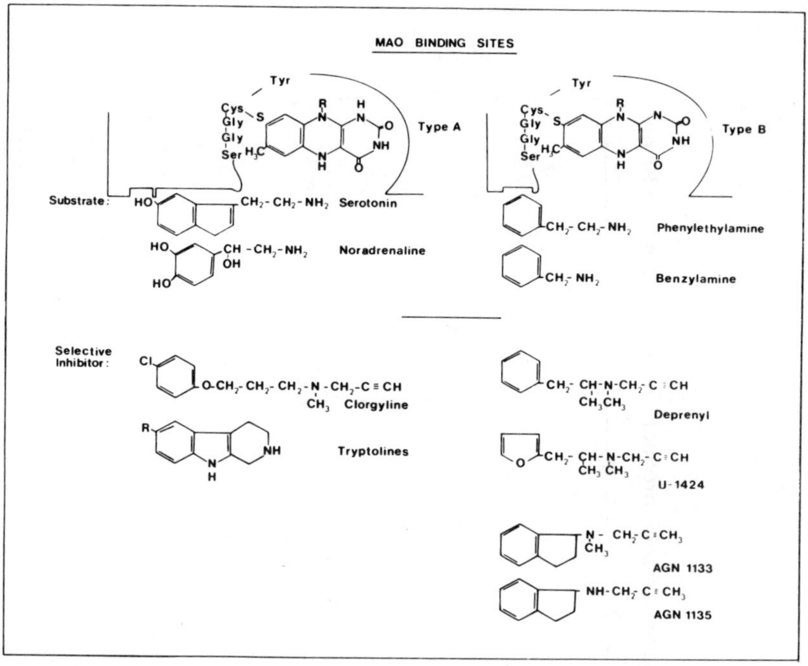

Fig. 4. The binding sites, substrates and selective inhibitors of MAO type A and B (Salach et al., 1979; Youdim & Finberg, 1980).

schizophrenic subjects have shown that while MAO activity in the platelets of control subjects remain reasonably constant, those of schizophrenics on CPZ have a small (30%) but signficantly ($P<0.01$) reduced platelet enzyme activity (Fig. 5) with both substrates by the 16th week of treatment. The results are not unexpected since in vitro CPZ and its metabolites are reversible inhibitors of human brain MAO A & B (Roth et al., 1979). We have confirmed these results using an enzyme, the platelet mitochondria MAO with PEA and 5-HT as substrates (Table 3). The in vitro inhibitory action of CPZ and its metabolites could be explained by the "stabilizing" and binding action of these drugs on biological membranes (Seeman, 1972), noting that MAO is associated with outer mitochondrial membrane (Schnaitman et al., 1967). The concentrations at which platelet MAO is inhibited by the above compounds in vitro (Table 3) can be achieved in man considering that patients receive up to 500 mg daily dose of CPZ (Hefez et al., 1980) and that they can be concentrated within the platelet presumably by an uptake process (Pletscher, 1978). Maickel et al. (1974) have shown that chronic treatment of rats with 2 mg/kg CPZ can result in brain levels of approximately

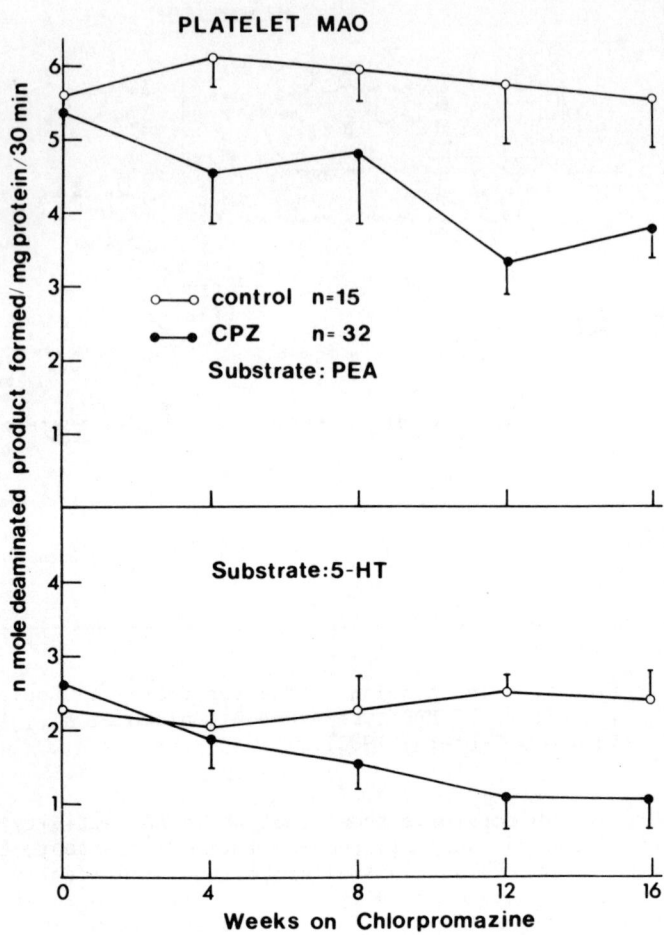

Fig. 5. Platelet MAO activity in drug-free first episode schizophrenic patients and matched controls. The platelets were isolated according to the method described by Youdim (1976) and MAO activity was assayed as described in Table 2 using serotonin (5-HT) and phenylethylamine (PEA) as substrates.

TABLE 3. Inhibition of Platelet MAO by Phenothiazines

	Percent Inhibition	
Drug (50uM)	5-HT	PEA
Chlorpromazine	42 ± 2	45 ± 3
Des-methylchlorpromazine	47 ± 4	49 ± 2
7-Hydroxychlorpromazine	40 ± 1	44 ± 4
8-Hydroxychlorpromazine	41 ± 4	39 ± 7
7,8-Dihydroxychlorpromazine	65 ± 7	56 ± 6

MAO activity toward 5-HT and PEA were assayed according to the method described in Table 1 in the absence or presence of 50 µM phenothiazine derivatives. All preparations were preincubated with or without the above drugs for 30 min at 37°C before the addition of substrates (Youdim, 1980).

30 µg/g (equivalent to 100 µM). Table 3 shows that concentrations far below this can inhibit MAO activity.

The present results show that in the pre-CPZ treatment, platelet MAO activity of first episode schizophrenic patients is not significantly different from their matched controls. However, chronic treatment of patients with CPZ results in lowered platelet MAO activity. Since most reports of reduced platelet MAO activity were observed in patients chronically treated with neuroleptics, results must be interpreted with caution. A large number of biological, methodological, environmental and dietary variables may be also responsible for the apparent changes in the platelet MAO activity in various psychiatric disorders. These factors must be systematically excluded and MAO activity compared to another outer mitochondrial membrane enzyme in order to implicate selectively lowered MAO activity. To date very few studies (Agarwal et al., 1980) have adhered to the above conditions.

IV. THE FUNCTION AND USE OF PLATELET MAO

The function of mitochondrial MAO may be related to its location in a particular organ or cell, thus: (a) it plays an important role in the intraneuronal inactivation and regulation of catecholamines and serotonin (5-HT); (b) in the intestine MAO inactivates the pressor amines, e.g. tyramine and dopamine, derived from their precursor amino acids by decarboxylation; (c) in the liver the enzyme may be responsible for controlling the blood levels of pressor amines and (d) blood vessel and lung MAO could have a crucial role in protecting systemic organs from the toxic effect of high circulating levels of vasoactive monoamines (Youdim et al., 1980b; Youdim & Finberg, 1980). However, no such function has been assigned to MAO in the platelet.

As one of its functions, the platelet in man may be responsible for the non-chemical inactivation of circulating 5-HT by the process of uptake and storage (Pletscher, 1978). Considering that the platelet MAO consists almost entirely of type B enzyme (Murphy & Donnelly, 1974) and that 5-HT is selectively inactivated by MAO type A, the MAO in the platelet, unlike that within the neuron, would not function to inactivate the 5-HT taken up by the platelet. This hypothesis receives support from studies with platelet uptake of 5-HT after inactivation of platelet MAO by irreversible MAO inhibitors. Pletscher (1978) has shown that total inhibition of MAO has no nett effect on 5-HT uptake by the platelet.

There are two functional possibilities that could account for the presence of MAO type B in the platelet. As discussed previously the platelet has the largest reservoir of 5-HT in the body. The preservation and availability of 5-HT for release into the peripheral tissues when needed for physiological homeostatus may be crucial. Secondly there are in the circulation non-polar amines such as phenylethylamine, tryptamine and their derivatives (Usdin & Sandler, 1976). These amines, which are substrates of MAO type B, can cross not only platelet membrane but also the blood brain barrier without the process of uptake. They have been implicated in the pathogenesis of schizophrenia (Usdin & Sandler, 1976), and since they have the ability to release dopamine from its binding sites within the brain there is a need for their inactivation (Sandler et al., 1976; Wyatt et al., 1976). In summary the function of MAO type B in the platelet may be considered to be (a) protection from chemical inactivation of 5-HT and (b) oxidative deamination of toxic type B and A - B amine substrates.

There is abundant evidence that MAO inhibitors are effective and specific anti-depressants, when given in adequate doses, for an adequate period of time to the correct type of patient (Pare, 1976). It is not known why some drugs are more effective than others. Since MAO exists in multiple forms (Youdim et al., 1971) it is now possible to speculate that the MAO inhibitor anti-depressant action may be related to the degree of inactivation of a particular form or forms of the enzyme in the C.N.S. Previous studies on human brains obtained at autopsy from geriatric patients with terminal diseases, and treated for their depression with different classes of MAO inhibitors, have shown that multiple forms of MAO were inhibited to various degrees and the inhibition was never above 70% (Youdim et al., 1972). Animal behavioural and biochemical findings of Green & Youdim (1975) do indicate that MAO is present in the brain grossly in excess of normal requirement by some 85%. This may be one reason why successful therapy of depressive illness and Parkinson's disease was difficult to achieve. The consideration that the human platelet

MAO activity, like that of the brain enzyme is of type B (Table 2 and Fig. 4), led us to monitor the platelet MAO inhibitory action of deprenyl (a selective type B inhibitor) during treatment of depressive illness and Parkinson's disease with the latter drug. It is evident that the drug daily dosage of 10 mg is sufficient to inhibit almost completely both platelet and brain MAO activity (Birkmayer et al., 1977; Riederer et al., 1978; Mendlewicz and Youdim, 1978). Of great interest is the correlation between the degree of inhibition of platelet MAO and therapeutic response to deprenyl. Patients having platelet MAO inhibition of 85% or more showed therapeutic response to deprenyl, while the drug was ineffective in subjects whose platelet MAO was inhibited by less than 85%. Thus it may be possible to use the platelet MAO activity as a peripheral marker for the therapeutic action of selective MAO type B inhibitors.

ACKNOWLEDGMENT

This work was supported in part by an Israel Center for Psychobiology (Jerusalem) Grant and a Technion Grant, 180-152 (Haifa). M.B.H.Y. is a holder of Research Achievement Award from Israel Center for Psychobiology. The authors would like to thank Mrs. B. Glanz for her technical assistance.

REFERENCES

Agarwal, D.P., Werner Goedde, H., and Schrappe, O., 1980. In Monoamine Oxidase, Structure Function and Altered Function (Eds. T.P. Singer, R.W. Von Korff and D.L. Murphy), Academic Press, New York. pp. 397-402.
Ball, S.E., Boullin, D.J., and Glenton, P.A.M., 1977. J. Physiol. (Lond.), 272, 98-99P.
Baumgartner, H.R., and Born, G.V.R., 1968. Nature, 218, 137-140.
Birkmayer, W., Riederer, P., Ambrozi, L., and Youdim, M.B.H., 1977. Lancet 1, 439-444.
Bleuler, E., 1911. Dementia praecox on the group of schizophrenia, translated by J. Zinkin (1950). International University Press, New York.
Born, G.V.R., and Michal, F., 1975. In Biochemistry and Pharmacology of Platelets. Ciba Foundation Symposium No. 35. (Eds. K. Elliot and J. Knight), Elsevier, Amsterdam, pp. 287-307.
Boullin, D.J., 1978. In Serotonin and Mental Abnormalities (Ed. D.J. Boullin), Wiley, Chichester, pp. 1-40.
Boullin, D.G., Orr, M.W., and Peters, J.R., 1978a. In Platelets, A Multidisciplinary Approach (Eds. C. de Gaetano and S. Garrattini) Raven Press, New York, pp. 389-410.
Boullin, D.G., Glenton, P.A.M., and Orr, M., 1978b. Brit. J. Pharmacol., 62, 537-542.
Boullin, D.J., Grahame-Smith, D.J., Grimes, R.P.J., and Woods, H.F., 1975b. Brit. J. Pharmacol., 53, 121-126.
Boullin, D.J., Grahame-Smith, D.G., Grimes, R.P.J. and Woods, H.F., 1975c. Brit. J. Clin. Pharmacol., 2, 37-41.

Boullin, D.J., Knox, J.M., Peters, J.R., Peters, M., Orr, M.W., Gelder, M.G., and Grahame-Smith, D.G., 1978c. Brit. J. Clin. Pharmacol., 6, 538-540.
Boullin, D.G., Woods, H.F., Grimes, R.P.J., Grahame-Smith, D.G., Wiles, D., Gelder, M.G., and Kolakowaska, J. 1975a. Brit. J. Clin. Pharmacol., 2, 29-35.
Brockington, I., Crow, T.J., Johnstone, E.C., and Owen, F., 1975. In Monoamine Oxidase and Its Inhibition. Ciba Foundation Symposium No. 39. (Eds. G.E.W. Wolstenholme and J. Knight), Elsevier, Amsterdam, pp. 353-370.
Feighner, J.P., Robins, E., Guse, S.B., Woodruff, R.A., Winolur, G., and Munoz, R., 1972. Arch. Gen. Psychiat., 26, 5763-5775.
Fowler, C.J., Callingham, B.A., Mantle, T.J., and Tipton, K.F., 1978. Biochem. Pharmacol., 27, 97-101.
Green, A.R., and Youdim, M.B.H., 1975. Brit. J. Pharmacol., 55, 415-422.
Heal, D.J., Green, A.R., Boullin, D.J., and Grahame-Smith, D.G., 1976. Psychopharmacology, 49, 287-300.
Hefez, A., Oppenheim, B., and Youdim, M.B.H., 1979. Israel. J. Med. Sci., 15, 618.
Hefez, A., Oppenheim, B., and Youdim, M.B.H., 1980. In Enzymes and Neurotransmitters in Mental Disease (Eds. E. Usdin, T.L. Sourkes M.B.H. Youdim), Wiley, Chichester, pp. 78-93.
Houslay, M.D., Tipton, K.F., and Youdim, M.B.H.. 1976. Life Sci., 467-483.
Johnston, J.P., 1968. Biochem. Pharmacol., 17, 1285-1297.
Knoll, J., and Magyar, K., 1972. Adv. Biochem. Psychopharmacol., 5, 393-408.
Maickel, R.P., Braunstein, M.C., McGlynn, M.L., Snodgrass, W.R., and Webb, R.W., 1974. In The Phenothiazines and Structurally Related Drugs (Eds. J.R. Forrest, C.J. Carr and E. Usdin), Raven Press, New York, pp. 593-602.
May, P.R.A., and Goldberg, S.C., 1978. In Psychopharmacology. A Generation of Progress (Eds. M.A. Lipton, A. DiMascio and K.F. Killam). Raven Press, New York, pp. 1139-1153.
Mendlewicz, J., and Youdim, M.B.H., 1978. J. Neural. Transmn., 43, 279-286.
Mills, D.C.B., and Roberts, G.C.K., 1967a. Nature, 213, 35-38.
Mills, D.C.B., and Roberts, G.C.K., 1967b. J. Physiol. (Lond.), 193, 443-453.
Murphy, D.L., and Donnelly, C., 1974. In Neuropharmacology of Monoamines and Their Regulatory Enzymes, Raven Press, New York, pp. 71-86.
Murphy, D.L., and Wyatt, R.J., 1972. Nature (Lond.), 238, 225-226.
Oppenheim, B., and Youdim, M.B.H., 1979. Brit J. Pharmacol., 66, 94-95P.
Oreland, L., 1980. In Monoamine Oxidase, Structure, Function and Altered Function (Eds. T.P. Singer, R.W. Von Korff and D.L. Murphy), Academic Press, New York, pp. 379-388.
Orr, M.W., and Boullin, D.J., 1976. Brit. J. Clin. Pharmacol., 3, 925-928.
Pare, C.M.B., 1976. In Monoamine Oxidase and Its Inhibition. Ciba Foundation Symposium. No. 39. (Eds. G.E.W. Wolstenholme and J. Knight). Elsevier, Amsterdam, pp. 271-296.

Pletscher, A., 1978. In *Essays in Neurochemistry and Neuropharmacology*, Vol. 3. (Eds. M.B.H. Youdim, W. Lovenberg, D.F. Sharman and J.R. Lagnado), Wiley, Chichester, pp. 49-102.

Pletscher, A., 1980. In *Platelets Cellular Response Mechanisms and Their Biological Significance* (Ed. A. Rotman), Wiley, London. (see this volume).

Riederer, P., Youdim, M.B.H., Rausch, W.D., Birkmayer, W., Jellinger, K., and Seemann, D., 1978. *J. Neural. Transmn.*, 43, 217-226.

Roth, J., Whittmore, R., Shakarjian, M., and Eddy, B., 1979. *Commun. Psychopharmacol.*, 3, 235-244.

Salach, J.I., Detmer, K., and Youdim, M.B.H., 1979. *Mol. Pharmacol.*, 16, 234-241.

Sandler, M., Carter, S.B., Goodwin, B.L., and Ruthven C.R.J., 1976. In *Trace Amines and the Brain* (Eds. E. Usdin and M. Sandler), Dekker, New York, pp. 233-282.

Schnaitman, C., Erwin, V.G., and Greenawalt, J.W., 1967. *J. Cell. Biol.*, 32, 719-735.

Schneider, K., 1959. In *Clinical Psychopathology* (4th edn.). Grunett and Strantton, New York.

Seeman, P., 1972. *Pharmacol. Rev.*, 24, 583-655.

Sudilovsky, A., Gershon, S., and Beer, B., 1975. *Predictability in Psychopharmacology: Principal and Clinical Correlations*. Raven Press, New York, pp. 1-217.

Tipton, K.F., and Youdim, M.B.H., 1976. In *Monoamine Oxidase and Its Inhibition*. Ciba Foundation Symposium No. 39. (Eds. G.E.W. Wolstenholme and J. Knight), Elsevier, Amsterdam, pp. 393-403.

Tipton, K.F., Houslay, M.D., and Mantle, T.J., 1976. In *Monoamine Oxidase and Its Inhibition*. Ciba Foundation Symposium. No. 39. (Eds. G.E.W. Wolstenholme, J. Knight), Elsevier, Amsterdam, pp. 5-32.

Usdin, E., and Sandler, M., 1976. *Trace Amines and the Brain*. Dekker, New York.

Wyatt, R.J., Murphy, D.L., Belmaker, R., Cohen, S., Donnelly, C.H., and Pollin, W., 1973. *Science*, 179, 916-918.

Wyatt, R.J., Gillin, J.C., Stoff, D.M., Majo, E.A., and Tinklenberg, J.R., 1977. In *Neuroregulators and Psychiatric Disorders* (Eds. E. Usdin, D.A. Hamburg and J. Barchas), Oxford University Press, New York, pp. 31-45.

Yang, H-Y.T., and Neff, N.Y., 1973. *J. Pharmacol. Exp. Ther.*, 187, 365-371.

Youdim, M.B.H., 1976. In *Monoamine Oxidase and Its Inhibition*. Ciba Foundation Symposium No. 39. (Eds. G.E.W. Wolstenholme and J. Knight), Elsevier, Amsterdam, pp. 404-406.

Youdim, M.B.H., 1979. In *Neuro-Psychopharmacology* (Ed. E. Saletu), Pergamon Press, Oxford, pp. 85-94.

Youdim, M.B.H., 1980. Unpublished data.

Youdim, M.B.H., and Finberg, J., 1980. In *Drug Receptors in the Central Nervous System* (Eds. Y. Dudai, V.I. Teichberg and U.Z. Littauer', Wiley, Chichester (in press).

Youdim, M.B.H., and Holzbauer, M., 1975a. In *Monoamine Oxidase and Its Inhibition*. Ciba Foundation Symposium No. 39. (Eds. G.E.W. Wolstenholme and J. Knight), Elsevier, Amsterdam, pp. 105-134.

Youdim, M.B.H., and Holzbauer, M., 1976b. J. Neural. Transmn., 38, 193-231.
Youdim, M.B.H., Collins, G.G.S., and Sandler, M., 1971. Biochem. J., 121, 34-36P.
Youdim, M.B.H., Ben-Harari, R.R., and Bakhle, Y.H., 1980. In The Metabolic Properties of the Lung. Ciba Foundation Symposium No. 87. (Eds. R.R. Porter and J. Knight), Elsevier, Amsterdam, (in press).
Youdim, M.B.H., Grahame-Smith, D.G., and Woods, H.F., 1976. Clin. Sci. Mol. Med., 50, 479-486.
Youdim, M.B.H., Collins, G.G.S., Sandler, M., Bevan Jones, A.B., Pare, C.M.B., and Nicholson, W.J., 1972. Nature (Lond.), 236, 225-228.
Youdim, M.B.H., Riederer, P., Birkmayer, W., and Mendlewicz, J., 1980a. In Monoamine Oxidase, Structure, Function and Altered Functions (Eds. T.P. Singer, R.W. Von Korff and D.L. Murphy), Academic Press, New York, pp. 477-497.

DISCUSSION (Condensed by the Editors from Recordings)

The first part dealt mainly with the role of platelets in the processes of hemostasis and thrombosis. It is now clear that only adhesion to certain surfaces will induce a change in the platelet which causes it to attach circulating platelets and form surface thrombi. There is as yet no answer, however, to the basic question of why on the exposed subendothelial tissue only a monolayer of platelet is formed which remains there and will not form a thrombus. Only platelets interacting with a fine enough fibre, whose surface is composed of collagen in triple helical conformation can induce thrombus formation. What is the rate and mechanism of thrombus formation? What is the effect of shear and the kinetic energy of the platelet on the interaction? On the question thus raised whether a platelet which has arrived at the injury site is or is not going to stick to a platelet monolayer already there, it was pointed out that there must be two kinds of adherent platelets, those which are inactive and those which are attached to a fibrous collagen surface. The use of collagen fibres as a model for the adhesion of platelets to the subendothelium was thus questioned. While studies of platelet-collagen interaction are relevant, factors such as the geometry of the adhering surface, hydrodynamic forces and other means of stimulating platelets should be borne in mind. It was agreed that knowledge and understanding of the events that take place immediately after injury and platelet activation is crucial. The need was stressed for new techniques to study platelet responses, such as shape change, membrane interactions and alterations and phosphorylation, all of which occur within a few seconds. For these purposes, photoaffinity probes having a lifetime of milliseconds should prove to be very useful. Instruments based on laser beams, to study fast shape change processes, were mentioned and preliminary studies in this direction are already in progress.

The last part of this discussion dealt with the role of calcium in the stimulation of platelets. Though there is no doubt that calcium plays a key role in platelet activation, the exact mode of its participation is far from being understood. In view of the report that calcium accumulating vesicles were isolated from platelets, it was agreed that a calcium accumulating system does exist in platelets but the origin of this system has not yet been defined. The importance of the dense tubular system as a calcium source was challenged.

Among the membrane components likely to be the receptors for platelet stimulation, the surface glycoproteins are especially favoured. The methods of labelling, separation and characterization of the platelet membrane macromolecules and their identification as receptors were discussed.

The involvement and importance of platelet membrane glycoproteins in various diseases, such as Glanzmann's Thrombasthenia, Bernard-Soulier Syndrome and Montreal Syndrome, were discussed. The interaction of thrombin with platelet membrane was considered in particular. The interaction of thrombin with its receptor seems to involve a stoichiometric reaction and does not follow an enzyme-substrate mechanism. Membrane glycoprotein V is hydrolyzed in the thrombin-platelet interaction and must thus be involved. The correlation between thrombin binding, the degree of hydrolysis and the degree of platelet activation has not, however, been elucidated.

The question of the existence of a thrombin receptor was challenged, in fact. It was argued that there are apparently far more receptors (or binding sites) for thrombin than are needed for activation. A question which remains to be answered is thus the purpose of these spare receptors.

The use of photoaffinity labels as tools in the study of membrane structure and function was discussed. The possibility of designing a probe that will penetrate into the membrane to a controlled and desired depth was suggested.

An interesting point raised in the discussion concerned the interaction of actin with the platelet surface as a result of activation. The contradicting evidence whether or not actin becomes exposed was discussed without being resolved. The use of labels, such as iodonaphthyl azide, and of antibodies to actin was considered, but no definite conclusion was reached. It was agreed that actin might be adsorbed in small quantities to the membrane of intracellular granules. Such actin molecules might then appear on the platelet surface as a result of secretion from the granules. It was reported that actin has a tendency to "stick" very tightly to the platelet membrane. It is clear, however, that the intracellular changes which follow activation of platelets with ADP and thrombin involve the microtubule and microfilament system.

ADP-dependent fibrinogen binding to human platelets was discussed extensively. Preliminary results involving photoaffinity labelling of the fibrinogen binding site were presented. The interaction of fibrinogen with platelets seems to be hydrophobic in nature and involves internalization. The role of calcium in the ADP-dependent fibrinogen binding was emphasized. The possibility that calcium might serve as a bridge between fibrinogen and platelet glycoproteins was considered. It was suggested that calcium ions might mediate an electrostatic effect on the platelet surface. It was agreed that while calcium is necessary it is not sufficient for fibrinogen interaction with platelets.

Similarities between fibrinogen and thrombin binding were pointed out. Fibrinogen binding increases when the temperature is lowered, i.e. when membrane fluidity decreases. Similarly, the binding of thrombin to fixed platelets is higher than to unmodified ones. Both processes seem to involve passive modulation but, at least in the case of fibrinogen, clustering is not a prerequisite for binding.

One of the reasons for amine storage is the relatively low pH inside the granules; amines such as serotonin, dopamine and mepacrine tend to move into these granules as a result. While catecholamines do not produce an optical shape change, they do affect platelets morphology. Evidence was brought that serotonin can cause a shape change at concentrations as low as 10^{-15}M compared to the usually reported value of 10^{-7} to 10^{-6}M. The meaning of serotonin-induced shape change at such low concentrations is unresolved.

Altogether, the role of serotonin in platelets function was questioned. Several possible reasons for the existence of serotonin in platelets were suggested. These include the removal of serotonin from the circulation, in order to eliminate its possible vasoconstriction effect and possible cerebral damage as a result of high sensitivity to serotonin. The usefulness of platelet monoamine oxidase as a model for monoamine oxidase of the central nervous system was challenged.

Author Index

A

Abrahams, S.L.   201, 210
Adelstein, R.S.   140, 196, 198,
  214, 228, 229, 231, 251, 261
Agarwal, J.P.   297, 301, 303
Aledort, L.M.   206, 211
Agin, P.P.   91, 93, 108, 117,
  122, 123, 124, 125, 126, 130,
  131, 133, 138, 140, 141, 162,
  167
Akkerman, J.W.N.   257, 261, 262
Alexander, B.   158, 166
Alfrey, C.P.   5, 8, 12
Ali, I.U.   64
Allen, D.J.   288
Ambrozi, L.   303
Ames, G.F.   120, 128
Amos, L.A.   171, 177, 187
Anaya-Galindo, R.   155
Anderson, E.R.   161, 166
Anderson, W.Jr.   198
Andersson, L.C.   107, 116
Antoniades, H.N.   249, 261
Ardaillous, N.   140
Arfors, K.E.   8, 10, 12
Asch, A.   140, 199
Ash, J.F.   192, 200
Ashwell, G.   108, 118
Assimeh, S.N.   64
Aster, R.H.   121, 129
Atherton, R.M.   225, 231
Atkinson, J.P.   231
Axelrod, J.   288

B

Baenziger, N.L.   90, 92, 231
Bakhle, Y.H.   306
Ball, S.E.   296, 303
Balleisen, L.   56, 57, 60, 63
Barber, A.J.   61, 64
Barenholtz, Y.   96, 105
Barnes, M.J.   57, 63
Barrow, D.A.   104
Bartholini, J.   271, 276
Barylko, B.   225, 229
Baver, J.S.   246, 261

Baumgartner, H.R.   8, 12, 15,
  17, 18, 19, 20, 21, 22, 23,
  24, 25, 26, 27, 28, 52, 57,
  59, 63, 65, 130, 280, 288,
  292, 303
Beachey, E.H.   52, 60, 63, 65
Beer, B.   305
Begent, N.A.   8, 12
Behnke, O.   171, 172, 184, 187,
  189, 195, 198
Belamarich, F.A.   11, 12
Bell, R.L.   131, 139, 203, 208
Belville, J.S.   229
Ben-Harari, P.R.   306
Benis, A.M.   8, 15
Bennett, W.F.   215, 225, 228,
  229
Bennett, J.S.   155, 161, 166
Bentz, H.   64
Bensusan, H.B.   52, 54, 61, 64
Bercovici, T.   107, 110, 116
Bereziat, G.   205, 208
Bergqist, D.   10, 12
Berlin, R.D.   95, 102, 103
Berliner, L.J.   149
Bernard, J.   26, 128
Berndt, M.C.   131
Berneis, K.H.   240, 244, 246
Bettelheim, F.A.   54, 64
Bettex-Galland, M.   135, 139
Bevan Jones, A.B.   306
Bharadwaj, B.B.   65
Bieri, V.   106
Billah, M.M.   202, 203, 209
Bills, T.K.   69, 74, 202, 208
Bing, D.H.   149
Birkmayer, W.   303, 305, 306
Bjerrom, O.J.   128
Blasberg, P.   14
Bleuler, E.   291, 303
Blikstad, I.   192, 198
Blout, E.R.   103, 104, 105
Bodevin, E.   26
Böhme, E.   214, 229
Bolhuis, P.A.   27

Bolin, R.B.   127, 128
Bolton, C.H.   10, 12
Booyse, F.M.   96, 103
Borchard, R.E.   263
Borise, G.G.   188
Born, E.V.R.   3, 4, 5, 6, 7, 10, 12, 14, 70, 74, 290, 291, 292, 303
Bornstein, P.   52, 64
Borochov, H.   96, 102, 154, 155
Borrelli, J.   158, 168
Boullin, D.J.   289, 290, 291, 292, 295, 296, 297, 303, 304
Bourguinon, L.Y.W.   200
Bouvier, C.A.   91, 92
Bowles, D.J.   115, 116
Boxer, D.H.   118
Brass, L.F.   52, 54, 64
Braunstein, M.C.   304
Bray, D.   135, 139, 192, 195, 198
Bredoux, R.   27, 129, 130
Brinkley, B.   64
Brinkley, B.R.   188, 198
Brockineton, I.   297, 304
Brodie, G.N.   90, 92
Broekman, M.J.   66, 166, 199, 263
Brooker, J.   222, 230
Brooks, C.   56, 59, 64
Brot, F.E.   251, 261
Brouet, J.C.   140
Brown, C.H.   5, 13
Brown, J.C.   114, 117
Brownstein, M.   288
Bruderer, H.   271, 276
Brudzynski, T.M.   140
Budzynski, A.Z.   167
Bunting, S.   27
Burkard, W.P.   271, 276
Burns, R.E.   184, 187
Butcher, A.D.   61, 65
Butler, A.M.   75, 206, 209
Butruille, Y.   20, 26
Buu, N.T.   287
Byers, S.O.   4, 13
Bygrave, F.L.   68, 74

C
Cabantchik, Z.I.   107, 116

Caen, J.P.   20, 21, 27, 60, 63, 64, 66, 96, 104, 114, 117, 119, 121, 122, 124, 126, 128, 129, 130, 140, 162, 165, 167
Cahen, D.H.   286, 288
Callingham, B.A.   304
Calne, D.B.   246
Calvo, F.   104
Campbell, I.C.   243, 244
Cande, W.Z.   190, 199
Cantacuzene, D.   245, 246
Cantour, C.R.   188
Capano, M.   75
Capitanio, A.   281
Carafoli, E.   68, 72, 74
Carlier, M.F.   180, 187
Carlsson, L.   195, 196, 198, 199
Caro, C.G.   4, 12
Carruba, M.O.   278, 288
Carter, S.B.   305
Cartron, J.P.   127, 128
Carvalho, A.C.A.   19, 28
Castaldi, P.A.   128
Castle, A.G.   171, 174, 176, 180, 182, 184, 187
Cazenave, J.P.   57, 64, 77, 114, 115, 116, 140, 262
Chahil, A.   246
Chaplin, D.   90, 92
Charo, I.F.   147, 149, 165, 166
Charo, T.   251, 261
Chediak, J.   122, 128
Chernoff, A.   166, 199, 288
Cherry, R.T.   101, 103
Chesney, C.McI.   54, 59, 64
Cheung, W.Y.   181, 187, 214, 229
Chiang, T.M.   52, 60, 63
Chignard, M.   70, 75, 204, 208
Chong, G.   65
Chuang, H.Y.   151, 155
Claesson, H.E.   251, 261
Clementi, F.   74
Clemetson, K.J.   115, 116
Cimo, P.L.   76
Cockburn, J.   8, 12
Cohen, I.   69, 72, 75, 165, 166
Cohen, P.   77
Colantuoni, G.   5, 8, 12
Cole, R.D.   190, 199
Coleman, R.   96, 103

Coligan, J.E. 90, 93, 129, 262
Coller, B.S. 165, 166
Collins, G.G.S. 306
Coleman, R.W. 155, 156
Colombani, J. 140
Colombani, M. 140
Compans, R.W. 117
Condeelis, J.S. 196, 197, 200
Constantinidis, P. 4, 8, 13
Conti, M.A. 198, 214, 229, 259, 261
Cooke, R. 259, 263
Cooper, R.A. 96, 102, 103, 105
Copley, 21
Corash, L. 245
Corbin, J.B. 215, 218, 229
Costa, J.L. 233, 234, 236, 237, 238, 239, 240, 241, 243, 244, 245, 247, 254, 261, 286, 287
Cottrel, B.A. 261
Craig, S.W. 91, 92
Crawford, N. 91, 93, 171, 174, 176, 181, 182, 184, 187, 188, 236, 246
Creveling, C.R. 239, 245, 246
Cross, M.J. 7, 13
Cross, J. 12
Crow, T.J. 304
Crowther, P.E. 155
Cuatrecasas, P. 202, 203, 209, 210, 258, 260, 262
Culp, L.A. 64
Cumming, J. 118
Cunningham, L.W. 57, 59, 61, 66
Cusak, N.J. 14
Cushing, R.J. 245

D
Dabbous, M.K. 64
Dabrowska, R. 132, 139
Daniel, J.L. 132, 140, 198, 214, 225, 229, 249, 259, 261
Daneelmaier, C.A. 250, 257, 261
Daprada, M. 236, 244, 245, 246, 268, 275, 277, 278, 279, 281, 283, 284, 285, 286, 287, 288
Dautigny, A. 140
Davey, M.G. 131, 133, 140, 149, 261
Davidson, M.M.L. 199, 213, 230
Davidson, R.L. 105
Davies, T. 230

Dawson, G. 108, 110
Day, H.J. 234, 246, 262
Dearnley, R. 7, 12
Dedman, J.R. 188
De Gaetano, G. 96, 103
De Gier, J. 106
De Gos, L. 27, 129, 130, 138, 140
De Meyts, P. 154, 155
Demopoulos, C.A. 69, 75
Deranleau, D.A. 75, 77
De Rosier, D. 196, 199
Desjardins, J.V. 230
Destree, A.T. 64
Detmer, K. 305
Detwiler, T.C. 69, 75, 132, 140, 143, 144, 146, 147, 149, 150, 155, 166, 208, 209, 234, 245, 255, 261
Devis, G. 76
De Vries, 72, 75
Deykin, D. 54, 64, 69, 77, 96, 103, 105
Diegle, T.A. 91, 92
Dinerstein, R.J. 76
Dingle, J.T. 54, 64
Dobson, C.M. 245
Domino, L.E. 247
Domino, E.F. 247
Donnelly, 290, 296, 297, 302, 304
Doolittle, R.F. 250, 261
Dounie, H.G. 9, 14
Drabikowski, W. 74
Drillings, M. 166, 199
Driver, H.A. 261
Dubler, D. 70, 75, 77
Duguid, J.V. 3, 13
Dupuis, D. 119
Dustin, 171
Dvilansky, A. 95, 116, 155

E
Ebert, M.H. 246
Edgington, T.S. 76, 166, 167
Eanes, E.B. 239, 246, 247
Edds, K.T. 195, 196, 198
Edelman, G.M. 191, 199, 200
Eddy, B. 305
Ediddin, M. 95, 103
Edwards, H.H. 131, 141, 199
Egan, J.J. 27, 28, 130, 167

Eipper, B.A. 184, 187
Eisler, T. 236, 246
Ellison, J.J. 199
Emmines, J.P. 77, 130, 247
Emmons, P.R. 10, 12
Engvall, E. 61, 66
Erwin, V.J. 305
Estensen, R.D. 205, 209, 211
Evans, G. 66, 206, 209
Evans, P.M. 153, 155

F
Faile, D. 52, 64
Farr, A.L. 278, 287
Fauvel, F. 60, 64
Feagler, J.R. 90, 92, 141, 145, 146, 150, 156
Feighner, J.P. 291, 304
Feinberg, H. 76, 161, 166
Feinman, R.D. 69, 75, 140, 144, 147, 149, 150, 155, 166, 234, 245, 255, 261
Feinstein, M.D. 214, 230
Fenton, J.W.II 143, 146, 147, 150
Fera, J.P. 95, 102, 103
Ferris, B. 63, 65, 117, 129
Feuerstein, I.A. 288
Fietzek, P.P. 64
Finalyson, J.S. 149
Feinberg, J. 299, 302, 305
Firkin, B.G. 20, 23, 92
Fisback, B. 27
Fischer, T. 6, 14
Flavin, M. 188
Fleischer, G. 95, 110, 116, 155
Foidart, J.M. 27
Ford, J.D. 66
Forst, R. 14
Foulks, J.G. 7, 12, 161, 166
Fowler, C.J. 297, 304
Fox, C.F. 104
Fox, J.E.B. 131, 140, 199, 213, 215, 219, 220, 225, 230
French, J.E. 127, 130
Friedman, L.I. 20, 27
Friedman, M. 4, 8, 13
Friis, R.R. 104
Frojmovic, M.M. 13, 54, 58, 61, 62, 63, 65
Fuchs, P. 95, 103
Fujiwara, K. 141
Fukami, M.H. 166, 233, 235, 246, 247, 249, 257, 261

Fuller, G.M. 190, 199
Fulton, C. 191, 199

G
Gaarder, A. 5, 13
Gabbiani, G. 92
Gahwiler, B.H. 275
Galetti, P.M. 5, 14
Gahmberg, C.G. 107, 108, 116
Ganguly, P. 133, 140, 146, 149
Gartner, T.K. 90, 92, 96, 103, 128
Gaskin, F. 188
Gates, R.E. 108, 116
Gay, S. 19, 26, 63
Gelder, M.G. 304
George, J.N. 75, 81, 82, 83, 88, 89, 90, 91, 92, 93, 96, 103, 107, 112, 113, 116, 117, 119, 124, 126, 128, 166, 231
Gerrard, J.M. 69, 71, 75, 91, 93, 201, 202, 203, 204, 205, 206, 207, 209, 211, 234, 247
Gerber, E. 231
Gerbes, R.J.
Gergely, P. 181, 187
Gershon, S. 305
Gey, K.F. 271, 276
Gillin, J.C. 305
Gitler, C. 107, 110, 116, 189
Gjemdal, T. 27
Glaser, T. 166
Glaser, J.H. 261
Glenton, P.A.M. 303
Glomset, J. 3, 14, 96, 105
Glusa, E. 214, 230
Glushak, C. 13
Glynn, M.F. 66
Goldberg, L.I. 239, 246
Goldberg, C.G. 290, 291, 304
Goldsmith, H.L. 10, 13
Goodman, D.W.S. 288
Goodwin, B.L. 305
Gordon, J.L. 52, 54, 57, 61, 63, 64
Gordon, R.K. 64
Graf, H. 229, 268, 272, 275
Graff, G. 75, 206, 209
Grahame-Smith, D.G. 303, 304, 306
Grand, C.W.M. 95, 103
Grand, M.E. 61, 65

Grand, R.A.   158, 159, 162, 165, 166, 167, 168
Green, A.R.   302, 304
Greenberg, J.P.   61, 64, 127, 128, 165, 166
Greengard, P.   188
Greenwalt, J.W.   305
Grimes, R.P.J.   303, 304
Gross, R.   96, 103
Gross, M.J.   8, 12
Gryglewski, R.   27
Guccione, M.A.   64, 128, 166
Guilmette, K.M.   103
Guse, S.B.   304

H
Hagen, I.   27, 108, 117, 121, 122, 126, 128
Hagen, L.   90, 93, 121, 122
Hakomori, S.I.   108, 116
Haley, B.E.   216, 230
Hamberg, M.   11, 13, 15
Hammond, S.A.   192, 200
Hanahan, D.J.   75
Handin, R.   141
Hardisty, R.M.   96, 103, 119, 124, 129
Harfenist, F.J.   64, 129, 166, 167
Harker, L.A.   96, 103
Harper, J.F.   222, 230
Harris, H.E.   192, 199
Harrison, M.J.G.   10, 13
Hart, R.F.   279, 287
Hartshorne, D.J.   139
Hartwig, J.H.   192, 196, 199, 200
Harwood, R.   61, 65
Hasitz, M.   155
Haslam, R.J.   10, 13, 73, 75, 132, 140, 196, 199, 213, 214, 215, 216, 218, 221, 224, 225, 228, 230, 231, 259, 261
Hathaway, D.R.   214, 228, 229, 231, 259, 261
Haudenschild, C.   8, 12
Hawkey, C.M.   61, 65
Haynes,   61
Heal, D.J.   296, 304
Hebda, P.A.   247
Hefez, A.   289, 291, 293, 296, 299, 304
Heggeness, N.H.   200
Hellem, A.J.   5, 13, 22, 26

Hellums, J.D.   5, 8, 12, 13
Helmkamp, R.W.   109, 117
Henkart, P.   95, 105
Henry, K.J.   64
Herchuelz, A.   76
Hermansky, F.   206, 209
Heyn, M.P.   103
Hildenbrand, K.   104
Hilgartner, M.W.   168
Hirsch, J.   77
Hitchcock, S.E.   192, 199
Holmberg, L.   23, 26
Holme, R.   260, 261
Holmsen, H.   140, 164, 166, 229, 233, 234, 235, 236, 246, 247, 249, 250, 251, 253, 254, 256, 257, 261, 262, 263
Holzbauer, M.   296, 297, 305, 306
Honegger, C.G.   274, 275, 276
Hopkins, G.E.   263
Horne, W.C.   99, 103
Hornebeck, W.   66
Hauslay, M.D.   297, 304, 305
Hovig, T.   171, 187, 261
Howard, M.   20, 23
Hoyer, L.W.   26
Huang, T.W.   19, 132
Huang. E.M.   140, 208
Hubbard, A.   117
Hugues, J.   5, 13
Hui, S.W.   245
Huitorel, P.   180, 187
Hunt, R.C.   114, 117
Hutton, R.A.   96, 103
Hwo, S.Y.   188
Hynes, R.O.   64

I
Inbar, M.   105
Inceman, S.   128
Ingerman, C.   206, 210
Isler, H.   275

J
Jackson, C.M.   140
Jacobelli, S.   247
Jacobs, M.   180, 187
Jaffe, E.A.   23, 26, 263
Jaffe, R.   54, 64
Jakabova, M.   75, 166, 231

Jamieson, G.A. 21, 27, 61, 64, 117, 124, 126, 128, 129, 130, 151, 152, 155
Jeanneau, C. 128
Jean Veau, C. 26
Jellinger, K. 305
Jenkins, C.S.P. 27, 116, 117, 130
Jennings, L.K. 131, 141, 197, 199
Jesse, R.L. 77
Jiminez, S.A. 59, 65
Johnson, G.J. 204, 208, 209, 210
Johnson, M.M. 27, 28, 129, 130, 167
Johnson, R.J. 235, 246
Johnson, S.M. 104
Johnstone, E.C. 304
Johnston, J.P. 298, 304
Jones, B.M. 153, 155
Jonsen, J. 13
Joy, D.C. 239, 245, 246
Jung, S.M. 117, 151

K
Kafka, M. 244
Kane, R. 199
Kang, A.H. 52, 60, 63, 65
Kaplan, K.L. 66, 165, 166, 198, 199, 263, 288
Käser-Glanzmann, R. 67, 71, 73, 75, 76, 164, 166, 220, 221, 231
Katzman, R.L. 60, 65
Kattlove, H. 158, 166
Kaulen, H.D. 71, 76, 96, 103
Kay, W.W. 65
Keely, S.L. 229
Kefalides, N.A. 19, 27
Keller, H. 27
Kennerly, D.A. 139, 203, 208
Kerlavage, A.R. 231
Kerr, F.W.L. 288
Kettler, R. 277
Kim, S.-J. 168
King, R.G. 21, 26
Kinlough-Rathbone, R.L. 3, 14, 64, 77, 116, 129, 132, 140, 166, 167, 208, 210, 234, 235, 246, 251, 253, 262, 263
Kinoshita, T. 129
Kirby, E.P. 140
Kirk, K.L. 245, 246
Kirkpatrick, J.P. 70, 76
Kirschner, M. 188
Klee, C.B. 229

Klug, A. 187
Knoll, J. 304
Knox, J.M. 304
Knuchel, H. 283, 287
Kochwa, S. 21, 28, 206, 211
Kocsis, J.J. 210
Koh, T.L. 64
Kohli, J.D. 246
Kopin, I.J. 246
Kowalski, E. 66
Krebs, H. 246
Krick, T.P. 204, 209
Krivit, W. 164, 168, 171, 188, 209
Kronic, P. 59, 65
Ku, C.S.L. 96, 106
Kuchel, O. 287
Kuhn, K. 54, 60, 63, 64
Kunicki, T. 119, 121, 126, 129
Kurylo, E. 65

L
Laemmli, U.K. 120, 129
Lages, B. 235, 246, 250, 262, 288
Lagnado, J.R. 188
Lahav, J. 61, 65
Lake, C.R. 246
Laki, K. 92, 93
Lambert, E. 128
Landis, B.H. 149
Lapetina, E.G. 202, 203, 209, 210, 258, 260, 262
Larrieu, M.J. 27, 117, 128
Laub, F. 189, 191, 192, 193, 195, 199
Laubscher, A. 267, 268, 272, 274, 275, 276
Launay, J.N. 277
Lavine, K.K. 90, 93
Lawler, J.W. 90, 93, 124, 129, 249, 262
Lebowitz, E.A. 259, 263
Le Breton, G.C. 71, 76, 161, 166
Leclerc, J.C. 128
Le Couedic, J.P. 75
Legrand, C. 129
Legrand, Y.J. 27, 60, 64
Leis, L.A. 204, 209
Leland, S. 13
Lentz, B.R. 99, 104
Leonard, B.F. 8, 15, 20, 27

Leroy, E.C.   5, 15
Lesznik, G.R.   166, 199
Leong, N.L.   258, 263
Levine, R.   263
Levitzki, A.   154, 155
Levy, J.   76
Levy-Toledano, S.   21, 26, 27, 121, 128, 129, 130
Lewis, J.T.   96, 104
Lewis, P.C.   89, 92, 103, 116, 128
Lindberg, U.   198, 199
Linck, R.W.   184
Lincoln, T.M.   229
Linden, C.D.   96, 104
Linder, S.   109, 112, 113, 118
Livne, A.   95, 116, 155
Lloyd, J.V.   131, 140, 258, 263
Lockwood, A.R.   188
Loewenstein, W.R.   190, 200
Lombart, C.   155
Lorez, H.B.   236, 246, 284, 285, 287
Lowry, O.H.   278, 287
Lucy, J.A.   102, 104
Luduena,   176
Lundblad, R.L.   141
Louvard, D.   200
Lüscher, E.F.   27, 67, 68, 69, 72, 75, 76, 77, 92, 116, 117, 131, 133, 135, 139, 140, 164, 166, 231, 249, 261
Lynch, G.   229
Lynham, J.A.   140, 199, 213, 214, 215, 224, 225, 228, 230, 259, 261
Lynn, W.S.   201, 210
Lyons, R.M.   81, 82, 88, 90, 93, 117, 131, 140, 214, 215, 224, 225, 231, 259, 263

M
MacIntyre, D.E.   57, 63
Magyar, K.   304
Maher, D.M.   239, 245, 246
Maickel, R.P.   299, 304
Majerus, D.W.   90, 93
Majerus, P.W.   90, 92, 93, 139, 140, 141, 145, 146, 150, 156, 203, 207, 208, 210, 231, 263
Majno, G.   92
Majo, E.A.   305
Malaisse, W.J.   70, 76

Malaiss-Lagae, F.   76
Malmsten, C.   251, 261
Malmström, K.   75
Mandelkow, E.   199
Mannucci, P.M.   26, 287
Mantegazza, P.   278, 288
Mantle, T.J.   304, 305
Marches, S.L.   117
Marchesi, V.T.   107, 117
Marcum, J.M.   117, 151, 181, 188
Marcus, A.J.   96, 104, 141, 201, 202, 203, 210
Margreth, A.   74
Marguerie, G.A.   74, 76, 161, 162, 166, 167
Markey, F.   198
Markwardt, F.   230
Martin, G.R.   27, 133
Martin, B.M.   140, 144, 145, 146, 150, 151, 155
Marx, R.   54, 60, 63
Mason, R.G.   155
Massini, P.   67, 69, 71, 72, 73, 76, 131, 140
Mautner, V.   64
Maxey, B.   128
May, P.R.A.   290, 291, 301
McCarty, D.J.   247
McClenaghan, M.D.   230
McConnell, H.M.   95, 96, 103, 104, 105
McConnell, R.T.   201, 210
McGill, M.S.   199
McGlynn, M.L.   304
McIntire, L.V.   76
McPherson, J.   166, 168
Means, A.R.   188
Mely-Goubert, B.   99, 104
Menashi, S.   61, 65
Mendlewicz, J.   303, 304, 306
Merits, I.   287
Meyer, D.   26
Meyer, F.A.   51, 54, 56, 57, 58, 61, 62, 63, 65
Meyers, A.M.   249, 253, 263
Michaeli, D.   52, 60, 65
Michal, F.   290, 291, 303
Michel, H.   26, 128, 130
Michell, R.   131, 140, 258, 263
Miletich, J.P.   90, 93, 132, 140

Miller, E.J. 19, 26
Mills, D.C.D. 10, 13, 204, 210, 291, 296, 304
Milton, J.G. 10, 13
Miniom, F.C. 90, 92, 103, 128
Minkes, M. 69, 76
Minter, B.F. 236, 246
Mitchell, R.H. 71, 77
Mitchell, J.R.A. 10, 13
Mittal, C.K. 221, 231
Miyata, T. 66
Moake, J.M. 5, 8, 12, 76
Mohammed, S.F. 155
Molinoff, P.B. 286, 288
Molish, I. 261
Moncada, S. 24, 27, 201, 202, 203, 210
Moore, A. 126, 127, 129
Moore, B.M. 104
Moore, S. 3, 14
Morgan, R.K. 81, 82, 88, 90, 91, 93, 103, 117, 128
Morgenstern, E. 77
Morinelli, T. 167
Morrison, M. 116
Mosesson, M.W. 66, 263
Muenter, M.D. 288
Muggli, R. 17, 18, 27, 52, 54, 56, 59, 63, 65
Munoz, R. 304
Murad, F. 221, 231
Murer, E.H. 261, 263
Murphy, E.A. 14
Murphy, D.B. 188
Murphy, D.L. 233, 243, 244, 245, 246, 254, 261, 286, 287, 288, 290, 296, 297, 302, 304, 305
Murray, B.A. 64
Mustard, J.F. 3, 8, 14, 52, 64, 65, 66, 73, 77, 116, 127, 128, 129, 131, 140, 158, 161, 165, 166, 167, 209, 210, 246, 262, 263, 288
Muszbek, L. 92, 93

N
Nachman, R.L. 26, 63, 65, 108, 115, 117, 126, 127, 129, 140, 250, 163
Näf, U. 69, 76
Nachmias, V. 137, 140, 171, 189, 190, 195, 199

Nathan, I. 93, 96, 97, 101, 116, 154, 155
Neff, N.Y. 298, 305
Nelson, E.B. 279, 287
Nelson, R. 246
Nicholau, C. 95, 104
Nicholson, W.J. 306
Nicolson, G.L. 95, 96, 101, 102, 104, 119, 129, 191, 199
Niedzwiecka-Namyslowska, I. 66
Niewiarowski, S. 133, 140, 161, 162, 165, 167
Nikaido, K. 120, 128
Nilsson, I.M. 26
Nishizawa, E.A. 206, 209, 263
Nossel, H.L. 5, 15, 288
Nugteren, D.A. 202, 210
Nurden, A.T. 21, 26, 27, 61, 63, 65, 66, 96, 104, 114, 117, 119, 121, 124, 126, 127, 128, 129, 130, 162, 165, 167
Nylen, M.U. 239, 246

O
O'Brien, J.R. 162, 167
Oesterhelt, D. 103
Okumura, T. 27, 124, 126, 128, 129, 130, 152, 155
Olsen, T. 90, 93, 117
Olsen, R.W.
Oppenheim, B. 293, 296, 304
Orci, L. 76
Ordinas, A. 57, 69, 117, 151
Oreland, L. 297, 304
Orloff, K.G. 52, 60, 65
Orr, J.L. 64, 166, 291, 292, 303, 304
Osborne, N.N. 284, 288
Osterud, B. 90, 93
Østvold, A.C. 262
Owen, F. 304
Owren, P.A. 13

P
Paasonen, M.K. 288
Packham, M.A. 3, 14, 52, 64, 65, 66, 77, 116, 128, 129, 140, 166, 167, 206, 208, 209, 210, 262
Padgett, G.A. 263
Pai, K.R.M. 129, 167
Painter, R.H. 64

Pantaloni, D. 180, 187
Papahajopoulos, D. 96, 104
Pardo, J.B. 91, 92
Pare, C.M.B. 302, 304, 306
Pareti, F.I. 287
Park, C.R. 229
Parker, J.C. 10, 14
Parola, A.H. 95, 101, 103, 104, 105, 116, 155
Pastan, I. 61, 66
Payling-Wright, H. 4, 14
Peerschke, E.I. 157, 158, 160, 161, 162, 164, 167, 168
Paulus, J.M. 288
Peller, J.D. 204, 209
Perkins, M.E. 64
Persson, T. 198
Perry, B.W. 64, 77, 129, 166, 167
Pert, J.H. 168
Peters, J.R. 303, 304
Peters, M. 304
Peters, P.D. 77, 247
Peterson, D.A. 75, 165, 206, 209
Peterson, J. 168
Pettigrew, K.D. 245
Pfueller, S.L. 68, 77, 92, 116
Phillips, D.M. 199
Philips, D.R. 21, 27, 61, 62, 63, 66, 90, 91, 92, 93, 103, 108, 116, 117, 122, 123, 124, 125, 126, 128, 130, 131, 133, 135, 138, 140, 141, 162, 167, 190, 196, 197, 199
Pickett, W.C. 69, 77
Picotti, G.B. 236, 246, 268, 275, 277, 278, 279, 281, 283, 284, 285, 287, 288
Pidard, D. 119
Pifer, D. 64
Pinkard, R.N. 75
Piras, M.M. 188
Piras, R. 188
Pletscher, A. 234, 236, 237, 240, 244, 245, 246, 267, 268, 271, 272, 274, 275, 276, 278, 283, 284, 287, 288, 290, 299, 302, 304
Plow, E.F. 76, 166, 167
Pollard, T.D. 137, 140, 141, 184, 187, 192, 197, 199
Porter, N.A. 210

Poste, G. 104
Potter, R.L. 218, 231
Potterf, R.D. 116
Poulsen, F.M. 245
Prasanna, H.R. 131
Pribluda, V. 109, 118, 189, 193, 199
Priel, Z. 54, 64
Prieur, D. 263
Probst, M. 128
Pudlak, P. 206, 209
Puett, D. 60, 66

Q
Quinn, P.J. 188

R
Rabin, D. 188
Radda, G.K. 97, 104
Rafelson, 96
Rand, M.L. 64, 128
Randall, R.T. 278, 287
Rao, G.H.R. 75, 201, 203, 204, 205, 206, 207, 208, 209, 210, 211
Rapaport, S.I. 90, 93
Rausch, W.D. 305
Ravazzola, M. 76
Reddington, M. 188
Regoelzi, E. 167
Reich, E. 117
Reimann, A. 104
Reimers, H.J. 64, 72, 77, 116, 128, 140, 208, 210, 262, 286, 288
Rendu, F. 246
Rennard, St.I 27
Renskers, K.J. 279, 287
Reveille, J. 245, 286, 287
Rhodes, J.A. 192, 200
Richards, F.M. 107, 118
Richards, J.G. 268, 272, 274, 275, 276, 284, 285, 287, 288
Richardson, B. 5, 8, 14
Riederer, P. 290, 303, 305, 306
Rieger, H. 6, 14
Rifkin, D.B. 114, 117
Rittenhouse-Simmons, S. 69, 77, 96, 105, 202, 210
Robbins, P.W. 103, 104
Robbert, L. 66
Robberts, G.C.K. 291, 296, 304
Robberts, R.M. 114, 117

Robey, P.G. 27
Robins, E. 304
Robkin, L. 262
Rohde, H. 27
Roosen, K.J. 261
Rose, B. 190, 200
Rosebrough, N.J. 278, 287
Rosenbaum, J.L. 188
Rosenfeld, C.I. 104
Rosenthal, S.L. 95, 104
Ross, G.D. 129
Ross, R. 3, 14, 96, 105
Ross, S.B. 271, 276
Roth, A.R. 76
Roth, G.J. 203, 207, 210
Roth, J. 299, 305
Roth, J.A. 279, 287
Roth, L.T. 76
Rothen, C. 70, 75, 77
Rothstein, A. 107, 116
Rotman, A. 107, 109, 112, 113, 115, 116, 118, 189, 193, 199
Rowntree, L.F. 8, 14
Rowsell, H.C. 8, 14
Rubenstein, J.L.R. 96, 105
Rubin, S.C. 218, 231
Rudolph, S.A. 188
Ruggeri, S.M. 26
Ruoslahti, E. 61, 66
Ruthven, C.R.J. 305
Ryan, G.B. 92

S
Saavedra, J.M. 278, 288
Sakariassen, K.S. 24, 27
Salach, J.I. 297, 299, 305
Salama, S.E. 199, 213, 216, 231
Salganicoff, L. 166, 233, 235, 246, 247, 261
Salzman, E.W. 23, 27
Samuelsson, B. 11, 13, 15
Sandler, M. 302, 305, 306
Santoro, S.A. 57, 59, 61, 66
Say, A.K. 230
Scarpa, A. 246
Scharf, R. 72, 77
Scher, C.D. 249, 261
Schmid-Schönbein, H. 6, 10, 14
Schmidt-Ulrich, R. 106
Schnaitman, C. 299, 305
Schneider, K. 291, 305
Schollmeyer, J.F. 93
Schultz, G. 229, 231

Schultz, K. 231
Schultz, K.D. 214, 231
Schrappe, O. 303
Scott, S. 210
Scrutton, M.C. 246, 262
Seachord, C.L. 263
Sears, D.A. 89, 92, 109, 116, 117
Seeger, R.C. 89, 93
Seeman, P. 11, 14, 299, 305
Seifried, H. 245
Seligsohn, U. 166
Sen, R. 241, 247
Senger, D.R. 64
Senye, A.F. 77
Setkowsky, C.A. 262
Setkowsky-Dangelmaier, C.A. 254, 262
Shafer, B. 245
Shaeffer, B.E. 104
Shakarjian, M. 305
Sharp, D.E. 7, 8, 12
Sharp, R.R. 247
Sharpless, N.S. 288
Shattil, S.J. 96, 102, 105, 151, 154, 155, 156
Shaw, J.O. 215, 224, 225, 231
Shelanski, M. 174, 188
Sheppard, B.L. 127, 130
Shepro, D. 247
Sherry, J.M.F. 139
Shetrline, P. 177, 188
Shigekawa, B.L. 188
Shinitzky, M. 95, 96, 101, 102, 103, 105, 154, 155
Shinoya, T. 8, 14
Shmuckler, M. 153, 156
Shulman, R.G. 247
Shuman, M.A. 146, 150
Sigel, E. 75
Siegel, M.I. 201, 210
Silber, S.A. 245
Silcox, D.C. 234, 247
Silliman, A. 199
Silver, M.J. 74, 96, 105, 202, 206, 208, 210
Silver, R.B. 190, 200
Simoneit, L.W. 11, 12
Simons, E.R. 54, 56, 59, 61, 64, 103
Singer, S.J. 191, 192, 199, 200
Sinha, A.K. 154, 156

Sixma, J.J. 27
Sixma, F.F. 261
Skaer, H.K.B. 119, 130
Skaer, R.J. 72, 77, 128, 130, 234, 247
Skonieczna, M. 66
Slayter, H.S. 90, 93, 129, 262
Slichter, S.J. 96, 103
Sloboda, R.D. 184, 188
Sly, W.H. 261
Smith, B.A. 105
Smith, F.B. 263
Smith, H. 187
Smith, J.B. 74, 96, 105, 202, 203, 206, 208, 210
Smith, K.K. 64
Smith, M.A. 245
Sneddon, J.M. 96, 105
Snodgrass, W.R. 304
Snyder, S.M. 278
Solatunturi, E. 288
Solum, N.O. 21, 27, 90, 93, 117, 128
Somers, G. 76
Sonder, S.A. 149
Sonnichsen, W.J. 146, 149
Sopata, I. 66
Souroujon, M. 95, 96, 102, 104, 105
Spaet, T.H. 25, 27
Stahl, P.D. 261
Stanford, N. 76, 139, 140, 203, 208, 231, 263
Stark, H. 245
Staros, J.V. 107, 118
Steck, T.L. 108, 118
Steers, E.Jr. 117
Stehbens, W.E. 4, 14
Stemerman, M.B. 19, 27
Stenman, S. 19, 27
Stenzel, K.H. 66
Stewart, G.J. 246, 263
Stocken, W.J. 70, 77
Stocker, K. 140
Stoddard, S.F. 75, 205, 206, 209
Stoff, D.M. 305
Stossel, T.P. 192, 196, 199, 200
Storm, E. 246
Stürzebecher, J. 230
Sudilovsky, A. 291, 305
Sueden, P.H. 229
Sullender, J. 140, 199

Sultan, Y. 26, 128
Sussman, I.I. 28, 130
Svensson, J. 11, 13, 15
Swanson, R. 65
Sweetman, H.E. 235, 247

T
Tainer, J.A. 201, 210
Takaji, T. 261
Tan, S.W. 143, 146, 147, 150
Tan, L.P. 188
Tanaka, Y. 245
Tanner, M.J.A. 108, 118
Tarasov, E. 117
Tailor, D.L. 192, 196, 197, 200
Tailor, E.W. 187
Tailor, K.M. 278, 288
Tailor, S.S. 218, 231
Teale, F.W.J. 99, 105
Tence, M. 75
Terfivainen, H. 246
Termine, J.D. 245, 246
Thomas, C. 135, 139, 192, 198
Tillack, T.W. 90, 92, 117
Tilney, L. 199
Tilney, L.G. 137, 141, 192, 196, 200
Timpl, R. 19, 27
Tinklenberg, J.R. 305
Tipton, K.F. 297, 298, 304, 305
Tobelem, G. 26, 27, 126, 128, 129, 130
Todrick, A. 243, 244
Toh, B.H. 92
Tollefsen, D.M. 131, 133, 141, 145, 146, 150, 151, 156
Townsend, D. 205, 206, 209
Tranzer, J.P. 283, 287
Traub, W. 52, 64
Trelstad, R.L. 19, 28
Tschopp, Th.B. 17, 18, 21, 24, 25, 26, 27, 28, 130
Turesson, I. 26
Turitto, V.P. 8, 15, 17, 18, 21, 22, 24, 26, 28
Turner, S.R. 210
Tyle, G.M. 286, 288

U
Ugurbil, K. 235, 238, 239, 240, 247

Urban, C.L.   61, 64
Usdin, E.   302, 305

V

Valensi, T.   26, 128
Valeri, C.R.   245, 247
Vallee, R.B.   188
Van Deenen, L.L.M.   106
Van Den Bovenkamp, G.J.   8, 13
Vanderkooi, J.   105
Van Dijck, P.W.M.   95, 106
Vane, J.R.   27, 201, 202, 203, 210
Van Leeuwen, E.F.   121, 130
Van Lenten, L.   108, 118
Van Moorik, J.A.   130
Vargaftig, D.B.   69, 75, 77, 204, 208
Vecchione, J.J.   245, 247
Verkleij, A.J.   106
Verma, S.P.   106
Verrier-Jones, J.   118
Ververgaet, P.H.J.Th.   106
Vilaire, G.   161, 166
Von Berlepsch,   278
Von Dem Borne, A.E.G.Kr.   130
Von Riesz, L.E.   130
Von Rokitansky, C.   3, 15

W

Wagner, D.D.   64
Wallach, D.F.H.   95, 96, 106
Walton, K.W.   3, 15
Walz, D.A.   149
Wang, C.L.   56, 59, 66
Wasiewski, W.W.   146, 149, 150
Wasserman, B.K.   66
Webb, B.C.   188
Webb, R.W.   304
Weber, G.   106
Weber, J.C.   239, 247
Weeds, A.G.   192, 199
Wehmeier, A.   14
Weihing, R.R.   197, 200
Weil-Malherbe, H.   279, 288
Weingarten, M.D.   188
Weise, V.   246
Weisman, Z.   54, 56, 58, 65
Weisenberg, R.   70, 77
Weiss, H.J.   17, 20, 21, 22, 24, 26, 28, 96, 106, 124, 130, 158, 167, 206, 211, 233, 235, 236, 246, 249, 262, 285, 288

Weiss, G.   141
Weiss, A.   224, 231
Weksler, B.B.   66, 117
Weng, K.   192, 200
Werner, G.   71, 77
Werner-Goedde, H.   303
Whetzel, N.   246
White, G.C.II   141
White, J.G.   68, 70, 71, 75, 77, 93, 102, 106, 122, 130, 132, 135, 141, 159, 160, 162, 164, 167, 168, 171, 173, 188, 189, 200, 201, 202, 203, 204, 205, 206, 207, 208, 209, 210, 211, 233, 234, 247, 259, 263
Whittmore, R.   305
Williams, D.C.   90, 91, 92, 103, 128
Williams, V.M.   93
Willis, A.L.   203, 210
Wilner, G.D.   5, 15
Winolur, G.   304
Witkop, C.J.   206, 207, 209, 211
Witte, L.D.   288
Wize, J.   66
Wojtecka-Lukasik,   59, 66
Woodruff, R.A.   304
Woods, H.F.   303, 304, 306
Workman, E.F.Jr.   131, 133, 140, 141
Wright, K.L.   104
Wu, K.K.   96, 106
Wyatt, R.J.   297, 302, 304, 305

Y

Yahara, I.   191, 200
Yamada, K.M.   61, 66
Yamada, S.S.   61, 66
Yandrasitz, J.   247
Yang, H.-Y.T.   298, 305
Youdim, M.B.H.   289, 290, 293, 296, 297, 298, 299, 300, 301, 302, 303, 304, 305, 306
Young, N.J.   181, 188
Yuan, B.O.   114, 118
Yung, W.   13

Z

Zabinski, M.P.   149
Zambotti, F.   278, 288

Zeltzer, P.M. 89, 93
Zieve, P.D. 153, 156
Zoller, M.J. 218, 231
Zonnevels, G.T.E. 130
Zucker, M.B. 61, 66, 158, 159, 160, 162, 164, 165, 166, 167, 168, 249, 251, 263
Zucker-Franklin, D. 91, 93, 132, 135, 140
Zürcher, G. 278, 286, 287

Subject Index

A
Acid hydrolyses (glycosidases), 250
Actin, 81, 87-89, 91, 191-196
  antibodies against, 89
  binding protein, 135, 192, 195
  mobilization of, 197
  polymerization of, 132, 135, 136
α-Actinin, 91
Actomyosin, 196, 198, 259
ADP, 206, 208
  effect on platelets, 68, 98, 100, 251, 252
  induced platelet aggregation, 82, 84, 85, 89, 90, 97, 127, 194, 260, 289
  induced shape change, 258
  in storage granules, 5, 7, 10, 214, 235
  receptor, 290
Amines, 233
  metabolism, 290
  storage, 277, 290
Anti-coagulation, 22, 23
Arachidonic acid, 11
  metabolism, 201-205, 208
Arsanilic acid
  diiodo diazo, 107
Aspirin, 25, 194, 206, 253
Atherosclerosis, 3, 15
ATP
  consumption, 234, 235, 257, 258
  in storage vesicles, 234, 235
  tumbling rate, 240

B
Bernard-Soulier syndrome, 20, 124-126
Benzoquinolizine (RO4-1284), 269
Benzylamine, 298

C
Calcium
  dependence of microtubule polymerization on, 190
  role in platelet activation, 67-74, 249
Calmodulin, 131, 181, 190, 259
Capping, 191
Catecholamines, 267, 268
Catechol-O-methyltransferase (COMT), 278

Central nervous system (CNS), 272-275
Cerebral Vasospasm syndrome, 29
Cerebrospinal fluid (CSF), 29
Cerebrovascular
  disorder, 29
p-chlormethamphetamine, 270, 271
Chlorpromazine, 290-298
Chlortetracycline
  fluorescence of, 253
Cholesterol
  phospholipid ratio, 151
Chymotrypsin, 148
Colchicine, 179, 191
Collagen, 11, 19, 30, 68, 71
  arginine in, role in interaction, 59
  chemical determinants on, 58
  dependence of activation on surface curvature of, 54
  dependence of adhesion on surface curvature of, 56
  effect of ADP on adhesion to, 58
  glycoproteins I, II and III mediating interaction with, 61
  interaction with soluble collagen adsorbed to surfaces, 54
  membrane binding sites for, 61
  physical determinants of, 53
  platelet shape in interaction with, 57, 58
  proline/hydroxyproline of, role interaction, 58
  structure and composition of, 52
  triple helical conformation of, role in interaction, 55, 57, 60
Concanavalin A, 190
Contractile activity, 69
Cross-linking agents, 152
Cyclic 3',5'-adenosine
  monophosphate (cyclic AMP), 69, 164, 204, 213-231
Cytochalasin B, 162, 164, 197
Cytochrome C, 275
Cytoskeleton, 135, 137, 138, 189, 191

D
Dense body (dense granules), 68, 72, 227, 249
Dense tubular system, 67, 71
Dictyostelium discoideum, 191
4,6-difluoroserotonin, 239, 240
Dihydroprostacycline, 25
Dinitrophenyl-β-alanine hydrazide labelling with, 112
1,6-diphenyl-1,3,5-hexatriene (DPH), 97, 98, 101
DNA, 193
DNAse I, 192-196
L-dopa, 272
Dopamine, 236, 238, 242, 268-272, 289-291, 297
Dyenin, 190

E
Endocytosis, 250
Endothelial cells, 3
Endothelium, 3, 8, 29, 31
Epinephrine, 289, 290
Erythrocytes, 9-11
Ethidium bromide, 193
Exocytosis, 194, 268

F
Factor IV, 249
Factor V, 249
Fibrin, 260
5-fluorodopamine, 240
Fibrinogen
  specific binding of, 127, 157-168, 249
6-fluoro-serotonin, 240
Fluphenazine, 233, 289, 292

G
Glanzmann's Thrombasthenia, 21, 119-123, 138
β-glucuronidase, 251
Glycocalicin, 152
Glycoproteins, 20, 21, 62, 83, 84, 86, 90, 119-130, 134, 138, 139, 197
  isolation of, 111
  labelling of, 103
  receptors, 152
Glycosidases, 250
Granules (storage)
  dense, 249, 256, 257, 259
  α-, 198, 249, 256, 257, 259

Gray platelet syndrome, 122-124, 126

H
Haemorrhage, 4
Heparin, 274, 275
Hermansky-Pudlak syndrome, 206
Hirudin, 146
Histamine, 272, 277

I
Imipramine, 268
Immunoelectrophoresis, 121
Iodonaphthylazide, 110
Ionophore (A-23187), 68, 153, 179, 205, 213, 224, 242, 243, 253-255

L
Lectins, 152
Lidocain
  treated platelets with, 137
Liposomes, 151
LSD, 272, 273

M
Magnesium
  in storage vesicles, 233-247
Membrane fluidity, 102
  dynamic changes, 96
Meningitis, 30
Methysergide, 272
Microfilaments
  organizing center, 191
Microtubules, 171-188, 191
  associated proteins, 175, 177, 183, 184
  organizing center, 191
Migraine, 30
Mitochondria
  release of Ca^{+2} from, 72
Monoamine oxidase (MAO), 289, 296, 297
  inhibitors, 290
Myelin basic protein, 274
Myosin
  phosphorylation of, 132, 135, 259

N
Nerve ending, 289
Neuroleptics, see chlorpromazine

Norepinephrine, 268-271, 289, 290
Normethanephrine, 277
Nuclear magnetic resonance (NMR), 233, 235, 237

O
Octopamine, 277

P
Parkinson's disease, 289, 302
Passive modulation, 154
Pathogenesis, 29
Phenothiazines, 296, 301
Phosphatidic acid (PA), 258-260
Phosphatidyl inositol (PI), 131, 202, 258, 259
Phospholipase A, 11, 202, 203
Phosphorylation, 213-231
Polylysine, 274
Polyornithine, 274, 275
Prostaglandins, 11, 69, 203
  PGD_2, 202
  PGE_1, 136, 201-211, 213, 221, 224, 227, 273, 274
  PGE_2, 202, 203
  $PGF_{2\alpha}$, 202, 203
  PGG_2, 71, 202-206
  PGH_2, 71, 202-205
  PGI_2 (prostacycline), 24, 25, 29-31, 132, 136

Q
Quinacrine (mepacrine), 236-238, 242

R
Release (see also secretion), 69, 100, 249-263
Reserpine, 238, 242, 268, 278
Ristocetin, 124, 162
  induced platelet aggregation, 23
Rotational mobility
  of membrane glycoproteins, 101

S
Schizophrenia, 289-306
Serotonin, 11, 206, 249, 270, 272, 277, 289-302
  in storage vesicles, 233-247
  release of, 100, 136, 168, 169
  uptake of, 267

Secretion (see also release), 82, 249
  thrombin induced, 86, 87
Shape change, 7, 29, 70, 97, 98, 184, 272, 281
  inhibitors, 273
Shear rate, 21, 22
Shear stress, 6
Sodium nitroprusside, 221
Spectrin, 195
Storage pool disease, 21, 249, 277, 279
Storage vesicles (see granules), 234, 235, 249
Subarachnoid haemorrhage, 30
Subendothelium, 17-19, 21, 29
Sulfanilic acid
  diiodo diazo, 81, 82, 85

T
Temperature
  effect on platelets, 157-168
Thrombasthenia, see Glanzmann's Thrombasthenia
Thrombin
  binding, 145, 151, 153
  induced activation, 11, 71, 81, 82, 87, 88, 97, 131, 136, 194, 196, 203, 257
  receptor, 133, 143, 145, 146, 253
Thrombogenesis, 4
Thrombospondin, 249
Thromboxane
  A_2, 5, 10, 11, 68, 69, 202-206, 208, 251-253
  B_2, 202
Thrombus, 18, 19, 23
Tubulin, 171-190
Tyramine, 242, 270, 271
Tyrosine hydrazide
  diiodo, 109

V
Von Willebrand factor (VWF), 20, 21, 23, 24, 124, 165